To Chandra

Mo

Persp

Secon

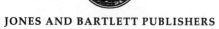

JONES AND BARTLETT PUBLISHERS
Sudbury, Massachusetts
BOSTON   TORONTO   LONDON   SINGAPORE

World Headquarters

Jones and Bartlett Publishers
40 Tall Pine Drive
Sudbury, MA 01776
978-443-5000
info@jbpub.com
www.jbpub.com

Jones and Bartlett Publishers
Canada
2406 Nikanna Road
Mississauga, ON L5C 2W6
CANADA

Jones and Bartlett Publishers
International
Barb House, Barb Mews
London W6 7PA
UK

Library of Congress Cataloging-in-Publication Data
Edgar, Stacey L.
    Morality and machines : perspectives on computer ethics / Stacey L. Edgar.—2nd ed.
        p. cm.
    Includes bibliographical references and index.
    ISBN 0-7637-1767-3
    1. Electronic data processing—Moral and ethical aspects.   I. Title.
QA76.9.M65 E34 2002
174'.90904—dc21

                                                        2002022110

Editor-in-Chief: J. Michael Stranz
Production Manager: Amy Rose
Marketing Manager: Nathan Schultz
Associate Production Editor: Tara McCormick
Editorial Assistant: Theresa DiDonato
Production Assistant: Karen C. Ferreira
Manufacturing Buyer: Therese Bräuer
Composition: Northeast Compositors, Inc.
Text Design: Jeff Cosloy
Cover Design: Diana Coe
Printing and Binding: Malloy Lithographing, Inc.
Cover Printing: Malloy Lithographing, Inc.

Intro: Earth, http://www.nara.gov/exhall/picturing_the_century/century/century_img89.html; Ch 1: "Then, Gentlemen, it is a consensus," The New Yorker Collection, 1985, Charles Barsotti from cartoonbank.com; Ch 3: "The Single Standard of Morality," The New Yorker Collection, 1982, Peter Steiner from cartoonbank.com; Ch 6: Solar Eclipse, http://www.jpl.nasa.gov/images/solar_corona.jpg, Courtesy of NASA/JPL/Caltech; Ch 7: "On the internet no one knows you're a dog," The New Yorker Collection, 1993, Peter Steiner from cartoonbank.com

This book was typeset in Quark 4.1 on a Macintosh G4. The font families used were Rotis Sans Serif, Rotis Serif, and Formata. The first printing was printed on 50# Thor Offset.

Printed in the United States of America

06 05 04 03 02   10 9 8 7 6 5 4 3 2 1

Preface

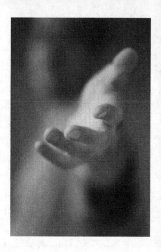

Piracy, privacy, robots, artificial intelligence, hacking, cyberporn, cybersex, viruses, worms, Trojan horses, wiretapping, communications decency, censorship, war games, Star Wars (now called Ballistic Missile Defense), information superhighways, cyberterrorism, the Internet (and its uses for good and evil), technostress—all are part of today's computer world. The computer has made many significant changes in our lifestyles. No one—not even a self-styled "Unabomber" recluse who wishes to destroy much of modern technology—is unaffected by these changes, changes that raise serious social and moral issues. Computers can enhance some areas of human concern, such as efficiency, but they also have the potential to worsen other problem areas, such as inequality. This book arose out of a realization that the advent of the computer has created new moral problems and given a new spin to old, persistent ones. The book points out what these areas of concern are and lays a basis for attacking these problems.

Computers are new; ethics has been around since humans began thinking clearly and communally. The intersection of these two areas provides a very exciting and challenging realm that must be entered and made livable if we are to have any hope for the future. This book is unique in that it takes seriously the need to lay a sound ethical basis for dealing with these new problems. The first two chapters of the book take on various positions that challenge the possibility of ethics, and meet them head-on with counterarguments. The possibility of a viable ethics having been defended, Chapter 3 examines the most promising approaches to ethics, so that the explorer in the new realm will have the appropriate tools and, if necessary, weapons at hand. At the end of the chapter, suggestions are given for approaching any ethical problem. Once armed, the adventurer is ready to investigate the various parts of the new country, described in the remaining chapters of the book.

Computer ethics is important to everyone. Those who will be professionals in areas involving computers have a responsibility to be aware of the moral issues computers raise and to be knowledgeable about how to find viable solutions for them. But everyone in today's society is affected by computers. We should all learn about their possibilities to improve conditions and about the dangers they present. The purpose of this book is to acquaint readers with these potentials and give them an ethical basis from which to approach them. To take an analogy from a well-known computer game, there are dungeons to explore and dragons to slay (or befriend). Welcome to the great adventure!

Acknowledgments

I want to thank my classes in computer ethics, in which we learned and discussed much together and which gave structure and content to this book. My special thanks go to Jerry Erion (now a Ph.D. teaching philosophy) and Maureen Neary (now playing a crucial role in a New York City publishing company), for their substantial help in tracking down interesting references and examples, and to Laura Sythes (now an editor), for her good advice and a sympathetic shoulder. Thanks to Dave Merli and Andrew Terjesen, who are doing graduate work in philosophy, for their help in proofreading the first draft of this book.

Among the reviewers, I especially thank Terrell Ward Bynum (Department of Philosophy, Southern Connecticut State University), Sterling Harwood (Department of Philosophy, San Jose State University), Walter Maner (Department of Computer Science, Bowling Green State University), and James H. Moor (Department of Philosophy, Dartmouth College). Their many insightful comments, criticisms, and suggestions made this a much better book.

Special thanks go to my editors, Michael Stranz and Amy Rose, who were a constant source of encouragement and direction on this project. Being able to call and talk to them at any time, about any problem, was a great boon. I felt that they really cared about this project, which kept me going even when things were difficult.

I am grateful to the State University of New York–Geneseo for giving me the opportunity to develop and teach a new, groundbreaking course in computer ethics, out of which this book arose.

Stacey L. Edgar

Contents

Chapter 7   **Privacy   253**

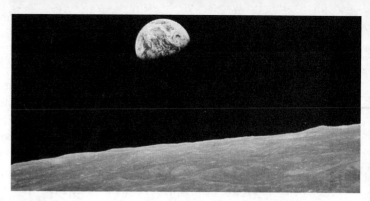

Introduction

 COMPUTER ETHICS?

Over the past few decades, new conditions have given rise to new ethical problems. Business ethics has become a discipline dealing with the many facets of today's world—from the proliferation and power of global corporations and a volatile stock market subject to "insider trading" and computer programs that buy and sell in vast quantities. Advances in genetics have raised new problems for medical ethics—from stem cell research to "death with dignity" to the abortion question. Threats to the environment due to increased industrial productivity, depletion of natural resources, and the population explosion have created a new set of ethical concerns generally called *environmental ethics*. These areas are generally referred to as *applied ethics*—that is, clusters of problems and issues that raise new moral dilemmas and to which we must apply our best moral judgments.

Computer technology is another area in which amazing changes have occurred in the past four decades. In the span of a few years, the computer has changed our lives tremendously—the way we do business, the way we shop, and the way businesses and government agencies keep records and analyze data. Such changes can affect our privacy, our jobs, and perhaps even our freedom.

Countless innovations due to computers—from the word processor to stunning breakthroughs in mathematics and science—are extremely beneficial, however. For example, the Apollo mission to the moon would not have been possible without computers; similarly, space stations and missions to Mars and Jupiter would not have gotten off the ground. Even these advances raise new questions regarding creativity, the nature of proof and truth in mathematics, the possibility of "artificial intelligence," and others we will discuss briefly, insofar as they have moral implications. But the most pressing questions in computer ethics relate to invasions of privacy, questions of ownership of intellectual property, professional responsibility, computer reliability (especially in potentially dangerous situations), computer crime (including embezzlement, software theft, computer viruses and other invasions of systems, and actual crimes *against* computers), a changing work environment, cyberterrorism, and insidious threats of government control reminiscent of Orwell's "Big Brother" in *1984*.

Areas of applied ethics may bring us new problems with which to grapple, but there have been no major breakthroughs in moral thinking and ethical theory to parallel the ongoing technological advances. In 1959, C. P. Snow wrote of the "two cultures"—roughly the scientific community and that of the humanities—and the problems arising because of the lack of communication between them. Henry M. Boettinger, assistant comptroller at AT&T, wrote in 1970, "The humanists must enter into a dialogue with the scientists, not as amateur, negative, do-gooder dilettantes, but as equal partners in a modern form of the Socratic dialectic" (Boettinger, 1970, p. 46).

Joseph Weizenbaum, computer scientist at MIT, wrote of the "two cultures of the computer age," which he feared could become a radical split into those who enjoy the benefits of the new technology and a high standard of living, and "the remaining and potentially very large segment of the population [who] will drift further and further away from playing anything but the most menial and irrelevant roles and will fall behind at an increasing rate" (Weizenbaum, 1969, p. 57). He predicts that if these two "cultures" are allowed to come into existence, they "may render each other into waste."

If knowledge and information translate into power, then it is possible that a few will have the power and many will be isolated from it. Thus, a gap could develop both between rich and poor (financially) and between those rich and poor in information technology and the corresponding power. This is a serious issue, partly addressed in Chapter 11. The solution to the threat must lie in education and fair access to computer capabilities.

Over the past two and a half millennia, we have seen amazing advances in science and technology, but only small and generally recent strides in our collective understanding in the moral and social realms. Only recently have the evils of slavery and discrimination been widely recognized, and as recently as 60 years ago, it took a Hitler to bring the horrors of genocide forcefully before the average human consciousness.

It is the advances in science that have generated many of our "new" moral and social problems, and it will take some hard thinking and action to solve them. Representatives from the "two cultures" must work together to meet these problems. Members of the scientific community must bring a greater technical understanding of the underpinnings of the technologies involved; those from the humanities must bring a basis on which to make moral judgments and choose social and political alternatives well. There has been considerable insight along these latter lines over the past 2,500 years, and it would serve us well to take this critical work into account rather than try to start from scratch ourselves. We may face *new* (or at least *different*) problems, not exactly like any faced in the past, but the foundations of sound ethical judgment should be applicable to these as well. Today's scientist may not benefit greatly from a detailed study of Aristotle's theory of moving bodies, but today's moral thinker may learn much from Aristotle's writings on ethics. Though there may be some specific new moral dilemmas that arise out of the modern milieu, approaches to ethical problems in general are the foundation to which we must turn.

Walter Maner, who is said to have been the first to use the phrase "computer ethics," pointed out that the issues that arise in computer ethics fall into four categories:

1. The computer technology may *aggravate* certain traditional ethical problems (as, for example, creating new avenues for invasion of privacy).
2. The technology may *transform* familiar ethical problems into "analogous but unfamiliar ones," such as changing the criteria for owning an "original" (photo, literary work, etc.).
3. It may *create new problems* that are unique to the computing realm (such as computers making battlefield or other strategic decisions without human intervention).
4. In some cases (the authors say these are "rare"), the new technology may *relieve* existing moral problems. The example that comes to mind here, though not Maner's, is that computer analysis may allow more accurate projections of the future consequences of different choices—say, with regard to the environment or responses to terrorism—and thus allow a more informed moral choice to be made (Pecorino and Maner, 1985, pp. 327–28).

James H. Moor defined **computer ethics** as "the analysis of the nature and social impact of computer technology and the corresponding formulation and justification of policies for the ethical use of such technology" (Moor, 1985, p. 266). He points out that computers have created "new choices" for human beings. Since he defines computer ethics in terms of the *ethical use* of the technology, clearly we must begin by attempting to understand ethical criteria for making the best choices. Moor adds that "much of the important work in computer ethics is devoted to proposing conceptual frameworks for understanding ethical problems involving computer technology."

Computers are changing the way we humans make decisions, and even the sorts of activities that are considered valuable. We have moved from an agricultural to an industrial to an information society. Much of the information that is processed, and that transforms our lives, is "invisible" to the human senses as it is manipulated electronically. This *Invisibility Factor*, as Moor calls it, can lead to abuse in the form of tampering with computer programs or data, to unrecognized biases present in the programs that make important decisions, and to human loss of control and even lack of awareness of the complexity of what is going on in the computer manipulations, including whether they could be in error. Moor concludes: "We must decide when to trust computers and when not to trust them" (Moor, 1985, p. 275).

Thus, to deal with the problems arising in computer ethics, we will begin with an ethical foundation that looks to both past and current thinkers for guidance. One cannot deal effectively with a moral problem by just trying to *intuit* a solution, since such intuition may fail at other times, or be inconsistent, unless it is grounded in something more basic, such as a general rule for assessing moral situations. We will begin by examining a range of ethical positions and evaluating how satisfactory they are, so that we will have some basis for assessing the issues particular to computer ethics. One cannot go blindly into a maze of moral problems without some sense of how to solve them.

IS THERE REALLY A NEED FOR ETHICS IN COMPUTING?

The answer to this question is a resounding "yes!" The support for this answer will be found in Part Two of this book, in which the range of moral problems that are uniquely traceable to computer use is examined and evaluated. In an article that appeared in the *Chronicle of Higher Education*, Thomas DeLoughry (1988) stated that ethics is an area generally overlooked in computer science curricula, yet the Computing Sciences Accreditation Board has recognized its importance, requiring instruction in the "social implications of computing" as a criterion for accreditation. Unfortunately, in many cases the nod to computer ethics involves little more than instructors telling their students not to copy copyrighted software.

A recommendation of the ACM (Association for Computing Machinery) Computing Education Board stated that college computing programs share *values*, as well as attributes and curricula, and that "undergraduate programs should prepare graduates to understand the field of computing, both as an academic discipline and as a profession within the context of a larger society" ("Computing Curricula 1991," p. 72). Thus, students should be acquainted with the history of computing—the economic, political, and cultural trends that have shaped the discipline. They should be familiar with the "ethical and social issues" that are related to the field of computing.

The recommendation goes on to say that students must "develop the ability to ask serious questions about the social impact of computing and to evaluate proposed answers to these questions" (p. 73). It is the purpose of this book to do just that—to prepare a philosophical basis for asking the tough questions and evaluating answers to them, and then examine the various areas in which these questions arise. The recommendation continues to say that those working in the field must be able to anticipate the impact of various products on the environment, and ask what effect they will have on the "quality of life." They must also be aware of related legal rights, "and they also need to appreciate the ethical values that are the basis for those rights. Future practitioners must understand the responsibility they will bear, and the possible consequences of failure. They must understand their own limitations as well as those of their tools" (p. 74).

Dianne Martin, a professor of electrical engineering, and David Martin, former Director of the U.S. Office of Government Ethics and now in private law practice, wrote in 1990:

> Computers often alter relationships among people. Data communications can take place without any personal contact and at such high speed that the individual may not have time to consider the ramifications of a particular transmission. In addition, electronic information is more fragile than "hard-copy" paper information. New ethical dilemmas with competing rights and values have arisen due to the advent of high-speed, worldwide transmission; low-cost, mass storage; and multiple-copy dissemination capabilities. Precepts regarding proprietary rights, residual rights, plagiarism, piracy, eavesdropping, privacy, and freedom of expression should be examined and perhaps redefined. Advancements in computer technology were made under the naive assumption that efficiency was the main purpose or thrust, not moral values. Now the application of ethical principles to computer technology must take its proper place so that the ethical dimension is integrated into the concept of managing technology and the human relationships that accompany technological advancements (Martin and Martin, 1990, p. 24).

Here they have put perspective on the initial presumption that computing is morally neutral, the major areas of ethical concern, and the need for an ethical awareness to deal with the impact.

J. J. Buck BloomBecker tells of giving a speech entitled "Computer Crime: Career of the Future?" to discuss his work in the detection and prevention of computer crime and, unfortunately, having many of those who attended expecting a "how-to" lesson! (BloomBecker, 1986, p. 4). Donn B. Parker wrote that he had "polarized the academic community by making a statement that we are creating a new generation of computer criminals in our computer science departments. My position was based on the fact that the application of ethics had never been introduced into computer science departments. Some faculty members said they don't deal with ethics, only with computers" (Parker, 1982, p. 51). Of course, the implicit question is whether the two can be separated (whether technology in general is/can be morally neutral), which we will discuss in Part Two. Steinke and Hamann (1990, pp. 261–264) point out the responsibility of colleges and universities to act according to higher (ethical) standards rather than mere legal requirements, to set a "moral tone" for those they educate. Areas of special concern cited are those of the privacy of student records and illegal copying of software.

A number of articles and books deal with the importance of bringing ethical issues to the attention of those in the computer field—both students and professionals—but often the approach suggested is more of a "consciousness-raising" session than a serious consideration of moral issues. A case-study book that merely reports the opinions of a number of people presented with different scenarios—in which one must decide whether the actions taken were ethical, unethical, or not in the realm of ethics—does *not* deal with the ethical issues. Morality cannot be merely a matter of (current) consensus, for reasons we discuss in upcoming chapters. It is for this reason that we begin by laying a ground for moral judgments.

The National Computer Ethics and Responsibilities Campaign was launched in early 1994 with a short-term goal of talking about the major issues, and a five- to ten-year goal of actually changing attitudes in crucial areas. The campaign's principal sponsor is the Washington-based Computer Ethics Institute;[1] cosponsors include the Software Publishers Association, CompuServe, and the National Computer Security Association. The campaign has been to issue a "call to action" to make responsible computer use "a national priority." Part of the plan is to make information, resources, training materials, and sample codes of ethics available on the Internet, and to support educational efforts with the campaign. "We need to get people to ask: 'Is this the right thing to do?'" (Betts, 1994, p. 33). Some of the concerns addressed were the subject of a 1994 ACLU poll, and included the release of telephone records and health insurance records to an outside party, and the selling of credit-card information to mail-order companies.

Joseph Weizenbaum wrote with great insight in 1976: "[The teacher] must teach more than one metaphor, and he must teach more by the example of his conduct than by what he writes on the blackboard. He must teach the limitations of his tools as well as their power" (Weizenbaum, 1976, p. 277). In discussing expert systems and the wider area of artificial intelligence, we will examine the dangers of being too mesmerized by the "computational theory of mind," which can, with its deterministic and materialistic implications, lead to losing sight of what is of moral (and aesthetic) *value*. As Weizenbaum cautions, if we must teach only one metaphor, we run the risk of it swallowing up much that it does not adequately account for by deeming it either "meaningless" or "reducible" to the basic metaphor. Our concern in this book is with computer *ethics*, which goes beyond the realm of *what is* (*fact*) to the realm of *what should be* (*value*).

■ ENDNOTES

1. The Computer Ethics Institute is a group of concerned individuals from many areas, including business, education, religion, public policy, and computers. They are located at the following address:

> Computer Ethics Institute
> 11 DuPont Circle, NW
> Suite 900
> Washington, DC 20036

The Institute has formulated a set of guidelines for computer use:

Ten Commandments of Computer Ethics

1. Thou shalt not use a computer to harm other people.

2. Thou shalt not interfere with other people's computer work.

3. Thou shalt not snoop around in other people's computer files.

4. Thou shalt not use a computer to steal.

5. Thou shalt not use a computer to bear false witness.

6. Thou shalt not copy or use proprietary software for which you have not paid.

7. Thou shalt not use other people's computer resources without authorization or proper compensation.

8. Thou shalt not appropriate other people's intellectual output.

9. Thou shalt think about the social consequences of the program you are writing or the system you are designing.

10. Thou shalt always use a computer in ways that ensure consideration and respect for your fellow humans.

■ REFERENCES AND RECOMMENDED READINGS

Baird, Robert M., et al., eds. *Cyberethics: Social and Moral Issues in the Computer Age*. Amherst, NY: Prometheus, 2000.

Bergin, Thomas J. "Teaching Ethics, Teaching Ethically." *Computers & Society*, vol. 21, nos. 2, 3, and 4 (October 1991), 33–39.

Betts, Mitch. "Campaign Addresses Computer Ethics 'Void'." *Computerworld* 28, 21 (May 23, 1994), 33.

BloomBecker, J. J. Buck. "Computer Ethics: An Antidote to Despair." *Computers & Society*, vol. 16, no. 4 (October 1986), 3–11.

Boettinger, Henry M. "Humanist Values: What Place in the Computer Age?" *Financial Executive* (March 1970), 44–52.

Brown, Geoffrey. *The Information Game: Ethical Issues in a Microchip World*. Atlantic Highlands, N.J: Humanities Press, 1990, Chapters 1 and 9.

Brown, Geoffrey. "Is There an Ethics of Computing?" *Journal of Applied Philosophy* 8, 1 (1991), 19–26.

Bynum, Terrell Ward, Walter Maner, and John L. Fodor, eds. *Teaching Computer Ethics*. New Haven, CT: Research Center of Computing and Society/Southern Connecticut State University, 1992.

"Computing Curricula 1991." *Communications of the ACM* 34, 6 (June 1991), 69–84.

DeLoughry, Thomas J. "Failure of Colleges to Teach Computer Ethics Is Called Oversight with Potentially Catastrophic Consequences." *Chronicle of Higher Education* (February 24, 1988), A15, A18.

Ermann, M. David, et al. *Computers, Ethics, and Society*. 2nd ed. New York: Oxford University Press, 1997.

Floridi, Luciano. "Information Ethics: On the Philosophical Foundations of Computer Ethics." *Ethics and Information Technology* 1 (1999), 37–56.

Forester, Tom, and Perry Morrison. *Computer Ethics: Cautionary Tales and Ethical Dilemmas in Computing.* 2nd ed. Cambridge, MA: MIT Press, 1994, Chapter 1, Appendix B.

Hester, D. Micah, and Paul J. Ford. *Computers and Ethics in the Cyberage.* Upper Saddle River, NJ: Prentice-Hall, 2001.

Hollander, Patricia A. *Computers in Education: Legal Liabilities and Ethical Issues Concerning Their Use and Misuse.* Asheville, NC: College Administration Publications, 1986.

Johnson, Deborah G. *Computer Ethics.* 3rd ed. Englewood Cliffs, NJ: Prentice-Hall, 2001, Chapter 1.

Kizza, Joseph M. *Ethics in the Computer Age: ACM Conference Proceedings (November 11–13).* New York: ACM, 1994.

Maner, Walter. "Unique Ethical Problems in Information Technology." *Software and Engineering Ethics* 2 (1996), 137–154.

Martin, C. Dianne, and David H. Martin. "Professional Codes of Conduct and Computer Ethics Education." *Computers & Society* 20, 2 (June, 1990), 18–29.

Moor, James H. "If Aristotle Were a Computing Professional." *Computers and Society* 28, 3 (September 1998), 13–16.

Moor, James H. "Reason, Relativity, and Responsibility in Computer Ethics." *Computers and Society* 28, 1 (March 1998), 14–21.

Moor, James H. "What Is Computer Ethics?" *Metaphilosophy* 16, 4 (October 1985), 266–275.

Orwant, Carol J. "Computer Ethics – Part of Computer Science?" *Computers & Society*, vol. 21, nos. 2, 3, 4 (October 1991), 40–45.

Parker, Donn B. "Ethical Dilemmas in Computer Technology." In Hoffman and Moore (see Bibliography), 49–56.

Parker, Donn B., Susan Swope, and Bruce N. Baker. *Ethical Conflicts in Information and Computer Science, Technology, and Business.* Wellesley, MA: QED Information Sciences, 1990. A collection of interesting scenarios raising ethical dilemmas that arise in connection with computers.

Pecorino, Philip A., and Walter Maner. "The Philosopher as Teacher: A Proposal for a Course on Computer Ethics." *Metaphilosophy* 16, 4 (October 1985), 327–335.

Searls, Delmar. "Teaching Computer Ethics." *SIGCSE Bulletin*, 20, 3 (September 1988), 45–48.

Spinello, Richard. *Cyberethics: Morality and Law in Cyberspace.* Sudbury, MA: Jones and Bartlett, 2000.

Spinello, Richard, and Herman Tavani, eds. *Readings in CyberEthics.* Sudbury, MA: Jones and Bartlett, 2001.

Steinke, Gerhard, and Gilbert Hamann. "Ethics and Computers: Can Universities Set the Standards?" In *Advances in Computers and Information—ICCI '90.* New York: Springer-Verlag, 1990.

Stepp, Laura Sessions. "Ethics for Computer Use Top Industry's Concerns." *Washington Post,* 6 October 1990, p. 13.

Weizenbaum, Joseph. "The Two Cultures of the Computer Age." *Technology Review* 71 (1969), 54–57. Weizenbaum's social concerns for the computer age are further expressed in his book, *Computer Power and Human Reason* (San Francisco, CA: W. H. Freeman, 1976).

Wessel, Milton. *Freedom's Edge: The Computer Threat to Society.* Reading, MA: Addison-Wesley, 1974. Written by a lawyer for the American Federation of Information Processing Societies (AFIPS), it provides numerous insights that are still valuable almost three decades after it was published.

Wiener, Norbert. *The Human Use of Human Beings.* Boston: Houghton Mifflin, 1950, Chapters 1 and 2. The concerns of a brilliant mathematician and originator of the field of "cybernetics—the science of command and control in the animal and the machine." A few years after Hiroshima, Wiener is deeply concerned about maintaining the *human* part of *humanity* in a world increasingly reliant upon machines.

Witham, Larry. "High-tech Ethical Dilemmas Are Byproduct of Computer Age." *Washington Times,* 12 October 1990.

Part One

Ethical Foundations

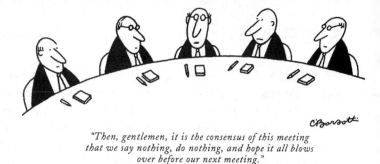

Chapter 1

Ethical Decision Making

*W*hat are the things that make human beings unique? Is it that they use complex language, do mathematics,[1] play games, have (or construct) religious systems, make conscious choices? A major element of human uniqueness is the fact that many humans act with respect and concern toward other humans, other living species, and even the environment. These actions are what we term *morality*. In some cases, they are done simply because of a strong feeling for others, but in many cases people who act morally are following principles that govern their actions.

Most human beings are social, gregarious by nature, as Aristotle noted; they tend to come together in communities. Aristotle said that humans are *political* by nature, since during his time they lived in community city-states, and the city-state in Greece was called a *polis*. In the *Republic*, Plato wrote about an ideal polis, a city that was proposed in thought and speech as a *model* for all good communities. In a community like Plato's, you would interact with other human beings. You generally are close to those who are *like* you—your family, who are close through blood ties, and your friends, who have the same interests and concerns as you do.

If there is not enough of everything material to go around—usually property and lovers—then you may also have enemies, those who want to take away what you have. This could include your land, your water, your flocks, your valuables such as jewelry or works of art, or your sexual part-ner(s). The ways in which you interact with these other human beings—

your friends, your enemies, and those to whom you are indifferent—are often governed by rules. These rules may be dictated by religious commandments, or the customs of your community, or the laws of the land, or your reason and common sense. Some rules or laws are arbitrary—such as "drive on the right side of the road"—but they are useful, since such a law prevents accidents. Other rules seem to have a deeper basis. Ethics examines the basis for principles of action and choice, where such actions and choices affect others.

Other animals do not act morally (*or* immorally); they seem to be strictly creatures of instinct, responding to pleasurable and painful stimuli, their behavior largely conditioned by these interactions. Humans, on the other hand, can *reflect* on what they are doing. They can think about the past, mulling over what they did and whether they should have done something else. They can *plan* for the future, mentally weighing different courses of action and their probable results.

The fact that humans have the use of language contributes much to this capability to evaluate actions. Memory, of course, is crucial as well, but other animals also have memory. Without language or some way to symbolize different events and then weigh them against one another mentally, memory would do little more than provide a kind of "instant replay," and allow for the continuity of experience. No comparisons could be made without memory, and no general principles could ever be discovered. It is interesting to note that computers have both memory and the use of language/symbolism. We will therefore consider whether they might ever be considered moral agents in our discussion of artificial intelligence.

Humans can mentally play with their memories, and look for common patterns among them; this gives rise to science and mathematics. They can also project some of these memory patterns onto future events, imagining what they might be like. This capability opens the door for them to make conscious **choices**: I could do A (like some pattern in my memory), or I could do B (like another pattern). The question then arises, which *should* I do? I could flip a coin, or go with how I feel at the moment, *or* I could evaluate the relative merits of A and B, based on my memories of past experiences. I could also look for some general principle for my choice of action; examples include "always keep to the right"—when trying to find your way out of a maze—or "punt on fourth down," or "do unto others as you would have them do unto you." The first two principles deal with practical means to reach some goal (they are of the form, "If you want X, do Y"); the third is an **ethical** principle that says "Do Z." The inquiry into such principles engages our mental capabilities.

Panayot Butchvarov, in his book *Skepticism and Ethics* (1989), makes a useful division of ethics into three parts:

1. The theory of good and evil—a metaphysical[2] inquiry into what they are, and whether and in what sense they may be said to exist.
2. The theory of right and wrong—an epistemological[3] inquiry concerned with our judgments that certain actions are right or wrong, and how such value is determined.
3. The theory of virtue and vice—an inquiry into the conditions under which we assign praise or blame. It includes moral education, the theory of punishment, and "certain aspects of the theory of distributive justice" (Butchvarov, 1989, pp. 29–30).

The term 'moral' generally refers to actions that are deemed worthy of praise or blame, and 'ethics' or 'ethical' refers to attempts to determine some general basis for choosing and judging moral actions.

A fundamental question for human beings is how we should live our lives. This generally involves trying to determine and secure what is **good**, and avoid what is **bad**. Thus the inquiry into what is good as a *goal*, or *end*, forms an essential basis for directing our lives. The good may not always be achievable, however. An *action* is considered **right** if it attempts to maximize good and minimize evil, and **wrong** if it does the reverse. Careful evaluation of actions, on which we base our judgments as to their rightness or wrongness, is what makes us moral, rather than amoral, beings. This evaluation is done based on some foundation, whether it is a "feeling" basis such as *caring* or *sympathy*, or a "rational" basis such as *calculating* the optimum choice among fundamental goods and evils. An act may be considered *right* even when all it does is choose the lesser of two evils, though it does not achieve the *good* end. If you must choose between saving the life of your child or your beloved pet, neither choice achieves the good, but one is more right (justifiable) than the other.

A creature that was totally passive, or completely reactive, would not be a moral being. Morality is defined by the process of making choices, and such choices should have a firm basis on which they are made. We will examine a variety of choice-making approaches.

MAKING MORAL DECISIONS

A moral decision is one that will affect others or yourself. The others are usually human beings, present or future, but could also be other living creatures, or the environment. Some examples of moral decisions are whether you or your lover should have an abortion, whether you support the death penalty, whether you should eat meat, whether you should recycle despite the inconvenience, or whether you should "blow the whistle" on the computer company that employs you and is defrauding the government. When you are faced with such a decision, there are five possible approaches you can take.

- *Make your decision based on your emotions, how you feel*
  Your individual feelings (or "intuitions") tell you what is best for you. The question is, can your feelings ever mislead you? Here are some examples.

  1. You feel the need of a serious drug, like heroin, to dull the pain of your failed romance. So you take it.
  2. You have an urge to steal something from a store, and no one is looking. Besides, it would give you a thrill. So you steal an expensive watch.
  3. You *want* your team to win the Super Bowl, and so you bet a large amount that you really can't afford, despite the many reasons that they probably won't win (injured quarterback, record of losses under pressure, etc.).
  4. Someone has done something very bad to you, such as lying in order to make you lose your job, which you need and love. You are furious, and want to kill the person. So you do.
  5. You feel that the Normandy invasion is a fake, so you don't send troops to meet it (Hitler in 1944). This mistake in intuition quite probably cost him the war.
  6. You *feel* that rerouting money from electronic transfers of funds into your own account is just a game that will let you show how clever you are (and make you rich at the same time), so you do it. After all, you never even *see* those you are stealing from, and they are probably insured anyway.
  7. You notice that there is a loophole in the security for the Internet, and so you let loose a *worm* program that keeps replicating itself and brings down close to 3,000 computers, because you *feel* that it would be a good way to point out the weakness of the system (Robert Morris, Jr., at Cornell in 1988).
  8. You are the manager in a data processing section of a large company. You made sexual advances to one of the employees in your

section and were rejected, so you trump up charges on the basis of which the employee is fired.

9. You are a physicist working on a top-secret project called the Manhattan Project. You believe that pure science is "value-free," and should be pursued for the sake of any new knowledge. The result of your work is the bombing of Hiroshima and Nagasaki on August 6, 1945.

- *Avoidance*

This might be called the "Que sera, sera" attitude—"What will be, will be." Avoid making a decision, try ignoring the problem or not taking it seriously, and maybe it will go away, or get resolved one way or the other without your involvement. This approach comes in a variety of forms.

The Undecided. Never make a serious decision, because if you do, you might make a mistake. If you don't make any decisions, you can keep your record clean of any errors. If you wait long enough, someone else will step in and make the decision, or the problem may go away, or it will be too late for you to make a decision because "nature" will have resolved the issue. In the *Inferno* (Canto III), Dante called such people "opportunists," and after death they raced round and round in the vestibule of Hell, going nowhere, since they had never taken a stand on anything in their lifetimes.

The problem with this is that you are never being moral at all; it is as if you are a plant, not a human being. But since you have the *capacity* to choose, since you *could* have made a choice, you can be faulted for not having done so. In religious terminology, you would never commit a sin of *commission*, but you are committing sins of *omission*—having failed to do something you should have done.

The Gambler. Leave the "decision" up to chance, or Fate. Again, that way, *you* can't be blamed. "It was just the fall of the dice!"

Example: Play "Russian roulette," because you do not really care whether you live or die, but you do not have the stomach to make a conscious decision one way or the other.

The Lazy, Irrational Coin-Tosser. In this category, someone is either totally indifferent, or too lazy to bother to pursue the basis on which a judgment should be made, so he makes a random, arbitrary choice.

Example: You are a general who decides you must shape up your troops by punishing them for slacking off. It would be too much trouble to research which soldiers were truly to blame, so you just decide to have every twentieth soldier shot as a warning.

The Rational Coin-Tosser. In some cases, you really cannot know enough to make an informed decision, or most of the available choices seem to put you at a disadvantage. Then the most sensible thing you can do is go for the 50–50 chance. There is a story about a biologist who had somehow offended the German leader Otto von Bismarck, and so was challenged by Bismarck to a duel. The man was given the choice of weapons. When he came to the field on the day set for the duel, he arrived not with a brace of pistols but with a pair of cooked sausages. He informed Bismarck that one of the sausages had been infected with trichinosis, which would cause the person who ate it to die a painful death. Bismarck was to pick and eat one of the sausages, and he would eat the other. Bismarck left the field.

Flipping a coin or choosing blindly is *not* making a decision rationally. Again, one is avoiding the moral responsibility, this time by leaving things to chance instead of to someone else, or to the inexorable progress of nature. It is a denial of the human **right** *and* **responsibility** to make choices. Surely in most cases you have some information, and perhaps some code of conduct, that would give you more good guidance than a chance fall of a coin would do. Even in the case of Bismarck and the sausages, the man challenged made an informed decision that he would stand less than a 50–50 chance if he had to confront Bismarck in any normal mode of combat. In that case, leaving it to chance was (rationally) his best bet.

- *Pass the buck*

    When you are confronted with a decision, but you really don't want to make it, there are various other ways to avoid taking responsibility for it, by shifting the blame elsewhere.

    1. **Find a scapegoat.** Always make sure that someone else is in line to take the fall if anything should go wrong; have a scapegoat ready and waiting in case things don't work out. This way, even if *you* make the decision, you can lay any flaws in the decision on someone (or something) else.

        a. *Blame it all on your parents.* "After all, I am just a product of my genes and my upbringing, neither of which was my fault!" Of course, then, your parents could pass the buck to *their* parents, and so on *ad infinitum.*

b. *Blame it on your teachers.* "They told me to do it! It's not my fault!" Teachers are occasionally confronted by students with bad exams who insist that the teacher told them to make certain moves in a proof (which are illegal), or that the teacher said a certain thing in class that they just put on the exam (wrong answer). The problem with these claims is that, in addition to the teacher being sure of *not* having said such things, no other students in the class thought so either.

c. *Blame it on your friend, or on the Devil.* "Charlie made me do it!", or "The Devil made me do it!"

d. *Blame it on your source.* By all means, never think for yourself. Always have someone else do it for you. Then if what you have done is brought into question, you can always transfer blame to the source for your decision. For example, if you are asked to write a program to control automatically the splash-down of a rocket, and you look at a model that does not take into account the rotation of the earth on its axis, you will blame the error on your source. However, if *you* are the one who failed to take the earth's rotation into account, *you* should be blamed. And, in any case, you were the one who *chose* the source.

2. **Go by the "book."** In other words, never make any *real* decisions on your own but always go with what precedent or authority says. That way *you* can't be blamed for anything.

a. *Blame it on your "boss."* Those who ran the concentration camps and the gas chambers in Hitler's Reich said afterward, in their "defense," that they were only following orders.

b. *Blame the law.* Hide behind the law whenever you can. This is another version of "never think for yourself." If you were asked, when segregation was still the law of the land, to make a decision as to whether the school you are involved in should be segregated, you would just say "Of course; that's the law," and think about it no further. And you would take no *responsibility* for the fact that what you were doing was not morally conscionable.

c. *As a general, you fight your battles by the book.* But armies that go "by the book" can be wiped out by a general with a brilliant *new* strategy. Note also that the general on the other side always knows what you will do, if you always fight by the book; but you will not know what he is going to do, which gives him a distinct advantage. (For example, think about Frederick the Great.)

    d. *Appeal to an authority (like Aristotle).* (Remember that authorities have been wrong.) Aristotle thought that the earth was at the center of the universe, as did philosophers and scientists through the Middle Ages. As late as the 1500s, people were burned at the stake or brought before the Inquisition for daring to suggest that the earth might *not* be at the center of the universe.

    Authorities disagree. What do you do then? For example, some scientists say that there are no problems caused by the depletion of the ozone layer, while others say that there are *real* problems out there. Who do you believe? Which authority do you follow? Are we back to flipping coins? Or should we look into *who* is making these claims—what credentials they have in their fields, who they work for—and, much more importantly, what *evidence* they bring in defense of their claims?

    The "book" or the law may be wrong, and need changing. In Sophocles' *Antigone*, King Creon's law is a *bad* law, and Antigone is justified in challenging it. In the United States, laws demanding segregation were *bad* laws and needed to be repealed. One should always ask "Is it a good law? Is it right?" before blindly following the "book." Sometimes older laws are simply not adequate to deal with new situations. We will see in Chapter 4 that the current laws for protection of property in this country do not adequately address problems arising in the software industry. Either the existing laws need a clear interpretation that fits them to these new cases, or the laws need to be broadened to cover them.

3. **Follow the crowd.** Another version of passing the buck is supposing that what the majority thinks is always the best thing to do. The question is, how often have the feelings of the majority been wrong?

    a. The witch-burning crazes.

    b. "Let's go with Alcibiades to Syracuse for a grand adventure!" (Said by the Athenians during the Peloponnesian War, a decision that cost them the war.) (See Thucydides, *The Pelopon-nesian War*, Book Six)

c. "The world is flat, Columbus. If you sail too far to the west, you will fall off of the edge."

d. Genocide in Hitler's Germany.

e. Slavery, and then segregation, of African-Americans in the United States.

f. "Women don't have souls; they are an inferior species." (Said by the male majority in power in many times and cultures, including present-day Afghanistan.) Is it true?

g. "Let's stick with building our mainframes; those small computers are just a fad!" (Said by management in some large computer companies of the past.)

Just as emotions can lead you astray, the views of many authorities or of the majority can do so as well. One should seek a more well-grounded way of evaluating choices.

- *Base the decision on caring, sympathy, or maternal love*
Though an ethics based on *sympathy* or *empathy* for other beings was put forward in 1740 by David Hume, it has received its greatest support recently from feminist ethics. An appeal to a fundamental caring relationship has more legitimacy than other emotional reactions we discussed earlier, but it still has problems in how it is to be used in making moral choices. For one thing, the range of those we care for may be too narrow to provide a basis for a general morality. Nel Noddings, in *Caring*, does not want to substitute *eros* (love) for *logos* (reason), but suggests it as a more basic approach to ethics.[4] We will not ignore the force of eros, or of sympathy, in our discussions, but it does not seem strong enough to be our primary approach. Perhaps what is needed in the long run is a combining of *eros* and *logos*, to put a moral "heart" into our ethical deliberations.

- *Find a rational criterion on which to base the decision*
Given the inadequacies of our earlier choices, this looks pretty good, but it still needs some work. What do we mean by 'rational' or 'reason'? If this is to be our guide in making good moral decisions, we had better have a good handle on it.

There are different views of **reason**, one which we will call the *ancient* view, and one the *modern* view.

VIEWS ON THE NATURE OF REASON

The Modern View of Reason

The **modern view** is that reason is a calculating device that (in the realm of "ethics") works in helping you satisfy your passions and desires. Your emotions tell you what you want, and reason figures out how to get it for you. Although a variety of thinkers, including some in the ancient world, held views that reduce reason to a calculating device,[5] this view is most clearly characterized by Freud.

Sigmund Freud (1856–1939) believed that the personality is composed of three systems: the id, the ego, and the superego. In a healthy individual, they work in harmony. The **id** is developed in infancy; acting on the *pleasure principle*, it attempts to relieve tensions and discomfort. It is demanding, impulsive, irrational, asocial, selfish, and pleasure-loving; it is the "spoiled child" of the personality, and always retains its infantile character.

The **ego** is the executive branch of the personality; it is created from the psychic energy of the id, but since the id cannot deal effectively with the external world, the ego acts on its behalf. The ego is governed by the *reality principle* (its contact and interaction with the "external world"–that is, the world outside of the individual personality). The ego serves the demands of the id, and intercedes with and manipulates the world outside to satisfy the desires and demands of the id. It is the calculating device that serves the passions.

The **superego** consists of the *ego ideal*, which embodies the goals that the child's parents held to be "good," and the *conscience*, which is the child's view of what its parents held to be "bad." Thus "good" is, according to Freud's model, only what your parents rewarded you for, and "bad" is simply that for which you were punished. The superego constitutes a person's "moral code," and it is derived from the views of the family and society.[6]

In *Civilization and Its Discontents* (1930), Freud begins by attacking organized religion as a "mass delusion" (Marx had called it the "opiate of the masses"). He writes that common religion has satisfied the need for a father figure who will continue to protect and guide us, and who will listen to our prayers and satisfy our wants.[7]

Many believe that religion provides the basis for ethics and that, without religion, people would behave like beasts. Freud disposes of religion[8] and puts nothing in its place as a basis for ethics. For him, reason (the ego) simply serves the id, and the superego (where one might think morality resides) is merely a conglomeration of the biases and customs imposed on the child by parents and society. There *is* another alternative, and that is that reason *can* provide a basis for ethics. It is this possibility that we will examine further.

The Ancient View of Reason

A number of ancient thinkers believed that reason does calculate and compare (as the moderns believe), but that it also can discover fundamental principles by which we can guide our lives, our judgments, and our actions. Plato taught that we should aspire to seek Truth itself, Beauty itself, the Good itself. These three Ideas, or Forms, would provide standards against which any claims to truth, or beauty, or goodness, must be measured. They must form the basis for any adequate logic and mathematics, aesthetics, and ethics, respectively.[9]

Plato has a compelling image in the *Phaedrus* of a charioteer and two horses as a metaphor for the human soul. This soul goes through many "lives" in seeking reality, and through that journey the charioteer must control the two horses pulling the chariot. One is gray in color, with blood-red eyes, and is always misbehaving and trying to upset the chariot. It is headstrong, and represents the desiring part of the soul. The white horse has a fine conformation, is obedient and strong, and tries to help the charioteer keep the chariot upright and on track; the white horse represents the spirited part of the soul. The charioteer is the reasoning part of the soul, and it is the job of that part to guide and direct the rest to the end of its journey.[10]

Aristotle believes that there are two kinds of intuitive reason whereby we discover the truth. One is that through which we discover the truth about particular things, through perception or observation, and which provides the ground for science. The other is that whereby we discover the first principles about relations among unchanging entities (forms or universals). Reason can tell us *where* we should be going as well as *how* to get there. Aristotle believes that reason can lead us to knowledge of first principles. It is reason, for example, which leads us to the indisputable truth of the Law of Non-Contradiction: something cannot both be and not be, in the same sense, at the same time. One needs only to clearly comprehend the statement of the principle, and then reason recognizes its truth. The Law of Non-Contradiction is a first principle from which the other truths of logic may be deduced.

Aristotle's account of reason is connected to his distinction between **means** and **ends**. The **end**, or purpose, of an action is the *reason* for doing it. (For example, my purpose in being a teacher is to help others to *understand* some fundamental issues, and ways in which they may be approached.) The **means** is simply the way in which one gets to the end. There may be a number of different means to an end, and reason will help you decide which means is the best. (To follow the example given, in teaching I can use lecture or class discussion, or a combination of the two; I can assign papers or give exams, or a combination; I can use an overhead projector or a chalkboard, or neither; I can assign readings or make everything based on the students' personal experience outside the classroom; and so on.)

Calculating reason (the only kind of reason the moderns say there is) can tell you the means for obtaining a certain end, and help you choose among various possible means to that end, but it cannot tell you *which* end you *ought* to pursue. If we had only calculating reason, then, we could make choices among means, but we would have no choice regarding ends. Presumably, then, they would be given to us by others (our parents, our state, etc.)—but how did *they* choose those ends? Perhaps someone might say that the ends are given to us by God. If that is the case, how does God communicate those ends to people? It could well be through their intuitive reason. If it is through *revelation* to other people, who then tell us, how do we decide between conflicting accounts of revelations?

Aristotle says that if we could reason only concerning means, which would mean that our only choices would be of means, then everything would be chosen because of something else, and this would go on without limit. If that were the case, all of our desires would be "empty and vain." Thus there must be some ends that we choose because they are good in themselves (like happiness), and our reason recognizes this. (See *Nicomachean Ethics* 1094a1–20.) We need intuitive reason to recognize appropriate ends, or else the calculating choices of means left to us will be meaningless. A calculating reason alone is not sufficient; we must be able to determine what ends or purposes are *best*.

A calculating reason, for example, might be able to tell you the most efficient and effective ways to make money, but it could not calculate for you *why* you should make money, or what is best to spend it on. A calculating reason could help you write an efficient computer program to control a "doomsday device" that would destroy all life on earth, but it cannot tell you whether or not you *should* build such a device. Calculating reason may tell you *how* to implement an "information superhighway," but it cannot judge whether it is a good idea, or what are the best ways in which it should be used.

Aristotle notes that the choice of ends (goals) is the most important thing in a human life. To "commit the greatest and noblest of things to chance" would be tragic. If all we could do was calculate effectively but we had no control over what we were calculating *about*, what purpose or meaning would life have?

Which View of Reason Is Correct?

Recall that the only important difference between the "modern" view (of a calculating reason) and the "ancient" view (of an intuitive reason) is whether we can discover first principles or not. Now it seems clear that we *can* and *do* discover first principles in logic (such as the Law of Non-Contradiction). Is this the only area in which we can discover first principles (and, if so, why)?

Can we discover first principles in mathematics, or do we just *invent* mathematics any way we like? The arguments appear to favor discovery. We know that "2 > 1" must always be true, and we can't just invent any relationship we like. We will discuss various positions on the foundations of mathematics in Chapter 4, when we examine them to ask what light they shed on the question of the ownership of mathematical truths, and how this relates to ownership of computer programs.

If it seems to you that I can make 1 greater than 2, without changing what the notation *means*, think about it more carefully. What is true in mathematics is not a matter of majority opinion. Most mathematicians are Platonists. They believe that mathematics discovers eternal relationships among eternal mathematical objects. There is also the phenomenon of what has been called "the unreasonable effectiveness of mathematics in science." It seems that some mathematical truths also mirror truths about the physical world (for example, the fact that harmonic chords in music can be represented as mathematical ratios). If mathematics consisted only of manipulating notation, then there would be no concepts that naturally belong to this discipline, such as number, negation, quantifier, inference, and the like. Once committed to those concepts, we cannot have the relations among them any way we wish.

Now if there can be knowledge of fundamental truths, of first principles, in logic and mathematics, why not in other areas as well? There are two possible kinds of first principles: (1) those that are intuited to be true and (2) those that are merely true by arbitrary convention (like the rules of a game). If the rules are not invented in logic and mathematics, why do some people want to claim that they are invented in ethics? We will examine some reasons that are commonly given for this belief, and assess them, in the next chapter.

■ ENDNOTES

1. Aristotle is reported, by Bertrand Russell, to have said that humans are rational because they can do sums.

2. *Metaphysics* is the study of what *is* (exists), what is *real*. The word comes from the name given (by subsequent editors, not by Aristotle) to Aristotle's work that comes (is catalogued) *after* his *Physics*. The term was first used by Nicolaus of Damascus, apparently referring to the position of that treatise in the edition of Aristotle prepared by Andronicus. (Sir David Ross, *Aristotle* [London: Methuen, 1964/1923], 13) Aristotle begins Book Alpha of the *Metaphysics* by saying, "All men by nature desire understanding" (980a 21). Thus metaphysics is a search for *wisdom*. At the beginning of Book Gamma, Aristotle says, "There is a science which investigates being qua being and what belongs essentially to it." (1003a 23) The Greek for "being qua being" is *on hei on*, that was later to prompt the name *ontology* for this science of being *as* being (that is, in its essential nature). José Benardete notes that Kant "characteristically understands metaphysics to comprise the three subdisciplines of rational (as contrasted with empirical) psychology, rational (as contrasted with physical) cosmology, and rational (as contrasted with revealed) theology, featuring respectively the soul, the world, and God" (José A. Benardete, *Metaphysics: The Logical Approach* [Oxford: Oxford University Press, 1989]). For Plato, metaphysics would be the study of the Forms or Ideas, the eternal, unchanging standard models for the particular entities we find in the sensible world (see Plato in general, and specifically *Republic* VI and VII). Metaphysics has come to include inquiry into personhood, the mind-body problem (these first two connect with Aristotle's *soul*); space, time, matter, and causality (connected with *cosmology*, or study of the world); freedom versus determinism (a combination of the first two categories); and the nature of *God*. Benardete includes artificial intelligence as a relevant inquiry in his book on *Metaphysics* (Chapter 19). The ethical element of metaphysics would involve persons and freedom.

3. *Epistemology* is the theory of knowledge. It investigates what knowledge is and the range of things we may be said to know, what are adequate grounds for claims to knowledge, the nature of truth, and the reliability of various claims to knowledge. A brief view of the relation between epistemology and ethics is given in the article by Richard B. Brandt on "Epistemology and Ethics, Parallels Between," in *Encyclope-*

dia of Philosophy, vol. 3, ed. Paul Edwards (New York: Macmillan, 1967), pp. 6–8.

4. See Nel Noddings, *Caring: A Feminine Approach to Ethics and Moral Education*, and Rosemarie Tong, *Feminine and Feminist Ethics*, Chapter 6.

5. Democritus (460–370 B.C.) believed that everything was explainable in terms of atoms bouncing around in an empty and infinite space (the void). Thus sensations of taste and color and the like are *in us*, and exist only "by convention"; that is, they do not tell us about how anything outside of us *really is*, since all we are sensing is the activity of the atoms *in us*. "It is necessary to realize that by this principle man is cut off from the real" (Sextus Empiricus, *Adv. math.* vii, 137). Thus sensations, emotions, and thought in general are just motions of atoms.

Thomas Hobbes (1588–1679) was a philosophical thinker who was influenced greatly by Euclid's *Elements* and the science of Galileo and Gassendi. He came to believe that everything (including human interactions and social systems) is explainable in terms of the motions of bodies. In the *Leviathan* (Part I, Chapter 9), he gives an account of the subjects of knowledge that places Science (knowledge of consequences) at the top, then divides that into Natural Philosophy (knowing the consequences of the accidental, random interactions of natural bodies) and Politics (Civil Philosophy), which examines the consequences of the interactions of the motions of "politic" bodies (i.e., political groups). Reasoning is just calculating.

David Hume (1711–1776) believed that all that is available to us is our perceptions. Given this basis, he drew out its consequences, which included the undermining of any notion that could not be tied to a corresponding impression. Wielding this "razor," Hume disposed of God, most of mathematics (that part dependent on the notion of the infinite, and being able to *know* the results of any long calculations), "substance," the void, causality, and the self.

An inactive (or, as Hume puts it, *impotent*) principle such as reason can never be the foundation for an active one such as morality, which excites passions, and produces or prevents actions. Reason just sits back and calculates; the moral sense gives rise to certain feelings and actions. He writes in Book II, *Of the Passions*: "Reason is, and ought only to be the slave of the passions, and can never pretend to any other office than to serve and obey them" (*Treatise*, Book II, Part III, Sect. iii).

6. Problems occur because society may disapprove of what the id demands, and thus the superego tries to prevent the ego from carrying out the demands. This leads to internal conflict, unhappiness, and often a "death wish." (See Freud, *A General Introduction to Psychoanalysis* [1917], and Calvin S. Hall, *A Primer of Freudian Psychology* [1954].)

7. Freud says: "The whole thing is so patently infantile, so foreign to reality, that to anyone with a friendly attitude to humanity it is painful to think that the great majority of mortals will never be able to rise above this view of life" (*Civilization and Its Discontents* [*C&D*], p. 21).

8. Freud also argues against the feasibility of the religious (and societal) dictum to "Love thy neighbor." He says that if I am supposed to love everyone equally, it makes my love of no worth whatsoever. I give it indiscriminately, with no regard to whether someone merits it or not. Further, I spread it too thin, so that there is not a meaningful amount for any one individual. In addition, "not all men are worthy of love" (*C&D*, p. 49; cf. p. 90). One should not be expected to love a Hitler, or a Saddam Hussein, or an Osama Bin Laden, or a Torquemada (the head torturer in the Spanish Inquisition). It is even more "incomprehensible" and impossible to be asked to "Love thy enemies" (*C&D*, p. 57). One's natural instinct is to want to see one's enemies hanged (see *C&D*, p. 57).

9. The path toward these eternal, unchanging Ideas may begin in illusions and distorted sensations, but it can move upward through the natural world, to the realm of science and mathematics, and finally to the Forms themselves. This is the upward journey that Plato described in the image of the Divided Line at the end of Book VI of the *Republic*. It is reason that helps us discriminate whether what we are entertaining at any given time is an illusion or reality.

10. In the *Republic*, where Plato is trying to design an ideal state (or *polis*), he finds (in Book III) that the state seems to have three parts, like the soul. There are the merchants, farmers, and craftsmen, who provide for the desires of the body; there are the soldiers, who bravely protect the state (they are the spirited part of the *polis*); and there are the leaders (the *guardians*), who keep the state stable and on track. It is clear that, in the harmonious state, each must do his or her proper job, and do it well for the benefit of all; it is in this, says Plato, that justice lies. It is also clear that the *reasoning* part of the state, the wise guardians, must be in control.

■ SHORT ESSAY QUESTIONS

1. Explain briefly the five basic ways one can make a decision that were discussed in the text. Can you think of any other ways to make decisions? Take a particular important decision in your life and try (in your imagination, and then write about it) each of the methods, and assess the quality of the results you could expect from each approach.

2. Scientists seem largely to support the modern view of reason as simply a calculating device. Can you think of anything within the realm of activity that scientists engage in that would provide an exception to this view?

3. What do you think of Freud's criticism of the rule, "Love thy neighbor"? (See endnote 8.) Can you give a rational defense of the rule against Freud's criticism, not just saying that it is what your parents said, or what your religion says?

4. Machiavelli is reputed to have said, "The end justifies the means." He used it to defend that the proper end (goal) for a prince of a state is to get power and keep it, and to use *any* means whatsoever (lying, cheating, stealing, killing, torturing, etc.) to do so. If ends are somehow simply given, and not seen to be good or bad, then is there any argument against Machiavelli's position based on the "modern" view of calculating reason? Machiavelli is sometimes called "the first modern man." Discuss.

5. Write a short essay to explain why you are going to college (or, if you are not in college, why you are doing your job, or avocation, or whatever occupies the major portion of your time). As you write, at each stage imagine there is a persistent child who keeps asking you, "But *why* do you want to do that?"

6. Would there be any problem if *everyone* were to adopt the position of "passing the buck" to someone else? Discuss.

■ LONG ESSAY QUESTIONS

1. Aristotle's argument about means and ends is very important. Show that you understand it by making up an example to explain it clearly to someone who has not read the discussion in the book, or Aristotle. At the end, evaluate whether you think Aristotle is right, and why you reached your conclusion.

2. You and your colleague have a heated disagreement about whether you should steal the formula that is the basis for another company's success. He argues that it will be relatively easy to steal it, and that it will be the most effective means of getting into the competitive market and getting rich. Further, getting rich will make you both very happy. You are unable to propose an easier or more effective way to compete in the market, but you want to argue against his position. What argument do you bring against him? Can you successfully argue against him and still stay within the modern view of calculating reason? If you need to go beyond it, to what do you appeal?

3. Does it seem that Freud borrowed his three-part personality from the tripartite soul that Plato discusses? Look for similarities and differences. This is a scholarly research topic and will take some effort and some additional reading.

4. Some ethics texts, as you can see from the "Recommended Readings" list, have titles like "Why Be Moral?" This is a good question with which to begin a study of morality. Without doing any further reading on your own at this point, try seriously to answer the question. Note that it seems to have two distinct aspects: (1) "Why should *you* be moral?" and (2) "Why should *others* (other than yourself) be moral?" Think about it, and come up with the best answer as you can. Do the two aspects of the question really stay distinct, or do they blend together?

5. Examine some congressional debates on a difficult issue, such as censorship of the Internet, or pornography, or wiretapping, or appropriation of funds for the Ballistic Missile Defense Organization. Much of this information is now available on-line as well as in your local library; for instance, the *Congressional Quarterly* is available by online subscription (for a fee), but it also has a free trial period (see www.cq.com). You can access the *Congressional Record* online at:

www.access.gpo.gov/su_docs/aces/ aces150.html

Another useful source of information, with an index, is at:

http://thomas.loc.gov/home/textonly.html

See how many instances you can find of approaches we discussed in this chapter to moral decision making, such as avoidance, passing the buck (various flavors), gambling, going by the book, following the crowd. Judge, in the light of our analysis and what you read in the proceedings, just how satisfactory, effective, or moral these attitudes are.

■ REFERENCES AND RECOMMENDED READINGS

Aristotle. *Nicomachean Ethics.*

Bahm, Archie J. *Why Be Moral?* 2nd ed. Albuquerque, NM: World Books, 1980.

Baier, Kurt. *The Moral Point of View: A Rational Basis of Ethics.* New York: Random House, 1965.

Brandt, Richard B. *A Theory of the Good and the Right.* Oxford, England: Clarendon Press, 1979.

Butchvarov, Panayot. *Skepticism and Ethics.* Bloomington, IN: Indiana University Press, 1989.

Donagan, Alan. *The Theory of Morality.* Chicago, IL: University of Chicago Press, 1977.

Foot, Philippa, ed. *Theories of Ethics.* New York: Oxford University Press, 1987.

Fox, Richard M., and Joseph P. DeMarco. *Moral Reasoning: A Philosophic Approach to Applied Ethics.* Fort Worth, TX: Holt, Rinehart, and Winston, 1990.

Frankena, William K. *Ethics.* 2nd ed. Englewood Cliffs, NJ: Prentice-Hall, 1973.

Freud, Sigmund. *Civilization and Its Discontents.* Trans. and ed., James Strachey. New York: W.W. Norton, [1930] 1961.

Freud, Sigmund. *A General Introduction to Psychoanalysis.* An authorized English translation by Joan Riviere was published by Permabooks, a division of Doubleday (New York) in 1953.

Gewirth, Alan. *Reason and Morality.* Chicago, IL: University of Chicago Press, 1978.

Gilligan, Carol. *In a Different Voice.* Cambridge, MA: Harvard University Press, 1982.

Hall, Calvin S. *A Primer of Freudian Psychology.* New York: Mentor (New American Library), 1954.

Hobbes, Thomas. *Leviathan: Or, The Matter, Forme, and Power of a Commonwealth, Ecclesiasticall and Civill.* 1651.

Hume, David. *A Treatise of Human Nature.* 1739.

Midgley, Mary. *Animals and Why They Matter.* Athens, GA: University of Georgia Press, 1984.

Nagel, Thomas. *The View from Nowhere.* New York: Oxford University Press, 1986.

Neilsen, Kai. *Why Be Moral?* Buffalo, NY: Prometheus Books, 1989.

Noddings, Nel. *Caring: A Feminine Approach to Ethics and Moral Education.* Berkeley: University of California Press, 1984.

Plato. *Republic. Phaedrus.*

Pojman, Louis P. *Ethics: Discovering Right and Wrong.* Belmont, CA: Wadsworth, 1990.

Prichard, H. A. *The Foundations of Ethics.* Oxford, England: Clarendon Press, 1939.

Rachels, James. *The Elements of Moral Philosophy.* New York: Random House, 1986.

Rawls, John. *A Theory of Justice.* Cambridge, MA: Harvard University Press, 1971.

Rosen, Bernard. *Ethics Companion.* Englewood Cliffs, NJ: Prentice-Hall, 1990.

Ross, W. D. *The Right and the Good.* Oxford, England: Clarendon Press, 1930.

Stevenson, Charles L. *Ethics and Language.* New Haven, CT: Yale University Press, 1944.

Tong, Rosemarie. *Feminine and Feminist Ethics.* Belmont, CA: Wadsworth, 1993.

Toulmin, Stephen. *Reason in Ethics.* London: Cambridge University Press, 1961.

Williams, Bernard. *Ethics and the Limits of Philosophy.* Cambridge, MA: Harvard University Press, 1985.

Chapter 2

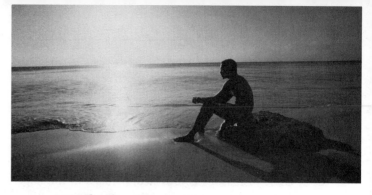

Is Ethics Possible?

SOME BAD REASONS FOR SAYING ETHICS HAS NO BASIS

There are some commonly held, and expressed, reasons given for doubting that there is any basis for deciding ethical issues. Most people have strong views about right and wrong in specific situations, but when they are asked to consider why they hold their views, they tend toward individual relativism ("what I feel is good *is* good") or skepticism ("there are no ethical truths"). Four arguments in support of ethical relativism are so common that they deserve special attention here. These arguments, and why they are unsatisfactory, are considered in the first part of this chapter.

Some people have developed more well-thought-out versions of ethical skepticism, and present arguments that constitute a more serious challenge to the possibility of a ground for ethics. Their arguments will be treated in the second part of the chapter, and the adequacy of these arguments will be assessed. One cannot just ignore ethical skeptics, for if they were right, there would be no point in our talking any more about ethics. If, however, we can see the flaws in the skeptic's position, we can then legitimately try to find an adequate basis for ethics. Once we have found a basis, we can apply it to real-world moral problems.

If this chapter strikes the reader as much ado about nothing, consider a discussion about why someone should not steal information from someone else's confidential computer files. Such a discussion can follow one of only three possible paths:

1. Every attempt to provide reasons for not stealing is met with another "why?", and so on ad infinitum. No reason is considered good enough to be the final reason.
2. A circle of reasons is provided, perhaps in the hope that if the circle is wide enough its circularity will not be noticed.
3. There *is* a final reason, where one is challenged to think of any alternative, or of a better alternative.

Skeptics claim that (3) is not an option, and that (1) and (2) are unsatisfactory (as they in fact seem to be). In effect, they argue that it is impossible to resolve ethical issues. The present chapter concerns the **possibility** of meaningful ethical inquiry. Chapter 3 engages in ethical inquiry.

Common "reasons" presented that claim to show that ethics is impossible include the following four.

1. **"Since people disagree about ethical issues, there can be no truth about these issues.** The people are just expressing their personal opinions, or their private rules. There is, however, no objective criterion for deciding their disagreements."

Criticism: People have disagreed about many issues in the past, yet there *was* an objective truth about these issues. They disagreed about whether the earth was flat, whether the earth was at the center of the universe, what was the correct value of pi, whether Fermat's Last Theorem was true, and numerous other issues, and in each case there was a truth that was unaffected by their views or their disagreement. It was merely a matter of determining what that truth was. Why should questions about whether women have value, whether slavery and genocide are wrong, whether animals have rights, whether a woman has a moral right to an abortion, what is the best life for a human being, or questions about property rights—in land, or in computer software—not also have answers that are objectively true, independent of personal biases?

The notion that there could be a private rule implies that it *cannot* be understood by anyone else, because the words or symbols of the rule supposedly refer to what is accessible only to the person—his or her own internal states or sensations. But the point of rules is for common agreement. How can I communicate the rules to myself? What information about the rules could I give myself that I do not already have?

How do you determine if you are following a rule correctly? By testing it against the understanding of others who use the rule. If there is no independent check on my use of a rule, then it can be whatever I want it to be. If, however, I can use a rule in any situation I like, with no check for whether I am using it correctly, it is not a rule, but just an arbitrary sound (that I can change equally arbitrarily). What check is there that I am obeying the rule? I could change the rule as I like, or conveniently forget the rule—but then it does not function *as a rule*. A "private rule" would not be a rule.

2. **"No one knows, or has ever known, the truth about morality, and so there is no truth about morality."**

Criticism: (a) This notion commits the fallacy (error) called an "Argument from Ignorance." This reasoning generally says either "Because no one has proved X to be true, it must be false," or "Because no one has proved X to be false, it must be true." Here you can plug in any number of propositions for X. If you use the claim "God exists" for X, then the first version is the argument of the atheist, and the second version is the argument of the theist. The same sort of argument cannot legitimately prove opposite truths (in this case, both that "God exists" is false and that "God exists" is true).

Another example of the Argument from Ignorance is that of the often-cuckolded husband, who innocently exclaims, "I never caught my wife cheating, so I know she is faithful." There are many cases of things that no one has *yet* discovered the truth about, but that may be discovered tomorrow or some day after that—for example, a cure for cancer, a cure for AIDS, whether there is life on Jupiter's moons. In 1988, someone could have honestly said, "No one knows whether Fermat's Last Theorem is true," but it would have been false to finish the sentence, "and no one will ever know, and so it must be false (or at least unknowable)." The proof was discovered shortly thereafter that Fermat's Last Theorem is true.

(b) The people making this claim most likely have not read all (or perhaps any) of the significant writings in ethics—Plato, Aristotle, Hume, Kant, Mill, and so on. If that is the case, how can the person legitimately claim to *know* that "no one has ever known" the truth about morality? Have they checked out all of the attempts to find the truth about morality? Can they show conclusively how each of these attempts has *failed*? If not, how can they be so sure (like the man with the promiscuous wife) that one of these attempts might not have hit upon the truth?

(c) One might also say that this claim commits another logical fallacy—that of "Hasty Generalization." Just because all of the attempts in the past have failed to reveal this truth, it would be wrong to infer that all future attempts will fail. Think of attempts to draw Excalibur from the stone (before Arthur tried), or the attempts of Penelope's suitors to string Odysseus' bow (before Odysseus, disguised as a beggar, succeeded).

3. A slightly less blatant claim, somewhat cowed by the last rebuttal: "Well, I really meant that **there are no moral principles on which everyone agrees**."

Criticism: (a) Is universal agreement the test of truth, or is there some other test of truth, such as the **correspondence** between a statement and reality, or the **coherence** of the claim with an accepted body of knowledge, or the **pragmatic** view that what is true is what works? How many examples can you think of where there was not universal agreement (or even *majority* agreement) on the truth of something that *was in fact true*? Begin with the examples of criticism in (1), such as the shape or position of the earth, pi, Fermat's Last Theorem. To these we might add:

> Not everyone agrees that murder, torture, and rape are bad.
>
> Not everyone agrees that smoking or heroin will damage a person's health.
>
> Not everyone agrees that there is a problem with the ozone layer.
>
> Not everyone agrees that the square root of two, or pi, are not rational numbers (yet there is a proof . . .); the people who do not agree simply don't understand anything but rationals.[1]

4. "But an objective good and bad, and absolute rules of morality, will rob me of my freedom, and I won't stand for that!"

Criticism: (a) The objectivity of good and bad would not rob anyone of the freedom to do what they want, to choose bad over good if they like. The appropriate parallel would be that a person is free to *believe* that pi = 22/7, even though this is not true. Pi is not equal to *any* rational fraction, but that objective truth does not restrict the freedom of anyone to believe what they want to believe. If, however, they want to get accurate answers when dealing with circular orbits for satellites, for example, *then* it does make a difference that their belief is wrong, and will give erroneous results.

(b) The freedom to believe does not change the truth about pi one bit; if you (and most people in your time) believe that the earth is flat, that does not make it flat. You are free to hold mistaken beliefs. You are not free to invent laws of nature, or the relations among numbers.

SOME MORE THOUGHTFUL DEFENSES OF ETHICAL SKEPTICISM

The following positions are still not strong, but they are more plausible than the previous four. We will examine these as well, and look carefully into any weaknesses they may have.

1. **Freud says that morality is a matter of feeling.**

Freud, and others of some repute, say that morality is only a matter of how one feels. We have already looked at Freud's view that good and bad are merely what your parents rewarded or punished you for, respectively. What supports this position?

Criticism: (a) To say "Freud says . . .", so it must be so, is a form of logical error called an "Appeal to Authority." Just because someone viewed as an authority says something, that does not make it so. On what evidence does the authority base the claim? Is it good evidence? Authorities have made mistakes. Authorities disagree (then what should you believe?).

(b) The person holding (1) responds, "But Freud is a scientist!" Are all scientists automatically right in everything they say? Then why has science changed and improved over the past centuries? If all scientists were right, then one could never speak of *advances* in science. And are scientists good authorities in areas outside of science (such as art or ethics), *just because they are scientists*?

(c) One must distinguish between a (scientific) theory and the experimental confirmability of that theory. A theory that cannot be verified or falsified is *not* a scientific theory. Thus if I have a theory that God is a little green elf with glasses, that is not a scientific theory, because there is no way to confirm or disconfirm it. Similarly, Freud's theory of the three parts to the personality is not a scientific theory that can be verified or falsified by scientific evidence.

A scientific theory allows one to *predict* what will happen in certain circumstances. But Freud himself said that the predictive test could not be applied to his theory, because the system of the personality was too complex to calculate the resultant forces. Douglas Hofstadter suggests as much in *Gödel, Escher, Bach* when he says that we humans may be too complex to understand how we work.[2]

(d) Like (c), what kind of scientific observation could count *for* or *against* the claim that "morality is based on feeling"? Try to think of an experimental test. If you say, "I feel that kumquats are intrinsically good" (*for*), or "reason tells me that equal entities deserve equal treatment" (*against* the feeling hypothesis), neither of these statements are about observable scientific facts. Thus the theory cannot be scientifically verified or falsified on its own grounds; that is, it is based on feelings, and feelings are not scientifically (publicly) observable. That is, the theory is *not* scientific.

2. "Morality is like taste—it is in (the taste-receptors of) the beholder. Who is to say for anyone else that vanilla ice cream is better than pistachio?"

Criticism: (a) Are war, torture, rape, and murder merely matters of taste? Is the fact that some people like them and some don't all there is to it?

(b) Are life, health, the absence of pain, knowledge, and mathematical truth merely matters of taste? Do some people prefer cancer to good health, being brutally tortured to a day at the beach, "5" as a solution to "2+2"? And even if a few people chose "5," would that "matter of taste" affect the true answer?

(c) When the skeptic asks "who is to say?", he is trying to undermine the possibility of any rational discussion of these issues, yet in raising his question he is attempting to engage in a rational discussion of the possibility of ethics. He cannot have it both ways.

(d) "It's a matter of taste" is essentially like saying "It's just how you feel;" the criticisms of morality as simply feelings are also valid against this version.

3. "Science has shown that we are all naturally and incurably selfish, and so we cannot help but go for what we think will make us feel good."

This position is referred to as **psychological egoism**. Psychological egoism is the observation made by psychologists that human nature dictates that humans always selfishly seek their own advantage as their main goal. This stance seems to be connected with the recognition of a strong primary drive in all animals for self-preservation. **Ethical egoism** is a moral position based on the psychological observation. Whereas the "scientific" observation only *describes* what is purported to be a fact of nature, the moral position *prescribes* a rule for moral conduct.[3]

Criticism: (a) Psychological egoism is another unverifiable and unfalsifiable hypothesis, and so it is *not* scientific. Hence the claim "Science has shown" is simply false. What would count as a scientific observation against (or for) the hypothesis? Those who make the claim try to cast every proposed counterexample as due to a kind of selfishness. If someone proposes Mother Theresa or Mahatma Gandhi as cases of unselfish actions, those defending the theory will claim that they both *really* acted out of selfish motives—to get attention, to be admired, or some such motivation. Neither the proposal nor the counterclaim is scientifically confirmable.

(b) Psychological egoism commits the fallacy of "vacuous contrast." For a concept (such as selfishness) to do some useful intellectual work, it must divide the world into cases that it covers and cases where it does not apply. According to the position, there can be *no* cases, not even imagined ones, that are *not* cases of selfish action. This absolutism renders the term 'selfish' empty—it does no useful work. The song lyric, "Everything is beautiful, in its own way," is the same kind of claim; it makes no useful distinctions.

(c) No evidence has been brought forward (and none *could be*) to support the strong claim that "science has shown."

4. According to Hume's doctrine of sympathy (empathy): Morality exists **only where there is a bond of sympathy between individuals.** This sympathetic feeling comes in degrees, and you have only a finite amount of it. Our resemblance to those people who are like us makes it easier for us to sympathize with, share in, their lives and their interests (or "sentiments"). Hume compares our sense of morality to our sense of beauty. When something (like a painting or a piece of music) causes pleasure in us, we deem it beautiful. Similarly, when a just action pleases us, we deem it virtuous; and when an unjust action (such as murder) displeases us, or gives us pain, we deem it a vice (Hume, *Treatise*, Book III, Part III, Sect. i).

Hume believed that all that is available to us is our perceptions. These perceptions are either *impressions* (sensations or reflections) or *ideas* (which are copies of impressions, though they may be arranged in new ways, by the imagination). Given this basis, he drew out its consequences, which included the undermining of any notion that could not be tied to a corresponding impression.

Claiming that there is no corresponding impression of "good" or "evil," Hume clearly would not turn to reason for a basis for ethics. He finds it instead in a kind of **feeling**, that of **sympathy**, among human beings. He argues that: "Moral distinctions are not the offspring of reason. Reason is wholly inactive, and can never be the source of so active a principle as conscience, or a sense of morals" (*Treatise*, Book III, Part I, Sect. iii). Reason is passive; it examines perceptions and determines their similarity or difference, but it is never the active source of a perception.

Criticism: (a) This is a purely descriptive theory. As such, it cannot be the basis of an ethical theory, which says what one *ought* to do. Hume himself makes this argument, that you cannot derive an *ought* from an *is*:

> In every system of morality which I have hitherto met with, I have always remark'd, that the author proceeds for some time in the ordinary way of reasoning, and establishes the being of a God, or makes observations concerning human affairs; when of a sudden I am surpriz'd to find, that instead of the usual

copulations of propositions, *is*, and *is not*, I meet with no proposition that is not connected with an *ought*, or an *ought not*. This change is imperceptible; but is, however, of the last consequence. For as this *ought*, or *ought not*, expresses some new relation or affirmation, 'tis necessary that it should be observ'd and explain'd; and at the same time that a reason should be given, for what seems altogether inconceivable, how this new relation can be a deduction from others, which are entirely different from it. (Hume, *Treatise*, Book III, Part I, Sect. i)

This is a good argument to show that you cannot go from strictly factual claims to moral claims about what someone *should* do, if you assume, as Hume does, that the only facts are those of Humean perceptions. There is no basis in the world of Humean perceptions for deriving prescriptive moral rules. Unlike *red* and *square, good* and *evil* cannot be found among these perceptions.

Hume says, as we have seen, that reason is passive, and could not be the source for an active principle of moral action. Therefore he concludes:

When you pronounce any action or character to be vicious, you mean nothing but that from the constitution of your nature you have a feeling or sentiment of blame from the contemplation of it. Vice and virtue, therefore, may be compar'd to sounds, colours, heat and cold, which, according to modern philosophy, are not qualities in objects, but perceptions in the mind. (Hume, *Treatise*, Book III, Part I, Sect. i)

Hume is perfectly content with this account of morality, as simply a factual report of how we feel and will feel. He says there *are* no oughts, only is-es. So the best we can do, philosophically, is to talk about the origins of the feeling of sympathy.[4]

If we are not satisfied with Hume's analysis, we have good reason to be disturbed. If Hume is right, then there *can* be no objective basis for morality, no way to resolve moral disputes (since different people simply feel differently) except by force. But we must deal with Hume's position, because it is a strong one. If we allow him his empiricist[5] starting point, then the rest of his argument follows with logical clarity. Not only are God, substance, infinity (and thus most of mathematics), personal identity, and causality wiped out, but now morality as well. If we hope to avoid these consequences, we must examine his starting point very carefully.

There are various non-empiricist accounts to which we can turn for help: Plato's supremacy of reason, which for him is an active, not a passive, faculty; Aristotle's conviction that reason can succeed in the search for first principles; and Kant's view of the possibility of *synthetic a priori* propositions (which we will examine in the section of Chapter 3 on Kantian ethics), which include mathematics, logic, laws of nature, moral laws, and metaphysical propositions about the soul, the cosmos, and God. Thus, as we look at these positions, we must keep in mind how they might help us to meet Hume's challenge.

Aristotle would say that, if Hume's claims here were true, we are facing the tragedy that what is most important in our lives *is* beyond our control. Yet Aristotle does not believe that this is the case, and spends considerable time in his various works discussing the search for first principles. It is through reason that we will discover such principles, whether they be the Law of Non-Contradiction, the necessity of a Prime (first) Mover to account for motion in the cosmos, or the fundamental principles of ethics.

(b) So the real question is, is Hume's view true? Compare it with the theory that we are all selfish, or with Freud's theory (to which it is very similar). Is there any possible scientific, controlled way to test this theory? If not, we may have to relegate it to the heap of failed (that is, unverified) theories. Or, at best, it will have no greater stature than any of the theories that compete with it, and perhaps less.

Biologically, what would the feeling of sympathy turn out to be? If it is just certain patterns of neural firings, could I simulate those patterns on a computer and thus give it "morality" in Hume's sense?

(c) Hume's theory of sympathy is not even obviously true, since I may give equal ("fair") consideration to people with whom I have no contact, or no similar traits or feelings (as in fair practices regarding housing, or education, or voting, or employment). If a person reserves all of his sympathy for one other person (and I have known one or two people like this), does that mean that he will act *immorally* (on Hume's grounds) to everyone else?

5. Cultural relativism: "All values are culturally based, and you can't criticize other cultures. Anthropology has shown us that different cultures have different value systems. Each value system is correct for its culture."

This awareness of cultural differences is not new in the last century or so. An example, often cited in textbooks on ethics, comes from Herodotus, *The Persian Wars* (Book III, Ch. 38):

> Thus it appears certain to me, by a great variety of proofs, that Cambyses was raving mad; he would not else have set himself to make a mock of holy rites and long-established usages. For if one were to offer men to choose out of all the customs in the world such as seemed to them the best, they would examine the whole number, and end by preferring their own; so convinced are they that their own usages far surpass those of all others. Unless, therefore, a man were mad, it is not likely that he would make sport of such matters. That people have this feeling about their laws may be seen by many proofs: among others, by the following. Darius, after he had got the kingdom, called into his presence certain Greeks who were at hand, and asked them what he should pay them to eat the

bodies of their fathers when they died. To which they answered, that there was no sum that would tempt them to do such a thing. He sent then for certain Indians, of the race called Callatians, men who eat their fathers, and asked them, while the Greeks stood by, and knew by the help of an interpreter all that was said, what he should give them to burn the bodies of their fathers at their decease. The Indians exclaimed aloud, and bade him forbear such language. Such is men's custom; and Pindar was right, in my judgment, when he said, "Law is king over all."

Herodotus noted many differences among the various cultures he visited. The Babylonians, he noted, buried their dead in honey (*Persian Wars*, Book I, Ch. 198). It seems clear in all these cases that, while the particular *means* chosen may differ, the *end* (or purpose, to invoke an Aristotelian distinction) in all of these cases is the same—to show honor and respect to the dead. Thus we may ask whether the *moral* basis is all that different, after all, in these different cultures.

In *The Moral Basis of a Backward Society*, Edward Banfield examines the "ethos" of a group in Lucania, a remote part of southern Italy. He puts forward the hypothesis that their morality is based on the principle: "Maximize the material short-run advantage of the nuclear family, and assume all others will do likewise" (Banfield, 1958, p. 83).

In *The Mountain People*, anthropologist Colin Turnbull finds in the Ik, a tribe in Uganda who seem to live in a Hobbesian state of nature, a people totally without human moral values.[6] One has to wonder how long a tribe holding such beliefs will survive.

Criticism: (a) Notice that the statement of cultural relativism contains within it an absolute moral principle: that it is morally *bad* to criticize other cultures, or not to respect their rights to their own views. At the very least, this is an inconsistency. What if some cultures felt that it was okay, and even *good*, to find fault with other cultures, and flaunt their customs? Cultural relativism would say that, since it is the value of that culture, that makes it right. But respecting the value in that culture would imply that the values in various cultures should not be respected, which would mean that we should *not* respect the value in that culture. Paradox! Contradiction!

(b) Accepting this view implies that no culture was ever mistaken about a value it held. Does that mean that slavery, the subjugation of women, genocide, etc., were right at the time they were held by some culture? If you reply that they were "right for that culture at that time," then you have a very weak sense of "right."

(c) It follows from (5) that it would be meaningless to ask whether one culture had a better view than another on some moral issue. But it is not meaningless to ask, for example, whether Hitler's Nazi Germany was wrong in its policy of exterminating the entire race of Jews.

(d) If (5) is accepted, it follows that cultures might change, but they could never be said to improve. Each stage of the culture would be said to be right. Thus it was right to have slavery (at one stage), and it was right to abolish slavery (at another stage). We should always be suspicious when a position leads us into contradictions.

(e) There could never be legitimate criticism within a culture, since what the culture was doing at the time must be "right" (according to the cultural relativism premise). This would make change in a culture rather unlikely.

6. **"The law is the only basis for morality."**

This is the view of Hobbes, and of Creon in *Antigone*. Hobbes argues that there are no societies without laws, and no morality without society. For him, morality coincides with following the laws of the state. Given his pessimistic view about human nature—that all humans are naturally selfish, aggressive, and without scruples—the only way to avoid humans killing each other off is to have them enter into an ironclad contract that they will do no harm—kill, steal from, and so on—to each other, and then give absolute power to some Leviathan to enforce the contract. Thus for Hobbes, what counts as just or moral action is that which obeys the laws of the state (which the Leviathan can make quite arbitrarily), and unjust or immoral action is any act that breaks the laws of the state.

John Rawls, in *A Theory of Justice*, is the modern proponent of social contract theory and the grounding of an ethical concept like justice in contracts and laws.[7] Rawls is concerned with *fairness*, and believes that rational fairness involves choosing and making the contracts with others that presume a "veil of ignorance": "they do not know how the various alternatives will affect their own particular case and they are obliged to evaluate principles solely on the basis of general considerations" (Rawls, pp. 136–137). He further assumes that all parties to the "original contract" are rational.

Criticism: (a) There can be society without law, and there can be morality without law. To see its possibility, one need only imagine it, and Jonathan Swift *did* imagine it in *Gulliver's Travels*. The society without law was that of the Giants of Brobdingnag in Voyage II, and the morality without law was found in the land of the Houyhnhnms in Voyage IV, where the peaceful horses lived in a "state of nature" such as John Locke had conceived. The other residents of the island, the Yahoos, were inferior creatures living in a Hobbesian state of nature, but they were easily controlled by the more rational Houyhnhnms.

(b) It is evident from history that there have been bad laws (and bad rulers). Yet on Hobbes' model there are no bad laws. To let the ruler and the laws determine what is just and right is to get things backward; what is just and right should determine the laws and who should rule. (See, for example, Plato's *Republic*, Aristotle's *Politics*, and Locke's *Second Treatise on Government*.)

(c) Those forming the contract, or the majority in a state, can unfairly exclude or exploit those who are not parties to the contract, or who are in the minority.

(d) Contracts can be (and often are) arbitrary. People can agree to do monstrous things (such as burn the "heretics" or the "witches"), or the contract can allow terrible things to happen to those who are not covered ("you're just a child, and children did not sign the contract, so you have no rights, and we can do whatever we like with you").

(e) Rawlsian contract theory presupposes that all relevant parties are capable of agreeing to the contract. Through most of human history, this restricts such contracts to males in the dominant group; morality surely has a wider scope than this. Mary Midgley suggests a list of nineteen categories of entities with which we might have moral relationships, or to which we might have moral obligations, that do not fit the contractual model.[8] These categories include the dead, posterity, children, the insane, the unborn, defectives, animals, artifacts, plants, God, and oneself.

(f) Butchvarov points out that Rawls's idea of rationality is one of calculating the effectiveness of various means to ends. Rawls writes: "a rational person is thought to have a coherent set of preferences open to him. He ranks these options according to how well they serve his purposes; he follows the plan that will satisfy more of his desires rather than less, and which has the greater chance of being successfully executed" (Rawls, 1971, p. 143).

Butchvarov further points out that Rawls says that humans enjoy exercising their capacities, but provides no argument as to which ends are rational (or good) to pursue.

> Rawls ignores another, far more fundamental notion of rationality in ethics, namely, that of the capacity to perceive intellectually, to understand, to grasp the intrinsic values of certain ends and to compare them. If there is such a kind of rationality, ignoring it would be like regarding a manifestation of rationality in deductive logic only the mastery of deductive techniques, and not also the grasp, understanding, and the rational acceptance of the truths of logic, of the *principles* of valid deductive inference (Butcharov, 1989, p. 37).

Concern only about means belongs to engineering; concern about ends is the business of ethics.

7. Sociobiology: "Ethics as we understand it is an illusion fobbed off on us by our genes to get us to cooperate" (Ruse and Wilson, p. 316). Our cooperation ensures the maintenance of the gene pool, DNA making more DNA, which is the only real purpose in this world. Ruse and Wilson (1989, p. 316) claim that "ethics is a *shared* illusion of the human race" (much like Freud's view of religion).

Where do Ruse and Wilson get their theory? They offer the following explanation:

> Our starting place is with the science. Two propositions appear to have been established beyond any reasonable doubt. First, the social behaviour of animals is firmly under the control of their genes, and has been shaped into forms that give reproductive advantages. Secondly, humans are animals (Ruse and Wilson, 1989, p. 314).

If humans are at all altruistic, it is only because altruism has worked out biologically. Groups made up of individuals who help each other (like ants in ant colonies) tend to survive, so the trait to help others survive is in the genetic code.

Criticism: (a) This is another "scientific" theory that cannot be confirmed or disconfirmed (which means that what they claim as a scientific theory is not science). Try to imagine a test case that would verify or falsify their claim.

(b) If we are all just acting out the programs written in our DNA, then there is no responsibility, no credit (or blame), and no such thing as *authorship*—thus there is no theory (since no one can choose to accept or reject it), and there are no authors of the marks on paper that claimed to be a theory.

8. Logical Positivism: "Every meaningful statement is either true by definition or verifiable by empirical observation."

This leaves no meaningful status for any statements about value, or religion, or the self, or general laws in mathematics or science. If statements about value, about what is good or right, are not meaningful, then there can be no rational ground for ethics; this is similar to Hume, and the same criticisms apply. Most logical positivists were emotivists in ethics, believing that a statement such as "X is good" is just a factual description of one's emotional state: "I like X." It might indicate further that "I want you to like X, too." [9] Thus, for the logical positivists, ethics should fall under psychology, and study why humans act "morally." [10]

Criticism: (a) If the Logical Positivists are right, then statements about the infinite (and thus much of mathematics), God, the soul, dreams, morality (all statements involving "ought" or "value"), all of space or all of time, or general laws of nature (such as Newton's Laws of Motion) are deemed meaningless by their principle. One can see why Kant wanted to demonstrate the possibility of synthetic *a priori* statements, which are neither true by definition nor scientifically verifiable.

(b) The statement, "Every meaningful statement is either true by definition or verifiable by empirical observation" (known as the Verification Principle) is not true by definition, and it is not verifiable by empirical (public) observation. Thus, on its own grounds, it is meaningless.[11]

 ## CODA

In this chapter we have examined four bad arguments put forward that ethics has no basis, and have looked carefully at eight somewhat stronger defenses of ethical skepticism and found good reasons to believe that these do not preempt a rational inquiry into nonemotive, nonconventionalist grounds for ethics; that is, we are not discouraged from pursuing the search for an ethics based on principles governed by reason. It is not enough, however, to show that no one has succeeded in eliminating the possibility of a nonarbitrary ground for ethics. It is quite reasonable to ask that the advocate of the existence of such grounds produce a case for such grounds themselves. Thus, in Chapter 3, we will examine critically the major efforts in the search for fundamental moral principles.

■ ENDNOTES

1. There is an interesting parallel that should be drawn here. In the dialogue *Meno*, Plato addresses the question, "Can virtue be taught?" This is a very important question, since it is desirable for all members of society to be virtuous; at the very least, it makes for a peaceful society. How can we instill virtue in everyone? Can we teach it in the schools? Can everyone get an inoculation against vice? Can one inherit a gene for virtue? Can it be instilled by lots of practice? Is there any other way to become virtuous?

   As with all interesting philosophical problems, there is no easy answer. It seems crucial, however, to determine what virtue *is* if we are to have a hope of answering the question. As the discussion proceeds, someone puts to Socrates the sophists' puzzle known as the Paradox of Inquiry. The Paradox deals with one's attempts to inquire after, to try to come to know, something new: "How will you look for it, Socrates, when you do not know at all what it is? How will you aim to search for something you do not know at all? If you should meet with it, how will you know that this is the thing that you did not know?" (*Meno*, 80d).

The Paradox of Inquiry challenges *any* attempt to inquire. Surely you would not inquire about what you already know, because you know it and have nothing to inquire about. So you must inquire (investigate) into what you do not know. But if you do not know it, how will you even begin to look for it, since you don't *know* what you are looking for? And if you were to stumble on it by accident, how would you *recognize* that you had found it, since you did not know what it was like? The sophists used this "debater's trick" to try to show the impossibility of knowledge of anything, and so to inflate the importance of what *they* teach—how to persuade, and dazzle, and confuse an audience so that you can get what you want.

Socrates takes on the paradox seriously; he does seek after truth and knowledge, and does believe that it is possible to find them. The story-like "answer" that Socrates gives to the paradox is that neither branch of the paradox ("horn of the dilemma") applies to a search for knowledge. You do not search for what you already know (now), but neither do you inquire after something of which you are totally ignorant. You know *in a sense*, or you will recognize it when you see it. What Socrates claims is that you knew it once, but you have forgotten it. Thus what is required is that you have to *remember* what you once knew. This is called Plato's **doctrine of recollection** (*anamnesis*).

The doctrine of recollection implies a series of past lives, and in the time between those lives the soul, having shed the prison of the body, has been able to "see" the Forms directly (see *Republic*, Book X, the "Myth of Er," which describes the time the soul is between bodily lives). This is a knowledge by direct acquaintance, in the way that you *know* that you have a pain in your tooth, because you are *directly acquainted* with that pain.

A myth is generally invoked by Plato when there is no immediately clear rational explanation of a phenomenon that certainly occurs. It is obvious that we *do* come to know what we did not know before; that is what **learning** is. So the question is, how do we do this, given the real difficulties the paradox presents? The answer is either that we did know it and just forgot (at the time of birth), and have to remember; or that we know it *in a sense* (perhaps there is some innate knowledge "wired in" at birth); or that reason will just be able to "see" that something is right when it is (it can *intuit* the difference between a right answer and a wrong one).

Think about how your mind works when someone explains something to you (a mathematical proof, or an argument that clearly proves something) and the truth finally "dawns"–it just "works," it somehow fits in with your reason, and you accept it. Just *how* this happens is not clear, and it is not certain that a more sophisticated science of physiology could explain it, either. Socrates proposes a *test* of his theory of recollection. Meno has a slave-boy who speaks Greek, but has never been taught any mathematics or geometry. Socrates poses to him the problem of how to double the area of a given square. He begins with a square of two units on a side (with area of four square units) and asks the boy what would be the length of the side of a square that had twice the area. The boy guesses–first double the length of the side, but that is easily shown to quadruple the area, and the boy readily recognizes this. Then he guesses a length in between the original and his first guess, a length of three units, but this is also shown to be too big.

Socrates then takes one of the original two-by-two squares in the larger (four-by-four) square they drew for the boy's first guess, and *draws* the diagonal of the square, which has the irrational length of two times the square root of two. That diagonal halves the area of the two-by-two square, creating a triangle of area two square units. If the diagonals are drawn in all four of the two-by-two squares, such as to create the sides of an interior square, it will be made up of four of those triangles of area two square units, which will give the desired new square of eight square units. Another way to look at this is that the four-by-four square was twice as big as the one we wanted; by cutting each of its four inner squares in half, we created a square half the size of the 16-square-unit square.

Socrates' point is twofold. First, the boy, though he had *no* previous training in mathematics (and we *all* start out that way) was able to recognize, with a little guidance, when his guesses were wrong, and also was able to recognize the right answer when he saw it, even though he did not know it, or know how to look for it, initially. Socrates attributes the recognition to recollection; it could have another explanation, but it *does* occur. We *do* come to learn things that we did not know before.

The second point is that the answer was something that could be *shown* (pointed to), but it could not be spoken, or given in an exact mathematical form. The square root of two is an irrational number, which means that it cannot be represented as the ratio of *any* two integers; such a ratio *could* be expressed in a nice finite mathematical language. The square root of two has an infinite, nonrepeating decimal expansion, which means it cannot be expressed accurately in any finite notation, or grasped completely by a finite mind. It *can*, however, be pointed out.

I believe that Plato's aim in this part of the dialogue is to show that virtue, as well, is not expressible in any simple, finite formula (such as "Always do X"); it is too complex for that. Thus it does not have a simple "pat" description such as many would like, so that they could get on about other, "more important" business. It may be, however, that virtue can be pointed to, it can be exemplified—and that Plato, in writing dialogues about the life of Socrates, has pointed to a paradigm of virtue, one that can be copied, even if it cannot be described completely in any finite language (just as the square root of two cannot be completely expressed in a finite mathematical notation).

2. Douglas R. Hofstadter, *Gödel, Escher, Bach: An Eternal Golden Braid* (New York: Vintage Books, 1980), p. 697.

3. This nice distinction between description and prescription is offered by Louis P. Pojman, *Ethics: Discovering Right and Wrong*, p. 200.

4. This treatment of Hume is not intended to cover caring and communitarian interpretations drawn from Hume's writings by some recent philosophers.

5. *Empiricism* is a philosophical position that the only knowledge we can have (if any) must come through the senses. Innate (inborn) ideas are denied, as well as any concept for which there is not a corresponding perception (such as infinity).

6. See Peter Singer's discussion of this book in his chapter on "Egoism, Altruism, and Sociobiology," in *The Expanding Circle*. This is also reprinted in Pojman, 1989, pp. 99–100.

7. Rawls' work on justice is very complex, and requires a much more detailed analysis than we can give it here. Thus the comments we do make only attempt to briefly take on the notion, put forward by Rawls, that laws and contracts are *it* with respect to justice (and other moral categories).

8. Mary Midgley, "Duties Concerning Islands," in Donald VanDeVeer and Christine Pierce, eds., *People, Penguins, and Plastic Trees* (Belmont, CA: Wadsworth, 1986), p. 161. The article appeared originally in *Encounter* LX (February 1983), 36–43.

9. Two early emotivists characterized the matter thus:

> "'Good' is alleged to stand for a unique, unanalysable concept... [which] is the subject matter of ethics. This peculiar use of 'good' is, we suggest, a purely emotive use. When so used the word stands for nothing whatever, and has no symbolic function... In the sentence, '*This* is good,'. . . 'is good'. . . serves only as an emotive sign expressing our attitude to *this*, and perhaps evoking similar attitudes in other persons, or inciting them to actions of one kind or another" (C. K. Ogden and I. A. Richards, *The Meaning of Meaning* [New York: Harcourt Brace, 1923], p. 125).

> A more extended version of this quote was used by Charles L. Stevenson in the frontispiece of his book, *Ethics and Language* (New Haven: Yale University Press, 1944).

10. Moritz Schlick, *Problems of Ethics*, trans. David Rynin (New York: Dover, 1962/1939), pp. 28–30.

11. A historical note: One of the major logical positivists, Moritz Schlick, who taught the principles of logical positivism in Vienna, including that all ethical statements are meaningless, was shot to death by one of his students in 1936.

■ SHORT ESSAY QUESTIONS

1. Is there a sort of continuum of matters of taste? Try to create a list of examples of things that are clearly a matter of taste, things that are clearly something more (like one's view on rape), and things that seem in between. Can you determine, from your lists, what the items in each of these three groups have in common? Can you determine what it is that *distinguishes* one group from the others? When you are finished, are there still three groups, or only two? If you still have an "in-between" group, is that where most interesting moral problems fall?

2. Is there any problem with the argument, in defense of ethical egoism, that *you* are always in the best position to know what is best for you? Use examples.

3. Do you agree with the claim that "morality is in the eye of the beholder," in the same sense that people claim that "beauty is in the eye of the beholder"? Discuss critically, drawing on the various positions covered in this chapter.

4. If our genes are merely "fooling us" into maintaining the gene pool, as Ruse and Wilson (1989) suggest, what becomes of ethics as a meaningful activity? Are there any ethical rules derivable from this position?

5. Discuss your reaction to Hume's position that all morality could be is a sympathetic feeling toward others. If you think there is something more, try to explain your view to Hume. How would he probably answer you?

■ LONG ESSAY QUESTIONS

1. It has been suggested that the main character from earth in Robert Heinlein's acclaimed science-fiction novel, *Stranger in a Strange Land*, is an example of an ethical egoist. Read the novel with this in mind, and provide a critical analysis of the claim. *Or* analyze Heinlein's *The Moon Is a Harsh Mistress* for examples of ethical egoism in a critical paper. (The suggestion about the ethical egoism to be found in these novels comes from James P. Thiroux, *Ethics: Theory and Practice*, p. 53.) Note also Heinlein's use of the Herodotus example of eating the dead in *Stranger*, where Mike has told the earthlings of this Martian religious custom (comparison is also made to a practice in certain earth religions, where wine and bread consumed are symbolic of the blood and body of a spiritual leader who has died); in both cases it is a sign of reverence. Note also the line (p. 122) about custom being king: "Never mind what they think in Kansas; Mike uses values taught him on Mars." A third essay topic could be an analysis of whether Mike, the Martian with the different customs, turns out to be the most *moral* (in an overall, not a local custom-bound, sense) of all of the characters in the book.

2. A good pair of articles evaluating ethical egoism on both sides is Brian Medlin, "Ultimate Principles and Ethical Egoism," *Australasian Journal of Philosophy* XXXV (1957), 111–18 [against]; and Jesse Kalin, "In Defense of Egoism" [pro]. Both articles can be found in either Louis P. Pojman, ed., *Ethical Theory: Classical and Contemporary Readings* (Belmont, CA: Wadsworth, 1989), pp. 81–98; or William P. Alston and Richard B. Brandt, eds., *The Problems of Philosophy* (Boston: Allyn and Bacon, 1974), pp. 204–219. Track down these two articles, summarize their major points, analyze their strengths and weaknesses, and come to a justified conclusion as to which is the better case.

3. Examine Peter Singer's chapter on "Egoism, Altruism, and Sociobiology," in *The Expanding Circle* (New York: Farrar, Strauss, and Giroux, 1981). Discuss his arguments in favor of ethical altruism from the "Prisoner's Dilemma" and the "sabre-tooth cat" attack. Do these provide a good basis for an ethical position (in this case, altruism—benefitting others even if at some harm or risk to yourself)? [The chapter is also reprinted in Louis P. Pojman, ed., *Ethical Theory: Classical and Contemporary Readings* (Belmont, CA: Wadsworth, 1989), pp. 98–105.]

4. Evaluate the argument put forward by Kurt Baier in *The Moral Point of View* (New York: Random House, 1965) against ethical egoism.

5. In James Rachels' book, *The Elements of Moral Philosophy* (New York: Random House, 1986), he discusses three arguments in favor of ethical egoism (pp. 67–73). Louis Pojman (in *Ethics: Discovering Right and Wrong*, pp. 47–48) mentions a fourth, which he calls the "Economist Argument"; here he parallels ethical egoism with Adam Smith's economic theory that unregulated self-interest will lead to overall prosperity for all (of course, it requires Smith's "invisible hand" to "explain" how it works!). Explain these four arguments in favor of ethical egoism, and assess how convincing they are.

■ REFERENCES AND RECOMMENDED READINGS

Baier, Kurt. *The Moral Point of View: A Rational Basis of Ethics.* New York: Random House, 1965.

Banfield, Edward C. *The Moral Basis of a Backward Society.* New York: Free Press, 1958.

Butchvarov, Panayot. *Skepticism and Ethics.* Bloomington, IN: Indiana University Press, 1989.

Herodotus. *The Persian Wars.* Trans. George Rawlinson. In *The Greek Historians*, ed. Francis B. Godolphin (New York: Random House, 1942).

Hobbes, Thomas. *Leviathan: Or, The Matter, Forme, and Power of a Common-wealth, Ecclesiasticall and Civill.* 1651.

Hofstadter, Douglas R. *Gödel, Escher, Bach: An Eternal Golden Braid.* New York: Vintage Books, 1980.

Hume, David. *A Treatise of Human Nature.* 1739.

Mackie, J. L. *Ethics: Inventing Right and Wrong.* Baltimore, MD: Penguin, 1977.

Nagel, Thomas. *The Possibility of Altruism.* Oxford, England: Clarendon Press, 1970.

Plato. *Meno. Gorgias.*

Pojman, Louis P. *Ethical Theory: Classical and Contemporary Readings.* Belmont, CA: Wadsworth, 1989.

Pojman, Louis P. *Ethics: Discovering Right and Wrong.* Belmont, CA: Wadsworth, 1990.

Rachels, James. *The Elements of Moral Philosophy.* New York: Random House, 1986.

Rand, Ayn. *Atlas Shrugged. The Fountainhead. The Virtue of Selfishness.*

Rawls, John. *A Theory of Justice.* Cambridge, MA: Harvard University Press, 1971.

Ruse, Michael, ed. *Philosophy of Biology.* New York: Macmillan, 1989.

Ruse, Michael, and Edward O. Wilson. "The Evolution of Ethics." In Ruse, 1989, pp. 313–17.

Sophocles. *Antigone.*

Swift, Jonathan. *Gulliver's Travels.*

Thiroux, Jacques P. *Ethics: Theory and Practice.* 3rd ed. New York: Macmillan, 1986.

Chapter 3

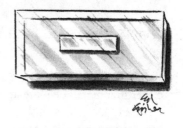

THE SINGLE STANDARD OF MORALITY
(IN ITS HERMETICALLY SEALED CASE AT THE
NATIONAL BUREAU OF STANDARDS)

The Search for a Basis for Ethics

*I*n Chapters 1 and 2, we looked at the importance of a fuller view of reason to the foundation of ethics, various commonly held beliefs that deny such a foundation, and a variety of considered arguments for adopting skeptical views about ethics. We concluded that a reason capable of discovering principles is crucial to ethical decision making, that common skeptical arguments about ethics are very weak, and that more sophisticated skeptical arguments are not strong enough to preempt a search for ethical principles. In this chapter we will look at some positions that offer hope for a rational foundation for ethics.

What follows is not a short history of ethical theory, but an attempt to organize and evaluate the array of efforts to find a rational foundation for ethics. The reader is encouraged not to think in terms of positions being either all right or all wrong. As in physics, a common failing of an ethical theory is to mistake a special case for the general case, as in "pleasure is the *only* good" instead of "pleasure is *a* good." There is merit in each of the positions presented, though none may yet provide the perfect view of ethics. We should learn what we can from each attempt, and perhaps in that way come closer to a more adequate approach.

Early materialist philosophies[1] led to relativism—colors, sounds, and the like are not *in* objects but rather are the motions of physical particles in the individual perceiver, and so "truth" about such things is *relative* to the perceiver. A group called the Sophists[2] ignored physical explanations, but taught a relativism—that each man is the measure of truth and good for himself. A variant on this sort of self-directed thinking is ethical egoism.

ETHICAL EGOISM

Ethical egoism is the view that one *should* attempt to maximize one's own happiness. **Individual ethical egoism** is the ethical position that the individual ("I") *ought to* act always to promote her ("my") best interest, regardless of other considerations. It might also be stretched to say, from my personal point of view as the individual in question, that everyone and everything ought to act or work in *my* best interest (though this is generally a view practically held by only a few, usually despotic rulers). **Universal ethical egoism** is the ethical position that all beings (or at least all human beings) ought to act in their own best interests, regardless of other considerations.

It seems that both individual and universal ethical egoist positions self-destruct. In a universe where all beings acted only to procure their own best interests, *regardless of other considerations*, they would soon wipe each other out. It is in fact this kind of universe that Hobbes envisions as the "state of nature," and he concludes that the only possible solution to avoid total annihilation is for the beings to join in a mutual contract (which they do only out of fear of death) to give some other being absolute power to keep them all to a nonaggression agreement. Is this a *moral* society? Let us now consider two arguments on behalf of ethical egoism.

1. **"One should take care of oneself and not worry about others, because one knows what is good for oneself but not for others."** You are in a unique position (epistemically) to know how you feel, what you think, and so on. Everyone else must rely on your behavior, or on what you tell them, to try to determine how you feel or what you think, but only you know for sure, directly, without any need for inference. Thus who better to make all decisions regarding your own best interests?

Criticism: Unlike psychological egoism, which is merely descriptive, this puts forward an *argument* making specific *why* your concerns should be only about yourself, because that is the only thing you know for sure. However, the argument is flawed.

(a) Often people do *not* know what is best for themselves. Knowing their own feelings (pleasures and pains) intimately does not necessarily make them the best judge of *how* to insure that in the future they will have lots of pleasures and no pains. Think of examples, such as your friend who is hopelessly in "love" with the wrong person, or the compulsive gambler or drinker, etc.

(b) Often people *do* know what is good for others. You can see that your friend has fallen for the wrong person; a doctor is the best judge of what treatment will make you well; a lawyer can provide a better defense for you in a court of law than you could do for yourself. (Note the old adage that even a lawyer who defends himself has a fool for a client—because he will not be *objective* and clear-headed when he is involved too closely.)

2. The Ayn Rand Morality: **"Only individuals are creative and, thus, only creative individuals are the ultimately valuable entities. Groups and group rules repress individual creativity; they are levellers. So it is the individual against the group, and the group ought to lose."** This is not a matter of emotion (feeling) or convention; it is a value-laden claim that only creative individuals are important, and they should be able to do whatever they want to exercise their creativity.

Criticism: (a) The interests of the individual, in most cases, cannot easily be distinguished from the interests of the group. People come together into groups (societies) for mutual protection and for companionship. Even the "loner" creative artist still depends on others for some things (including some form of patronage). Imagine trying to indulge your creative genius if you had to spend most of your time growing and harvesting (or hunting) your food, building your shelter, making your clothes and shoes, providing your own transportation, and protecting yourself from wild animals and marauding predatory humans. Try learning without books about what others have thought, and the latest advances in science. Human children need protection and care for a long period of their early lives (compared to most other animals), during a period when it would generally be too soon to tell whether they were creative geniuses or not.

(b) In *The Virtue of Selfishness* (1961), Ayn Rand writes: "The achievement of his own happiness is man's highest moral purpose." Thus if A's creative genius is to be an outstanding head of a major computer company, and B also wants the job, it is (according to Rand) A's *moral duty* to kill B. However, B may have the same moral duty (B is also a creative computer genius). This poses a problem, and Rand provides *no* way of resolving it in a moral fashion. The stronger will kill the (physically) weaker, independent of level of creative genius, and we are back to the rule of force.

Rand regards altruism as not knowing how to live your life, but only how to *sacrifice* it; she obviously disapproves of such self-sacrifice. Altruism is thus a vice for Rand, and selfishness is the highest virtue. She also claims (in *The Virtue of Selfishness*) that the self-interests of rational beings, *as rational beings*, will never conflict. Is this possible? Kant will argue that rational beings will agree on moral principles because of their rationality, but complete selfishness would never be one of those principles.

PLEASURE- AND PAIN-BASED THEORIES OF ETHICS

Epicurus developed the earliest "pleasure-pain" theory, which held that the good is pleasure, and that one's goal in life should be to maximize pleasure and minimize pain.[3] Despite the activities of some of his followers, Epicurus did *not* mean that we should live a life of constant orgies. He recognized that this would not lead to peace of mind. What he did advocate was to maximize long-term pleasure; the best way to do this was to emphasize the pleasures of the mind over those of the body, to lead a low-key, thoughtful, prudent life. Epicurus advised people to store up pleasant memories of past pleasures to have in reserve during bad times. Death was nothing to fear for the Epicureans; the body would just resolve itself into its basic elements (atoms), but remain part of nature. The "modern update" of Epicureanism is classical utilitarianism, a theory also based on the view that pleasure is good and pain is bad.

CLASSICAL UTILITARIANISM

Jeremy Bentham, in *Principles of Morals and Legislation* (1789), put forward an ethical theory that defined the greatest good as the greatest amount of pleasure for the greatest number of people. To live a moral life, one would thus try to maximize pleasure and minimize pain for the greatest number of people. To decide what to do when a moral choice arose, one would merely have to calculate the anticipated future pleasures and pains for all concerned, and make the choice that created the greatest amount of pleasure over pain.

When estimating these pleasures and pains, Bentham indicated that one should take into account the intensity, certainty (how likely they are), duration, "purity," and "fruitfulness" (how likely it is that they will lead to future pleasures) as well as how quickly they can be achieved. (Presumably, a pure pleasure would not be diluted by too many distractions.) Otherwise, for Bentham's theory, one pleasure was as good as another. If the total amount of pleasure is the same, "pushpin is as good as poetry," he remarked. (Pushpin is a simple children's game.)

In Bentham's "hedonic calculus," all you had to do was figure out the amount of pleasure (let us, say, measure it in pleasure units called "hedons") and the amount of pain ("anti-hedons" or negative hedons) for each choice, sit down, and do the calculation. The problem is how to figure out the probable number of hedons for each choice. Who is to be included in figuring the greatest good for the greatest number? Everybody? Will women be included in a male-dominated society? How about children? Slaves? Criminals in prison? Old people? All races, creeds, and colors? These are moral questions that a hedonic calculus will not answer, yet the answers must be determined in order to set up the calculus. Bentham seems to be caught in a catch-22.

Even if Bentham said "Okay. Include everybody," and we could facilitate the calculations with modern technology, there still would be problems. How are we to judge the amount of pleasure and pain for an event that has not happened yet? This could reduce to mere guessing, and our guesses could be far off.

We could do a "trial run." If the ethical question is whether or not to have capital punishment, we could run a test for six months where we had capital punishment, and then a test for six months where there was no capital punishment, and compare the results (normalizing for the number of people involved in both tests). We could have everybody in the country wired up to measure the amount of pleasure and pain hedons they were generating, and it would all be fed into a central supercomputer. At the end of the year, the supercomputer would tell us which was the moral choice (which one resulted in more pleasure over pain).

Of course, another problem would be that it would be difficult, if not impossible, to "control" the two six-month periods so that no other factors changed during that period. For example, if during the six months when capital punishment was in place, it turned out that the lotteries paid off, due to computer error, to half the population, then the pleasure total would skyrocket, and it would have nothing to do with the capital punishment issue.

One additional problem with Bentham's system is that it could justify any atrocity. If we imagine a sadistic society in which people get pleasure out of watching other people being tortured, then the intense suffering of a few people who were being tortured would provide a great amount of pleasure to a great number of people watching (in the arena, and over televised broadcast). Thus the torturing of these few people would be justified by the utilitarian principle. Slavery could also be justified by this principle.

John Stuart Mill (1806–1873) adopted Bentham's utilitarianism, with a difference. Mill said that some pleasures ("higher" pleasures) are better than others. Thus, for Mill, poetry would get a higher rating than pushpin, even though the total number of hedons generated were the same. "It is better to be a Socrates unsatisfied than a pig satisfied." This makes sense; few of us would willingly change our lives for that of a pig. On Mill's calculational scheme, the hedons for each action would first be multiplied by a weighting factor and then summed up and compared. Mill's contention that some pleasures are better than others invites a rational assessment of pleasures. In response to the question, "Which should I avoid?" or "Which should I cultivate?", the answer should not just be guided by raw "feels," or by quantity of physical pleasure or pain, but by reason.

In *Utilitarianism* (1863), Mill attempted to give a justification for the Principle of Utility ("the greatest good for the greatest number"). Either it is a first principle or it is derived. Initially, Mill tried claiming that it is self-evident. But a self-evident principle is one for which no alternative is conceivable. Alternatives to the Principle of Utility as a moral first principle are certainly conceivable; Kant has one in the Categorical Imperative (which we will discuss in the next section). Further, we have seen that the concept of the greatest happiness for the greatest number is vague; it raises questions. However, a self-evident principle must be clearly understood (like the Law of Non-Contradiction).

If it is not a self-evident first principle, then it must be derived. Mill attempts the derivation as follows. He says that the only evidence possible that something is desirable is that people actually do desire it. Since it can readily be shown that many people do desire pleasure, or happiness, then Mill concludes that it is desirable. Note, however, the slippery move here. Mill goes from the statement that "People desire pleasure (or happiness)" to "People *should* desire pleasure/happiness." He has added something to the conclusion that was not in the assumptions of the argument; he has added "should." But this addition is not logically valid. He has committed the error Hume pointed out (and was discussed in Chapter 2) of deriving an "ought" from an "is," and so his argument commits what is known as a *modal fallacy*. Thus he has not justified the Principle of Utility.

Mill has another problem as well. He wants to incorporate the feature that some pleasures are better than others into the theory. This does seem to improve Bentham's version, but how are we to know which are the better pleasures? Mill says they are the ones chosen by the competent judges. If I want to know who the competent judges are, so that I can go and check out what they choose, in order to know what the best pleasures are, how shall I identify them? Mill says they are the ones who choose the best pleasures. This has led us in a tight circle and has not answered the question. So there remains a problem of how one is to know what are the better pleasures, so that they can be properly weighted.

Despite all of its faults, classical Utilitarianism is a powerful ethical theory, and it has received a great deal of attention. It is a **teleological** theory, because of its concern with the *consequences* of actions. An act is good if it has good consequences (such as a maximizing of pleasure over pain). It gives us a kind of pseudo-scientific way to approach a moral problem. It makes use of reason in determining the morality of an action, one of the things we were looking for in a theory. Bentham and Mill are certainly correct in pointing out that pleasure is good and pain is bad; their problem may lie in supposing pleasure to be *the* good, and ignoring the existence of other goods.

Updated Utilitarianism

A utilitarianism that bases its judgments solely on pleasure and pain is *hedonistic*. Some theorists, such as G. E. Moore, have suggested that there are other goods that should be maximized, such as knowledge, friendship, health, aesthetic awareness; this is considered *ideal utilitarianism*. The calculations may proceed in the same way, but the emphasis has shifted away from pleasure.

A recent division has occurred between utilitarians who believe that the principle of utility is to be applied to particular *acts* and those who believe that moral choices are justified by an appeal to *rules* designed to maximize happiness.

Act Utilitarianism If our principle is "Choose the act that will create the greatest happiness/pleasure for the greatest number," then we are considered **act utilitarians**. Since each situation is unique, we judge that we must take each case on its own terms and assess what choice will satisfy our principle. We are not bound strictly by general rules such as "Keep promises," since we know that in a particular case keeping a promise may lead to overall greater pain for all than if we lie. J. J. C. Smart, a major proponent of act utilitarianism, points out that if we always act by following such rules, or by habit, we are not really *thinking* and *choosing deliberately*, yet deliberative choice is true moral agency. Smart offers this explanation:

> The act-utilitarian will, however, regard these rules as mere rules of thumb, and will use them only as rough guides. Normally he will act in accordance with them when he has no time for considering probable consequences or when the advantages of such a consideration of consequences are likely to be outweighed by the disadvantage of the waste of time involved.[4]

Thus, for the act utilitarian, one only appeals to "rules of thumb" when the decision is too pressing to allow for a careful consideration of consequences.

Rule Utilitarianism   If our principle is "Make a choice based on following a rule that has been justified by the principle of utility—that is, a rule that ensures the greatest good for the greatest number," then we are **rule utilitarians**. We believe that ethics simply *is* the complete set of such rules, which have shown their value over time. Law courts are rule-utilitarian, acting on the *precedents* that establish rules regarding what is criminal or punishable and what is not. We, as rule utilitarians, believe that the act utilitarians may undermine sound moral practice by their "seat-of-the-pants" choices, and that they (along with Bentham) could choose a heinous act just because it pleased the majority. Note that our rules are established based on assessments of the consequences of following the rule, and these consequences must be conducive to maximizing happiness.

Cost-Benefit Analysis   A modernized version of the Benthamite calculus shows up in the **cost-benefit analysis** advocated in today's management and government circles. For example, "On February 19, 1981, President Reagan published Executive Order 12,291 requiring all administrative agencies and departments to support every new major regulation with a cost-benefit analysis establishing that the benefits of the regulation to society outweigh its costs."[5] The prevailing view in these circles is that economists are in a position to make the "right" judgments in these cases, and anyone else is just voicing an emotive opinion. Mark Sagoff writes:

> It is the characteristic of cost-benefit analysis that it treats all value judgments other than those made on its behalf as nothing but statements of preference, attitude, or emotion, insofar as they are value judgments. The cost-benefit analyst regards as true the judgment that we should maximize efficiency or wealth. . . . [W]hat counts is what [people] are willing to pay to satisfy their wants. Those who are willing to pay the most, for all intents and purposes, have the

right view; theirs is the more informed opinion, the better aesthetic judgment, and the deeper moral insight.[6]

Clearly, there is more to knowledge, beauty, and the good than the power of the almighty dollar. It is a new version of the claim that "might makes right," only now it has become "money makes right." What is being put forward in all seriousness as an operating principle, even a "moral" principle, by many is in reality a strong example to show the weakness of utilitarianism, and of cost-benefit analysis. The fact that someone is willing to pay a great deal (in money or pain) for something or some advantage does not of itself make that valuable; one can cite so many cases showing the person blinded by greed or lust, having made a calculational error, suffering temporary insanity, etc.

Laurence Tribe, in the face of this onslaught of cost-benefit analyses, urges a return to the "great philosophical systems of our past" that were "grounded in the view that the highest purpose of human reasoning is to evolve a comprehensive understanding of mankind's place in the universe, not merely to serve as a detector of consistency and causality and thus as an instrument for morally blind desire."[7] His deep concern is with the destruction of nature and its replacement with plastic. If we allow personal desires to direct all acceptable judgments, then the beauty of the wilderness (in the Arctic and elsewhere) will give way to the profit motive, all neatly justified by a cost-benefit spreadsheet.

INTENTIONS, FREEDOM, AND UNIVERSALITY

Ethical theories that emphasize the intentions of a moral agent in acting are called **deontological** theories. They are in contrast with teleological theories like utilitarianism, theories in which the *consequences* are the deciding point in whether an action is moral or not. We will examine deontological theories next.

Stoicism

Like the Epicureans, a group called the Stoics[8] sought a rational guide to life in difficult times. They believed that the world is in constant change, but it is guided by an underlying *logos*, or reason. The Stoic goal was to make one's life as well-ordered (by a *logos*) as the universe. One should conduct one's life so that it is, as much as possible, in harmony with the order of Nature. Follow Nature, since you can't control it.

The Stoics believed that emotions should be repressed, that they are irrational and not within a person's control or understanding. "Reason leads me where I want to go, passion takes me wherever it goes." The word 'stoic' has come to mean one who is indifferent to emotion, and calmly accepts what comes.

What is right or wrong is your *intention*, since you can't completely control the consequences of your actions (other forces and chance may intervene); but you *can* control your intentions, and so that is where your moral responsibility lies. According to this theory, a **good will** is the crucial moral element in your life; you must recognize your duties to yourself and to others, and act on them. The Stoics involved themselves in activities that were good for others and for the state (to bring the laws of the state into agreement with the laws of nature, and help the order of the state mirror the order of the universe). So Stoic activity was largely "other-directed," whereas the Epicureans were "inner-directed," concentrating on their own lives.

The Theories of Immanuel Kant

Immanuel Kant (1724–1804) wanted the kind of certainty for his ethical system that is achieved in mathematics. In such a system, ethics would have a universality for all rational beings. If it were not *a priori*, then it would be dependent on local customs, circumstances, and other accidental unpredictable factors. Ethics should transcend custom, place, and bias. If we cannot attribute certainty to ethics, it becomes arbitrary and thus empty as a real guide to action. Kant's other philosophical work[9] provides a basis for his ethics, making it more comprehensible.

Kant's *Foundations of the Metaphysics of Morals* begins by arguing that the only thing that is good *without qualification* is a **good will**. Kant suggests taking any other thing that might be considered a good, such as knowledge, wealth, power, wit, and the like, and it quickly becomes clear that any of these, if improperly used, could lead to harm. Knowledge, for example, is good *if* it is used for good purposes; the expert knowledge of a master torturer, however, is not unqualifiedly good. Thus the only thing that can be seen to be good without any qualification needed is a good will (good intentions). It is good *in itself.*

The good will is not good because of what it accomplishes, but because of its intrinsic worth. Kant says that even if the greatest effort would fail in achieving the end set by the will, it would still "sparkle like a jewel" (*FMM*, 394). A good will does, of course, aim at producing good results; it is just that even if these good results do not happen (due to accident or sabotage), the will is no less good.

Since all physical organs are well suited to their purposes, the reason must be best suited to its purpose as well. But its function could not have been self-preservation (since animal instincts serve well enough for that), or to produce happiness (since instinct again is more effective, and sometimes reason even gets in the way of happiness). So the function of reason must be to produce a will that is good in itself.

Kant says that a human action is good only if it is done from a sense of duty. This does not mean that you can't enjoy doing it or it will have no moral worth; it just means that your enjoyment is completely irrelevant to the moral worth of the act. Animals act out of instinct to seek pleasure and avoid pain; their acts are not morally valuable. Only an action done rationally, out of a proper motive (of duty) is good.

The consequences of an action do not affect the merit of its intention. There are good and bad means to achieve what might be a worthwhile end, but only the effort undertaken with a good intention (and employing means that are not blameworthy) is good. It is generally agreed that it is good to give money to a worthwhile charity. However, Joe stole the money he gave to the charity, whereas Jen worked hard to earn the money she gave. Only the second action (Jen's) is morally good. This is the basis of Kant's attack on utilitarianism.

You could have three people who, on the surface, all acted the same (good) way, but only one whose actions were truly moral. Imagine three programmers who are working on programs to distribute federally available monies to needy children. All three do their jobs well, do not make more than the usual number of errors, and do not play around with diverting any of the money into their own personal accounts. Programmer A does not steal money because he is afraid of getting caught; programmer B is doing this job because she likes kids; programmer C is doing a good job because she has contracted to do the job, and it is her duty to fulfill that agreement. Only C's work, on Kant's view, has moral worth.

Note that, in the programmer example, no one can tell "from the outside" which person is acting morally. This is why Kant says that the moral law must be *a priori*, independent of experience, because experience and observation will not always be able to give us the criteria for the morality of actions.

It is difficult, if not impossible, to find real-life actions that are done *purely* from duty. It seems that other considerations, in the complexity of our lives, always creep in. This does not prevent us, says Kant, from using the idea of an action done purely out of duty as a model for moral actions.

Moral principles must be grounded purely *a priori*. Empirical considerations of self-interest and the like only impede moral progress. We must formulate our moral principles clearly and unambiguously, free of distracting situational details, before we attempt to apply them.

Imperatives   A *rational agent* is one who has the power to act and choose in accordance with a concept of law; this power resides in the will (or *practical reason*). Imperfect rational agents have *subjective* principles (or none at all); an *objective* moral principle is one on which all rational agents would agree and act upon *if they were being fully rational* (such actions are morally "good"). Imperfect beings sometimes act on objective principles, but they may be distracted by other considerations. To an imperfectly rational being, objective principles seem like constraints; they are commands. The explicit formulation of such a command is an **imperative** (such as "Always smile").

All imperatives include the word *ought*, which implies that the hearer of the imperative has a rational understanding of what it is that the principle commands. Given Kant's system, all such imperatives command *good* actions. A perfectly rational agent would view such principles as necessary, but not as commands. We (imperfect) humans would say "I ought"; the perfectly rational being says "I will." For the perfectly rational being (God, an angel), there is no earthly "pull" to be overcome. Recognizing what is good and doing it are necessarily tied together, with no hesitation or effort.

All imperatives are either *hypothetical* or *categorical*. Hypothetical imperatives postulate an end, and then specify a means to that end. They are of the form, "If you want A, then do B." A categorical imperative represents an action which is necessary in itself, and it commands that action. There are no "ifs" about it. All imperatives are formulas directing action toward some good. Everything that is possible through the efforts of a rational being can be viewed as the possible purpose or end of some will. Sciences have a practical component that specifies what is to be attained, and how it might be attained—these are imperatives of *skill*. There is no question about the good of the end; one is only concerned with what is effective in attaining it.

"If you want to cure X, give him Y." "If you want to poison X, give him Z." Both maxims are equally "good" (in the sense of being effective).

There is one *end* which can be presupposed to be had by all rational beings—their **happiness**. Any hypothetical imperative that deals with the means to be happy ("If you want happiness, do A") is a maxim of *prudence*. There is an imperative that is not based on any further end to be obtained, and which commands an action immediately. This imperative is *categorical*. It is not concerned with the material properties of the action or its results, but only with its form and the principle it follows (the imperative of morality).

For a maxim of skill, if you will the end, then you will the means to that end. This relation is *analytic*[10] (as in "every effect must have a cause"). In our earlier example for a specific case, if you want to poison X, then you *will* the use of means Z. Effect *poisoning X* is analyzed to contain *cause Z*.

In the case of the moral imperative, no obvious end is in view. It claims that any rational agent would necessarily act in a certain way *independent of the result*, simply as (*qua*) rational agent. The predicate specifying this action, however, is not contained in the subject "rational agent" and so cannot be reached by analysis of the concept. The proposition relating *rational agent* and the action is thus *synthetic*, but it asserts what a rational agent would *necessarily* do. This makes it a synthetic judgment *a priori* (again see endnote 10).

The problem facing Kant is to state the categorical imperative, which urges us to act in accordance with a universal law, a principle valid for all rational beings in virtue of their rationality. It tells us to accept or reject any particular maxim based on its universalizability. Can you will your action to be a universal law? If you can, then it is moral; otherwise it is not. The categorical imperative can be expressed in several ways:

- **Categorical Imperative 1: Act only according to that maxim by which you can at the same time will that it should become a universal law** (*FMM*, 421).

  Particular maxims ("don't lie"; "don't kill") gain their validity from the universal law.

  The Law of Nature. Kant is drawing an analogy between the universal law of morality and the universal (cause-effect) law of nature. As in scientific cases, we have a *test* for the moral law: can it be universally adopted? The application of this test requires a deep (empirically-based) knowledge of *human* nature.
- **Categorical Imperative 2: Act as though the maxim of your action were by your will to become a universal law of nature** (*FMM*, 421).

Duties may be toward self or toward others, and they may be perfect or imperfect. A perfect duty admits of no exceptions. In imperfect duties, some latitude exists in determining the range of application. A perfect duty to self is the prohibition of suicide. A perfect duty to others is not to make false promises. An imperfect duty to self is the rule that we should develop our talents; the choice/range of talents that should be developed is left open. An imperfect duty to others is benevolence; the range of ways is left open to our imagination.

The End in Itself. All rational action must have a principle *and* an end (purpose). Ends may be subjective or objective. If there were objective ends given by reason, they would be those a perfectly rational being *would* pursue, and an imperfectly rational being (like us) *ought to* pursue. Such ends could not be products of our actions, because that would make them *conditioned*; they must be *unconditioned* and have absolute value. They must be already in existence, and their existence alone must impose on us the duty to pursue them. These ends are *ends in themselves*—only rational agents can be such ends. If they did not exist, there would be no unconditional good, no highest principle of action (Categorical Imperative). It is thus *wrong* to use such beings as means and not as ends in themselves.

- Categorical Imperative 3: Act so that you treat humanity, whether in your own person or that of another, always as an end and never as a means only (*FMM*, 429).

Autonomy. A being is *autonomous* if it gives laws to itself; it is *heteronomous* if it gets its laws from others. The will not only is subject to the law, but prescribes the law (given by reason). We must follow a universal law of our own making, whose validity we recognize through reason. The moral law is the necessary expression of our natures as rational active beings.

- Categorical Imperative 4: Never choose except in such a way that the maxims of the choice are comprehended as universal law in the same volition (*FMM*, 440).

The Categorical Imperative excludes personal interest; it does not say, "I ought to do X *if* I want Y," but rather just "I ought to do X." A nice simplicity. A will that is not subject to law because of any interest is then autonomous; nothing external controls it (not even a hot-fudge sundae). Philosophies that explain morality in terms of interest(s) deny the possibility of morality. They put forward doctrines of heteronomy, where the will is bound by a law that has its origin in some end or thing *outside* of the will itself (putting the will in a kind of bondage). This can only give a hypothetical (and so nonmoral) imperative.

The Kingdom of Ends. "A rational being belongs to the realm of ends as a member when he gives universal laws in it while also himself subject to these laws." (*FMM*, 434) This comes directly from the Law of Autonomy. To the extent that rational agents are all subject to universal laws of their own making, they constitute a kingdom, or commonwealth. These laws command them to treat each other as ends in themselves.

- **Categorical Imperative 5: Act by a maxim which involves its own universal validity for every rational being** (*FMM*, 437).

The Concept of Freedom.[11] *Will* is a kind of causality exercised by rational beings. A rational will is *free* if it can cause something *without* itself being caused to do so by some external cause. *Natural necessity* includes nonrational beings that act only when they are caused to do so by something else.

A free will without law would be an "absurdity" (*FMM*, 446). A free will acts under laws, but not laws imposed on it by something else (since that would put it under natural necessity). Its laws must be self-imposed; this is **autonomy**.[12]

Freedom Must Be Presupposed. Morality requires freedom to choose. I am only morally *responsible* in cases where I do something (A), and I might have done otherwise (not-A). This freedom cannot be proved from experience (since then it would not be necessary). Reason, in order to *be* reason, must necessarily presuppose that it is not determined by outside influences; it must be the source of its own principles (otherwise its judgments could not be its own). A rational agent must presuppose its will to be free, or its actions could not be its own. Freedom is thus a necessary presupposition of all thinking and all considered action.[13] Kant has identified for us a fundamental good—freedom.

We have taken an extensive look at Kant's ethics because of its importance; it is also difficult to explain briefly. Kant's dealing with *rational* beings, rather than just human beings, makes the theory more universal than other theories, and broad enough that it could encompass artificially intelligent entities, should the need for consideration of moral duties toward them (and of them toward us) ever arise.

Kant's insights, however, did not preclude some difficulties for his position. First, it seems clear that a good will is not the *only* good; there are at least health, pleasure, and friendship, and Kant himself recognizes freedom as a fundamental good. Second, it is difficult to find maxims of action that can be universalized without exception. For example, it is easy to think of cases where an exception to "Never lie" would be the rational choice. Third, the Categorical Imperative has no moral *content*, and so *could* be used to universalize evil, or for trivial examples, such as "Tie your shoes," which are not moral. These difficulties may not be unsurmountable, however, with a little added thought and effort.

VIRTUE ETHICS

A fairly recent reaction to the inadequacies of Kantian and Utilitarian ethical theories has been a return to "virtue ethics," [14] which can be seen to have its origin in Aristotle. The main difference in virtue ethics is an emphasis on the nature of the good life for a human, and on good character. We will take Aristotle's views as representative of the position.

Aristotle's ethics is expressed primarily in two works, the *Nicomachean Ethics* and the *Eudemian Ethics*. The first is considered one of the most important works ever written on ethics, and it is the source of most of our exposition.

Aristotle begins Book I, Nature of the Good for Man, with the claim: "Every art, inquiry, and pursuit is thought to aim at some good; consequently the Good has been well defined as that which all things aim at." Some activities are done for the sake of something else (these are *means*); others are done only for their own sakes (these are *ends*). There must be some end for all of the things we do and, "if we do not choose everything for the sake of something else (for at that rate the process would go on to infinity, so that our desire would be empty and vain)," clearly this must be the good and the chief good. Happiness is an *activity* of the soul in accordance with human virtue. We thus must inquire into what this virtue is.

Intellectual virtue can be taught (Book VI), but moral virtue is a matter of *habit*. One becomes moral by practice, the practice of activities of the good character. We seek a mean between extremes (moderation, *sophrosyne*). One might write grammatically by accident (a monkey, for example, could type out a work of Shakespeare), but moral action cannot be accidental; it is *intention* that counts.

For an act to be **virtuous**, you must (1) *know* that what you are doing is virtuous; (2) *choose* the act; (3) *do* that act *for its own sake*; and (4) act according to a *fixed, unchanging principle*, or out of a *fixed character*. Virtue is not by luck or accident; it lies in states of character. It is difficult to be good! The decision rests, according to Aristotle, with *moral perception*; you have to "see" what is the right action, and then you most *choose* to do it.

Actions done by constraint, through true ignorance, or by compulsion are **involuntary**; they are not praiseworthy or blameworthy, since the source of the action is **external**. A **voluntary** action is one where the source of motion is from within. If someone holds your hand and, because he is stronger than you are, forces your hand holding a knife to plunge into someone else's heart, you are not responsible for the murder; the source of the action was not from within you, but external.

You are, however, responsible for bad actions you commit when, for example, you are drunk, even though you were not aware of what you were doing at the time of the act. You were responsible for *getting* drunk (the source of that action came from within you), and so you are responsible for all of the subsequent consequences of the action of getting drunk.

Choice relates to voluntary actions but not to irrational, emotional acts, or wishes, or those that are beyond your control. We deliberate about *means*, not about *ends*. The good end should be self-evident; reason comes in to figure out the best way to achieve the end. Notice that Aristotle, like Kant, takes freedom as a necessary presupposition for ethics. He does not attempt to give a rational proof of the existence of free will; it may well be that no such proof is possible (but then neither is a proof for determinism possible).

"The good man judges everything of this nature correctly, and thus the good man is the measure of all virtuous things." We are responsible for all of our voluntary actions, including bad habits. The good individual is the one who has developed good habits, and it should be our goal to recognize and cultivate such habits, to fulfill our human potential.

The intellect has the power to deliberate, but not to "do"; the origin of action is choice, and reason deliberates about the choice of means (but not about ends, or about the past).

You could *forget* a piece of scientific knowledge, or a mathematical proof, but you cannot forget the difference between right and wrong; there are constant reminders. It is a habit you have developed, just as how to ride a bicycle will come back to you quickly, even if you haven't done it for years. You would never say, "I forgot whether murder is right or wrong."

Aristotle says that the morally weak individual is like a city with good laws that does not use the laws (ignores them). The morally bad individual is like a city that follows bad laws. "Practical wisdom is the quality of mind concerned with things just and noble and good for man" (*Nicomachean Ethics* 1143b 21). "It is impossible to be practically wise without being good" (*N.E.* 1144a 36). Virtue is habit in conjunction with right reason.

Pleasure and pain are clearly recognized to be the steering principles of much of our action. Thus developing a good moral character relates to developing habits of taking pleasure in what we *ought* to take pleasure in, and being pained by evil.

Some say that pleasure is the good. But Plato has shown that pleasure cannot be the chief good, because a life in which pleasure is combined with prudence is superior to one of pleasure without prudence (a night of overindulgence is followed by a morning of hangover). There are destructive things we *ought not* to take pleasure in (such as torture), but some do; this pleasure cannot be the good, and so pleasure in general cannot be the good.

Pleasures are all desirable, but not to the same extent to everyone (water is not welcome to a drowning man). No one would willingly choose to live the life of a pig; thus there must be some higher good that humans seek. Happiness should be the most excellent activity in accord with virtue; thus it must relate to the best part of a human (which is the **intellect**). Contemplative activity is more continuous and self-sufficient than other human activities; it is most like the life of a god. Thus the best life for a human being, argues Aristotle, is the life of contemplation (of understanding).

In the *Eudemian Ethics*, Aristotle makes a comparison between good and being, a comparison that is taken up and elaborated as a basis for ethics by a modern writer, Panayot Butchvarov. Aristotle writes:

> For the good is [so] called in many ways, indeed in as many ways as being. 'Being', as has been set out elsewhere, signifies what-is, quality, quantity, when, and in addition that [being which is found] in being changed and in changing; and the good occurs in each one of these categories—in substance, intelligence and God; in quality, the just; in quantity, the moderate; in the when, the right occasion; and teaching and learning in the sphere of change. So, just as being is not a single thing embracing the things mentioned, the good is not either; nor is there a single science of being or the good. (*Eudemian Ethics*, Ch. 8 [1217b 25–34])

 ## THE FORM OF THE GOOD

We noted in Chapter 1 that the concept of the **good** is fundamental to ethics. We cannot determine what are right or wrong actions unless there are fundamental goods to be achieved, and evils to be avoided. We need to inquire whether the good exists independent of human thought, language, and desire, or whether it is merely whatever we say it is (relativism). We have already found some clues in the theories considered thus far—pleasure and freedom are accounted goods. However, if there are multiple goods, there must be something they have in common.

Plato and the Form of the Good

Plato wrote dialogues about many fundamental questions—the nature of knowledge, justice, friendship, courage, moderation, love, beauty, politics, naming, piety, loyalty, death, and the soul, among others. Plato believed in the existence of the eternal Forms, or Ideas (of Truth, Beauty, the Good, Knowledge, Justice, and the like) which represent the *standards* against which actual particular cases can be measured and judged. Of each concept investigated, he would ask, Is there *one* idea, or many? "Tell me what is the nature of this idea, and then I shall have a standard to which I may look, and by which I may measure actions" (*Euthyphro* 6e).

A geometrical example can be used to illustrate what Plato means by a Form. I can draw many different triangles on the board, and ask what they all have in common. Plato would say that what they have in common is the Form of Triangularity, which is something like the essential nature of triangles, or the set of defining conditions for what counts as a triangle. The concept of triangularity is not just the set of triangles that have been given the tag 'triangle' (which is what a position called *nominalism* claims). I can erase one or all of the triangles on the board, or go about destroying all triangles in the world, and the idea of triangularity will still remain the same. Nominalism also fails to explain how the idea of triangularity allows me to correctly identify *new* examples of triangles (or recognize that squares are not triangles) when they come along.

None of the triangles I drew on the board is a true geometrical triangle, since such a triangle would be bounded by three true geometrical lines, and Euclid tells us that 'line' is defined as "breadthless length." I can never draw a breadthless length with any earthly drawing instrument, but I can comprehend the idea of a true geometrical triangle. My pictures on the board are better or worse approximations to that ideal.

There are forms (or general ideas, or "universals") for all general terms, including 'dog', 'hair', 'mud', and the like, but the ones that Plato is most interested in are those that have to do with the truly human things, like virtue and knowledge. Of the forms, the highest is the form of the Good. All of the forms are good, including the form of the Good, and this makes it unique (the form of triangularity is not triangular, etc.).

No "pat" answer is arrived at in any of the dialogues to the main question being investigated, because these questions are so difficult. But all is not a waste of time. As Socrates notes at the end of the dialogue about knowledge, if "you should ever conceive afresh, you will be all the better for the present investigation, and if not, you will be soberer and humbler and gentler to other men, and will be too modest to fancy that you know what you do not know" (*Theaetetus* 210b). Socrates and the others have at least learned some things that knowledge (or virtue) is *not*, and so they will not have to go down those wrong roads again, but can try new paths; and learning what the idea *is not* brings us that much closer to finding what it really *is*.

Socrates often suggests that virtue and knowledge are closely connected. Virtue might be knowledge, but it may not be a kind of knowledge that can be "taught" (*Meno*) in normal ways of instruction, say, as the multiplication tables are taught. There are many examples of virtuous, just men who were never able to teach their sons virtue (Pericles, the great Athenian leader, is taken as a case in point). But perhaps virtue can be taught *by example*, to those who have a sharpened moral sense (analogous to having a natural intelligence). If one could persuade people, from the time they are young, to care for their souls and develop their proper excellence, they would all become just.

If we are to be moral, we must, as the "bottom line," come to understand the *good*. When Socrates (at the end of *Republic*, Book VI) is pressed to describe the nature of the Good, he replies that he cannot tell his friends about the Good directly and, even if he could, they could not understand it. So he says that he will try to get to it by *analogy*, by describing the "child of the Good"— that is, the Sun.[15] Socrates suggests that the Good itself is too fundamental to be defined or analyzed in terms of other things. Analysis always characterizes something in terms of its parts, and the Good may be simple (without parts).

Knowledge of the Forms is the meeting of the soul with reality. Plato describes, rather dramatically, the ascent to the realm of the forms (a mental climb) in the *Symposium*:

> One goes always upwards for the sake of this Beauty, starting out from beautiful things and using them like rising stairs: from one body to two and from two to all beautiful bodies, then from beautiful bodies to beautiful customs, and from customs to learning beautiful things, and from these lessons he arrives in the end at this lesson, which is learning of this very Beauty, so that in the end he comes to know just what it is to be beautiful. (Plato, *Symposium* 211c-d)[16]

Notice that the final phase is that the traveler *comes to know* just what beauty is. Again, knowledge is the key, here to aesthetics (beauty), as well as to ethics (virtue). The revelation is startling: "all of a sudden he will catch sight of something wonderfully beautiful in its nature" (*Symposium* 210e).

When Plato speaks of the understanding that follows instruction and long periods of study in the *Seventh Letter*, he speaks again of a sudden revelation ("the light dawns"): "suddenly, like a blaze kindled by a leaping spark, it [knowledge] is generated in the soul and at once becomes self-sustaining" (*Seventh Letter* 341d).

The form that the moral individual seeks is the highest of all—not Beauty, or Justice, but the Form of the Good. When this has been reached, knowledge of the good will guide all of the moral actions of this individual as clearly as solutions to mathematical equations will guide the traveler in space to her destination.

G. E. Moore and the Indefinability of the Good

George Edward Moore (1873–1958) is the philosopher of common sense. He picked up on Plato's suggestion that the good may be undefinable, and pointed out that many people for many years had been spinning their wheels trying to define "the good" when in fact it is too fundamental (basic) to be defined in terms of other things. To attempt to do so (to define good in terms of pleasure, for example) is, Moore says, to commit what he calls the "naturalistic fallacy." To the question "What is good?", Moore says he will respond "Good is good." To the question "How is good to be defined?", he responds that it cannot be defined (and that is that).

Moore compares "good" to "yellow" in that both are too fundamental to be defined in terms of anything else. Scientists may say that yellow has a certain wavelength, but that does not *define* yellow. The scientists would have to know (somehow) what yellow *was* before they could measure its wavelength. As the motto for the beginning of his book, *Principia Ethica*, Moore chose a quote from Joseph (Bishop) Butler: "Everything is what it is, and not another thing."

Notice how close Moore is to Plato's basic position. We cannot *define* yellow, but we can point out examples, and you can learn from these examples what yellow is. We cannot *define* (in a finite language or other symbolism) the square root of 2, but we can point to a line with that length. We cannot *define* virtue (goodness) in a simple formula, but we can point to examples of virtuous action. Perhaps, if you are attentive and are not "moral-blind" (analogous to color-blind for recognizing yellow), you will figure out for yourself what is good. If you are a rational being, seeing what good is will be sufficient incentive to make it the model (standard) for all your future moral actions.

Butchvarov and the Order of Goods

Panayot Butchvarov (*Skepticism in Ethics*, 1989, p. 63) pointed out that Moore's example of yellow being indefinable is not a paradigmatic case of indefinability. Such cases are those of what Butchvarov termed a "summum genus" (highest). Yellow is a species of color, but color is not a species of *another* genus except, perhaps, of the genus 'property' itself. Similarly, triangularity is a species of shape, but shape is a *summum genus*.

The best case for the indefinability of the good would be made by finding that the good is a *summum genus*. However, any genus ought to have species. In the case of the good, these species would be properties themselves, perhaps health, pleasure, knowledge, friendship, etc. This would explain, say, Hume's reluctance to admit the reality of the good. One cannot see the *summum genus* good any more than one can see the *summum genus* color. One can understand that orange is a color, but all one sees is orange. One can understand that health is a good, but all one literally observes is health. Similar remarks can be made for the *summum genus* evil. Plato, Moore, Butchvarov, and countless others would agree that ethics begins with the recognition that there are goods and evils in the world and that these are just as real as shapes.

Plato, Aristotle and others observed that knowledge and fortitude were among the goods. Epicurus, Bentham, Mill, and others observed that pleasure and satisfaction are goods. Modern ecologists and environmentalists find that health is a good not only for humans, but for other animals, for plants, and for ecosystems. The Stoics, Kant, and others recognized free choice, rationally directed, as a good. Countless writers, and humans in general, have recognized friendship as a good. Although none of these concepts are astounding, two difficulties have been raised for the position being developed.

First, there seem to be obvious cases where a so-called "good" is not good for humans. For example, although some drugs produce pleasure, they can kill. The point is well taken, but it confuses the concept of the good with the concept of right action. Taken all by itself, pleasure is a good thing; but in everyday life, hardly anything occurs all by itself. Sexual pleasure is a good, but unwanted pregnancies and venereal diseases are not. So, in real life, each person must calculate which action to take, given the possible goods and evils that are connected with that action.

The calculation would be impossible if there were no goods or evils. So there are two separate questions. (1) Which characteristics fall under the good (and which under evil)? (2) Given the best answer I can get to (1), what should I do? Question (2) is the issue of which action is the right action.

An action can be right, but not good. This is easily seen in a case where one must choose among several evils—for example, a case where one is forced to choose between killing a thousand innocent people or being killed. Whatever the choice, there is an evil outcome. Presumably, choosing to be killed is the right choice, but the act of being killed is not a good. Right action concerns calculation involving goods and evils. Recognizing goods and evils is a matter of classification, not of calculation. While we seem to have little difficulty in classifying many goods and evils, we often have great difficulty with calculations about what to do.

It is not unreasonable that in a given calculation concerning what to do we would want to maximize goods and minimize evils. This fact leads to the second difficulty for the view being developed. Are goods (and corresponding evils) equal in rank or is there a hierarchy?[17] The answer to this may seem to depend on what you are. It is unlikely that pleasure, knowledge, fortitude, and friendships are among the goods of plants, since plants do not seem to be capable of possessing such characteristics. Plants are capable of continued existence and health. Are these characteristics equally good to a plant? (I presume the plant cannot answer the question, but it doesn't follow that the question has no answer.) Continued existence is a necessary condition for either the healthy or the diseased state of plant. But continued existence in a healthy condition is the better of these alternatives. This suggests that health is a higher good than continued existence. Similarly, one could imagine a creature capable of pleasure but not friendship. Since there is pleasure in a friendship, one would find friendship to be the higher good.

The existence of evil complicates these remarks about a hierarchy of goods. Certain pains, with little hope of relief, might tempt one to forgo continued existence (living) and thus all other goods. However, it is generally recognized that there is a hierarchy of evils that corresponds to that of the goods—for example, pain for pleasure, ignorance for knowledge, hatred and animosity for friendship.

The view presented here of the basis for moral decision making, as noted, does not provide an easy formula for calculating the right thing to do. But it does offer the only nonarbitrary basis for evaluating anything. In some cases, it will show the absurdity of certain choices—for example, someone who destroys health and the prospects of continuing to live in order to make a lot of money and acquire many material things (neither of which is a basic good). Basic goods are sought for their own sake, not as a means of obtaining something else.

So the question we will ask as we proceed through this book is "What goods does this choice maximize and what evils does it minimize, and what is our best estimate of the choice's maximization of the good and minimization of evil?" This question is not intended to suggest that we expect perfection in human ethical decision making. It might be paraphrased as "Will this choice make things better or worse?"

CONCLUSION

Our search for a foundation for ethics was not intended to provide a bag of ethical theories from which you can draw as you wish, but rather to evaluate ethical theories to discover which parts of them make the most sense. For example, individuals seeking immediate gratification *could* pull short-range utilitarianism out of a bag, but the weaknesses of this position suggest that they *should not*. If one's desires are in control of the decision-making process, why go through the pretense of finding a "justification" of those desires? Any serious, nonrationalized ethical analysis will proceed from a foundation that best conforms to human experience and has best stood the objections raised against it. Major ethical theories, all of which contain certain difficulties, offer certain fundamental insights that we should not ignore. These insights should be in our minds when we make decisions about what to do.

Thus there are three approaches you might take regarding a basis for ethical analysis. The first is the "grab bag" approach—picking a theory to "fit the situation." As noted, the problem here is that you may well pick the theory that provides the answer you desire. Desires, and not rational principles, would ground this decision-making process.

The second approach is what might be called the "join some club" approach. That is, become a Kantian moralist, or a Benthamite utilitarian, or something else, and proceed. Typically, club joiners take the principles of the adopted position as sacred. This approach has the same difficulty as the "grab bag" attempt to offer a hypothetical foundation for ethics. That is, if one is a Kantian, the following analysis obtains, but if one follows Bentham a different analysis is forthcoming. The all-important question of *which* position you ought to adopt has been brushed aside. I would recommend against joining a club, since there is a third approach.

No major ethical theory is without widely known, easily seen principles that are relevant to human conduct. For example, the difficulties of classical utilitarianism do not undermine the validity of the observation that pleasure and pain should be important considerations in our deliberations. The criticisms of Kant's ethical views do not diminish the importance of a good will and the wisdom of considering others as one considers oneself, nor do the calculational complications of considering the full range of goods and evils entail that one should ignore this range in making moral judgments.

Chapter 2 was designed to show that no compelling reasons have been given to preclude a search for a rational foundation for ethics, and this chapter provided an introduction to the search. However, if you haven't undertaken the search, you will have no basis on which to conduct moral reasoning and thus no ground for making moral decisions. At the end of this chapter, it was argued that a sensible ethical theory would begin with recognizing fundamental goods and evils and a ranking of these. For example, health and friendship are basic goods, but it isn't unusual to find cases where someone has sacrificed health (or even life) for friendship.

Approaching Ethical Analysis

Any ethical analysis ought to proceed according to the following steps. First, make sure you know the relevant facts of the case. If you are considering possible future cases (to evaluate proposals) or fictional cases (to sharpen your powers of ethical reasoning), the relevant facts must be fairly detailed. Consider, for example, a fictional case put to a student who is asked to suppose that medical technology has made it possible for humans to halve their physical size in two generations. Should this be done? The student began to think of resources saved, decreased pollution, and so on. But she should have demanded more facts, such as, will the current human tendency to overpopulate continue? For if it does, the collision between human population growth and the capacity of the environment to support this growth would merely be postponed by a generation or so. However, if one adds, as a stipulated fact, that humans will suddenly adopt zero-population growth, the ethical analysis may change radically (as well as the urgency of the need to halve our size, with its attendant problems). This example clearly illustrates the need to establish the facts of any moral problem case.

Second, keep the *fundamental* ethical principles you have discovered clearly in mind. Many "consequentialist-based" ethical theories avoid specifying fundamental goods by using vague terms such as "beneficial" and "well-being." These theories leave open the question of how to decide what is beneficial and what counts as well-being. Other consequentialist theories, such as Benthamite cost-benefit analysis, base calculations on pleasure or satisfaction, but ignore the full range of goods (and evils) available to human beings. Duty-based theories, such as Kant's, make a good will the only good and/or require universalizability of moral maxims. But Kant's view seems too narrow; a good will is *a* fundamental good, true friendship is another one. The requirement of universalizability has two difficulties as *the* ethical rule: it is hard to find a maxim to which there should be no exceptions, and one *could* will evil for everyone, including oneself. Hegel's basic criticism of Kant's imperative was that it had no moral content. Finally, rights-based theories are not fundamental, since the concept of a natural right depends on the existence of goods. If nothing had any intrinsic value, there would be no real value. In such a case, it would be incoherent to talk of natural rights (Rights to *what? Why?*). Think about these things as you try to formulate the principles by which you will make decisions.

The third step in ethical evaluation is, keeping in mind the difference between a means to a fundamental good and that good itself, to identify which disputes in the case are concerned with means and which are over basic goods. You may find it useful to draw an analogy to other similar cases, which may help make the issues in your case more clear. For example, if you are addressing the question of whether you should "blow the whistle" on an employer who is deliberately allowing "rush-job" programs that have not been adequately tested to be delivered on a defense strategic decision-making project, because of a customer deadline, you may want to compare it with the case in which the Challenger disaster might have been averted if the "whistle" had been blown on the faulty O-rings and the launch postponed (see Chapter 9). The fundamental good of preserving courageous human life clearly outweighs the good of a deadline met and profit made.

The fourth step is to discover, or estimate as best you can, the impact of certain actions or proposals on the maximization of goods and the minimization of evils. Since real-life situations can be enormously complex, the fourth step will not be easy. Your deliberations may not be too difficult in cases involving one individual, or a small number of individuals, but they will be very hard in cases involving societies. Don't expect perfection or great precision here. However, you must try; otherwise nature will just take its course.

■ ENDNOTES

1. Socrates and Plato mark the first important Western thought about human value and knowledge, but they were preceded by a number of interesting and innovative thinkers who attempted to understand the world according to rational principles, and so deserve a brief mention in the account.

The pre-Socratic thinkers moved away from mystical explanations of phenomena to an attempt to find rational explanations that the human mind could comprehend. Most of them were materialists (their "first principles" were material—water or air or the *apeiron* or atoms) and talked in terms of names for forces (Love, Strife, Mind). The Pythagoreans looked to a more abstract first principle—the One—and sought for *mathematical* explanations of the universe (musical harmonies explainable in terms of mathematical ratios, and the "celestial spheres" creating a world-music by their motions). Democritus and Anaxagoras thought the observed phenomena could be explained in terms of what is not observable (atoms, or infinitely small homoeomeries). Xenophanes insisted that there is only one true account (in spite of differing opinions), as did Parmenides, who also demanded that contradictions be excluded from explanations.

Socrates' concern was that these physicalistic accounts made no provision for the uniquely *human* things—values, love, friendship, justice, courage, moderation, piety, knowledge. He sought to find explanations of the essential nature of such concepts in his discussions with others.

2. The Sophists were a group in Greece around the time of Socrates who taught the art of "persuasion" (that is, rhetoric). They took money for teaching people how to convince others (in the law courts, in debates, in buying and selling), how to be successful, given the customs of the *polis*. Their main concern was in winning, not in the truth, and so Socrates criticized them.

Protagoras was one of the major and most successful Sophists of the time. In a dialogue of that name, Protagoras says that he will teach Socrates' young friend "what he came to learn, which is how to exercise good judgment in ordering both his own affairs and those of the city, and how to be a man of influence in public affairs, both in speech and in action" (*Protagoras* 318e).

To this, Socrates asks whether Protagoras is talking about the art of politics, and of making men good citizens. Protagoras says yes, that is precisely his profession. But it is clear that what he means by a good citizen is a *successful* citizen, one who is rich and powerful, and knows how to win arguments by semantic tricks. For Socrates, the good citizen is the one who lives a just life and does his best for the *polis*.

Protagoras said that "man is the measure of all things" (an individual relativism). Truth is what is true for me, and you have your own truth, which is true for you. There is no idea of any possible objective truth that lies outside of our two beliefs. If we disagree, I can try to persuade you (using rhetoric); if that fails, we must fight. Socrates, on the other hand, uses argument to try to get at the objective truth.

In the dialogue *Theaetetus* (161b), Socrates attacks Protagoras' relativism: "Gratifying as it is to be told that what each of us believes is true, I am surprised that he does not begin his *Truth* by saying that of all things the measure is the pig, or the dog-faced baboon, or some sentient creature still more uncouth. He would then have addressed us in a manner befitting a great man, disdainfully, showing us that while we were admiring him as if he were a god, for his wisdom, he was no wiser than a tadpole, to say nothing of any other man." Socrates makes his point clearly: if each man is the measure of truth (for himself), why would anyone pay Protagoras to teach him anything?

3. During a time of unrest after the Peloponnesian War, several different philosophies having ethical aspects emerged. One was led by Epicurus (341–270 B.C.), who set up the "Garden" in Athens where his ideas were taught. Slaves and women were allowed to join the group (which was unusual at the time), but the Epicurean view of rationality led them to the idea of equality. The primary goal of their philosophy was not the truth, but to "heal the suffering of the mind."

They accepted Democritus' atomistic worldview because it freed them from the superstitions associated with worship of the gods. However, they needed a concept of free will (choice), which Democritus' system does not provide, and so they invented the notion of the "swerve." According to this theory, atoms go about bouncing randomly off other atoms, the results of the collisions following predictable paths; but occasionally an atom will "swerve" off its normal path, and this is when free will occurs. This is a bad account of free will, but at least they were trying.

4. J. J. C. Smart, "An Outline of a System of Utilitarian Ethics," in *Philosophical Ethics*, 2nd ed., ed. Tom L. Beauchamp (New York: McGraw-Hill, 1991).

5. Mark Sagoff, "At the Shrine of Our Lady of Fatima, or Why Political Questions Are Not All Economic," in *People, Penguins, and Plastic Trees*, eds. Donald VanDeVeer and Christine Pierce (Belmont, CA: Wadsworth, 1986), p. 230.

6. Sagoff, pp. 232–333.

7. Laurence H. Tribe, "Ways Not to Think About Plastic Trees: New Foundations for Environmental Law," in VanDeVeer and Pierce, 1986, p. 256.

8. A Phoenician merchant named Zeno (336–264 B.C.) came to Athens and established the Painted Porch around 300 B.C. (*stoa* is the Greek word for "porch"). The Stoics taught that one should live well or die (it was perfectly acceptable in Stoic philosophy to commit suicide if life became intolerable).

9. Immanuel Kant was born and lived in Konigsberg in East Prussia. He taught at the local university, and led such a well-regulated life that apparently people in the town would set their clocks by him. Kant wrote the *Critique of Pure Reason* (1781) to examine the limits of human reason. He found that human reason is troubled by certain (metaphysical) questions that reason itself will not allow it to ignore, but which reason is not able to answer. In the *Critique of Pure Reason* he presented a set of four Antinomies of Pure Reason—metaphysical questions for which human reason can present an equally convincing argument on each side. He proceeds to present these proofs (which he believes reason cannot deny) and concludes that, in these questions, reason leads itself into antinomies, or contradictions, and thus reason has met its ultimate limitation. Kant says, "I had to abolish knowledge in order to make room for faith."

Kant followed a line of Rationalists—Descartes, Spinoza, and Leibniz—who extolled the power of reason to resolve all issues. Gottfried Wilhelm Leibniz (1646–1716) is the paradigm rationalist, much as Hume is the paradigm empiricist. He was a German philosopher, scientist, historian, diplomat, and mathematician (a discoverer, independent of Newton, of the calculus). Leibniz used two fundamental rational principles to guide his system: (1) the Principle of Contradiction (whatever implies a contradiction is false); and (2) the Principle of Sufficient Reason (nothing exists without a sufficient reason why it is so and not otherwise). The fundamental elements of his universe are *monads*, which are more like individual minds than like Democritean physical atoms. This is the best of all possible worlds because God, like a super-mathematician, compared all of the possible worlds using a sort of minimax principle, and created the best one (since God has the perfect nature).

Leibniz believed that there are two realms: the realm governing the strivings of monads for perfection (grace), according to final (purposive) causes; and the realm of bodies governed by the causal laws of nature. The two realms, says Leibniz, are in perfect harmony, but they are distinct. Freedom is in the moral realm—a freedom to act according to a principle of the best. The pre-established harmony allows the two realms to operate as if they were two clocks running in perfect coordination, without ever interacting with one another.

Kant was initially very impressed by the work of Leibniz, and we can see traces of this influence in his mature work. However, when he was about 40, he read Hume, a philosopher who awakened him from his "dogmatic slumbers." Hume pointed out that causality is not self-evident, cannot be observed, and is not logically deducible from anything else. Yet causality is a principle fundamental to science. Kant observed that many other fundamental philosophical principles are in the same boat.

Kant wanted to see how much of Leibniz' pure rational system could be salvaged, given Hume's criticism. His monumental effort in the *Critique of Pure Reason* is to answer the question, "How are synthetic *a priori* judgments possible?" These judgments include the basic truths of mathematics, science, ethics, and metaphysics. (See note 10 for an explanation of the analytic/synthetic and the *a priori/a posteriori* distinctions.)

In essence, Kant wonders how we can come to know necessary truths (other than empty tautologies like "A is A"). He wanted to "insist on the authority of science and yet preserve the autonomy of morals." Kant conceived a new "Copernican revolution" in metaphysics. He made a revolutionary suggestion: Instead of assuming that our knowledge must somehow fit objects, what if we assumed that objects must fit our knowledge? If objects are *out there* (in the external world), we can have no knowledge of them. As the empiricist philosopher Berkeley pointed out, what we have are our *ideas*, and an idea can be like nothing but another idea—it cannot be like some material external *thing*. Yet our understanding follows rules, and we can examine these rules (like the Law of Non-Contradiction). Hume showed dramatically that if all we have is the world of particular perceptions, we can never know any necessary truths. Kant (and others) thought that they knew some necessary truths, so where could they come from? These truths are not *ana-*

lytic, since they tell us something about our experiences, though they aren't derivable from our experiences.

Kant postulated that there is a world "out there," full of entities of which we can have no knowledge. Such an entity he referred to as a "thing-in-itself" (*ding an sich*). My self ("transcendental ego") receives information from the things-in-themselves, and *structures* this input in various ways that create my world of experience. What we *can* come to know is the way in which experience is (necessarily) structured, given what kinds of beings we are. These rules are *a priori*, since they structure experience and so are prior (temporally and logically) to experience. Since this is not analytic knowledge, it is synthetic (we bring together the concepts of the content of experience and its form).

In trying to reconcile Leibniz' rational system (which provides rules for knowledge) with Hume's empiricism (which points to the limits on what we can derive from experience), Kant came up with a position that incorporated both: the rules of our understanding rationally structure experience, but our perceptions must give the understanding something to work with. Kant explained: "Thoughts without content are empty, intuitions without concepts are blind" (*Critique of Pure Reason*, B 75). Thus Leibniz' rationalism provides the structure for the thoughts, but Hume's empiricism provides the content to be structured.

10. An **analytic** statement is one in which the predicate (verb or adjective) is contained in the subject term of the statement, and thus only needs to be *analyzed out* to show the truth of the statement (like "A red rose is red"). A **synthetic** statement is one that is not analytic; that is, the subject does not contain the predicate. Thus the subject and the predicate term have to be brought together ("synthesized") by the statement. A statement is said to be **a priori** if its truth or falsity can be determined independently of experience (such as the probability of rolling a three with an unloaded die). An **a posteriori** statement is one that has to be verified or falsified through experience.

11. The Epicureans noticed a very important aspect about ethics. It is essential for one to have a free will in order to make moral choices—good *or* bad. The materialistic philosophy of Democritus purported to explain everything; thus "human" things such as love, value, and responsibility drop out of the account. If anything, they are just patterns of atoms in motion, but they have no special meaning or purpose. If this view (determinism) is true, then there is no point in talking about choices; there are none. Freedom is just an illusion, and all motions are determined by previous motions according to inexorable laws.

Materialism/determinism is undergoing a resurgence of popularity in recent years. Many who are writing today defend materialism, and the thesis that the mind is identical to the brain. Thus the processes of thinking are said to be reducible to mere patterns of brain activity. A recent version of this view is the "computational theory of mind"—that the mind/brain operates just like a computer, and by studying computer processes we can learn more about brain processes (and thus about the "mind"). Stephen Stich writes that "folk psychology" is outmoded and misdirected; we should get rid of all old-fashioned terms like 'consciousness', 'mind', 'intention', 'value', and the like. The problem is that any basis for ethics and responsibility is thrown out with them.

Ethics is about the principles for making moral choices. If there are no real choices, then we should stop talking about ethics and all do science. (Notice, however, that the word 'should' still is being used.) If we do not accept this consequence, then we must look more seriously into the concept of freedom (of choice) if we are to have a viable ethics.

Augustine, a medieval theologian and a saint in the Catholic religion, wrote *On the Free Choice Of the Will* early in his philosophical career. In Book Two, he takes on the problem of freedom of the will. Augustine asks, why did God give freedom of the will to humans, since it is by using this freedom that humans sin? It might seem that, since God gave the freedom to humans, then God is the cause of the sin. Augustine argues that this is not the case. He writes: "without it man cannot live rightly... Then too, if man did not have free choice of will, how could there exist the good according to which it is just to condemn evildoers and reward those who act rightly?" It is humans who sin, and God justly punishes the sinners. "Both punishment and reward would be unjust if man did not have free will" (*Free Choice of the Will*, II, i, 5). But God, because of God's nature, would not be unjust.

Thus God gave freedom to humans so that they could choose. A life without choice would not be a human life, but the life of an animal or a plant. But the gift of choice has two sides to it: a human may make the good choice, and turn toward the "City of God" (conversion); or a human may make the bad choice, and turn toward the earthly city of Babylon (perversion). Augustine, and many in the centuries after him, viewed humans as poised in a sort of "middle state," between God and the angels on the one hand, and the beasts on the other. A human's desires and bodily functions are the beastly part; the mind (and the soul) are the godlike part. It is infinitely better that God gave choice to humans than if God had not done so; but the blessing is a mixed one—it can be used for good or bad choices.

Freedom of choice is such a natural part of the way we view our lives that we seldom think about it, unless we are pressed. We make choices every day, about what to eat for dinner, whether to go to class or not, which route to take to a destination, who to spend our time with. Surely these are *real*, and not just *illusory*, choices. But the strong determinist position would deny that they are choices at all, and say that they are merely the results of causal chains of events of which we are not aware. It is just our DNA driving our actions, or influences from our childhood that we have forgotten that determined we would do A when we thought we *chose* A, or it's all just atoms bouncing around in the void.

There is no scientific test we can perform to determine whether there is free will or not. The convinced determinists will just tell us how each of our supposed choices was *really* this or that set of causal reactions. Under *freedom* we include freedom from constraint, but by free choice we mean much more than that. If the scientists offer us the Heisenberg Uncertainty Principle to try to make us feel better, that does not help at all, since it is just substituting a randomness for the causal chain reaction. But neither is what we mean by *free choice*.

You can initiate actions just by deciding to do so. You can decide to pick up your cup, or run down the street, or pet your cat, and then do it. No outside force produced your motion. And if it is some sort of "inner force" that physiology has not yet gotten a handle on, why is it that this physiological force does not always come out the same way under the same circumstances? Sometimes you pick up your cup, sometimes you do not. The determinists will assure you that this all is factored into the complete physiological account, but you remain unconvinced.

There is no proof on either side of the free will/determinism debate. It may seem that the scientists have the edge, because they are scientific. But we have already shown that there is no test that would confirm or disconfirm the determinist theory, any more than it would verify or falsify the free will theory; so neither is a *scientific* theory. The scientists/determinists imply that because they know how *some* things work, it is only a matter of time until they will know how *all* things work (including the mind), but any good student of logic knows that an inference from "some" to "all" is not valid.

The determinists claim that they have a *better* theory. But *value* terminology like "good" and "bad," "better" and "worse," and the like, are supposed to belong to outmoded folk psychology, and are to be avoided by all true materialists. If they can't claim a *better* theory on their own grounds, what exactly *can* they claim?

One should look at the consequences of each position. If the determinists are right, then there can be no such thing as *responsibility* in human affairs or anywhere else; it is all an illusion. The inference would be that *no one* ever in the history of human affairs has ever been responsible for anything. There might be physical causation that could be traced, but without a choice there can be no attribution of responsibility. To say that I am *responsible* for doing something implies that I could have done otherwise. If I had no choice, then my action (can I even still call it *my* action?) deserves neither praise or blame.

What are the consequences of the free will theory? They do not seem as radically unacceptable. The free will theory does not claim that *nothing* happens according to deterministic causal laws, only that there are some cases in which rational agents *choose* to initiate one action rather than another. The worst consequence of this theory seems to be that the determinist scientists would be frustrated that there was something they could not reduce to physics.

12. The principle of autonomy is *synthetic a priori*, and is reached only by bringing a third term (*freedom*) to the subject (*rational being*) and the predicate (*acting morally, that is, under universalizable law*) to connect them.

13. Kant attempts to justify freedom by an appeal to the *two standpoints*. The ideas that come to our senses are independent of our will, and so we assume that they come to us from objects outside of us. But we know these objects only through the ways in which they affect us; we cannot know how they are *in themselves*. We know only appearances, but behind these appearances we assume there exist *things in themselves (noumena)*.

The same distinction applies to my knowledge of myself. Through inner sense, I can know myself only as I appear, but behind the appearance I assume there is a real *noumenal* self. As I know myself through inner sense, and as capable of passively receiving sensations, I regard myself as part of the phenomenal world of sense. But insofar as I am capable of activity apart from sense, I am part of an intelligible world. I find in myself (and I must assume you do in yourself) a power of *reason*. We have a power of understanding that produces from itself such categories as cause and effect, and applies these concepts to bring some order to the phenomena of sense. Apart from sense, the understanding would think nothing at all ("concepts without percepts are empty"). Reason, on the other hand, spontaneously produces concepts which go beyond sense altogether. In virtue of this, we conceive ourselves as belonging to the *intelligible world* and as subject to laws that are grounded in reason alone.

But we still have a sensuous nature, and so must regard ourselves as belonging to the sensible world and subject to the laws of nature. This leaves us with two standpoints from which to view ourselves. As rational beings, we conceive ourselves as belonging to the intelligible world, with wills independent of external causes; as beings of sense, however, we are part of the sensible world. As rational beings, we act on the presupposition of freedom, from which follows autonomy; the law we set ourselves is the categorical imperative.

I am a member of both realms; my will is subject to the influence of sensuous desires. This is why the categorical imperative is to me a *command*, telling me to follow reason and not desire.

We cannot prove that freedom exists; we certainly cannot point out the *cause* of a free action—that would be the height of the ridiculous. What we can do is *defend* the concept of freedom against the attacks of those who claim that freedom is not possible (Aristotle called this "negative demonstration"). To consider rational beings from only one point of view (as part of the natural world) is to deny their freedom, but recognizing that there must be things in themselves that lie behind (give rise to) appearances opens the door to freedom. The laws governing *noumena* need not be the same as those for *phenomena*.

Kant makes a very telling parallel between the two realms that supports the presupposition of freedom. Causality cannot be proved, any more than freedom can. Causality is a necessary presupposition of any scientific inquiry, and that is sufficient justification for its use. The necessity of freedom for morality justifies *its* use.

14. One of the major works is Alasdair MacIntyre's *After Virtue* (University of Notre Dame Press, 1977). Others include James Wallace's *Virtues and Vices* (Cornell University Press, 1978), Philippa Foot's *Virtues and Vices* (Blackwell, 1978), Peter Geach's *The Virtues* (Cambridge University Press, 1977), and a rash of new books on specific virtues, such as Terrance McConnell's *Gratitude* (Temple University Press, 1993), George P. Fletcher's *Loyalty* (Oxford University Press, 1993), and J. R. Lucas' *Responsibility* (Clarendon Press, 1993). In addition, a recent top-selling popular book is William J. Bennett's *The Book of Virtues* (Simon & Schuster, 1993), which includes separate chapters on self-discipline, compassion, responsibility, friendship, work, courage, perseverance, honesty, loyalty, and faith.

15. Consider sight, which is something good in itself and also good for its consequences (it keeps you from bumping into things). For sight to occur, there must be an object to be seen, an organ for seeing (the eye), and a source of light, which is the Sun. The Sun is both the cause and nurturer of the things in the world which are seen, and also of the entity that sees. These things could not exist without the life-giving power of the Sun, and they could not be seen without its light.

Similarly, the Good (which is the cause of the Sun and of all good things), makes possible the knowledge of the Forms (the objects of knowing) by the intelligence. The Good "illuminates" the Forms so they can be "seen" by the "eye of the soul"—that is, the mind. The Good makes possible the realm of the Forms and the realm of souls or minds that apprehend them.

16. Plato, *Symposium*, trans. Alexander Nehamas and Paul Woodruff (Indianapolis, IN: Hackett, 1989), p. 59.

17. Butchvarov suggests a hierarchy of goods:

1. Existence (necessary to all other goods; intrinsically good).

2. Life (the corresponding good is health).

3. Sentience (he says only perverse moral thinking would suggest that one sacrifice oneself for an oak tree); the corresponding good is bodily pleasure.

4. Conscious desire—the good is satisfaction (sensual pleasures have location in space; intellectual pleasures do not).

5. Intellect (the corresponding good is theoretical knowledge).

6. Will (its good is courage or fortitude); Aristotle defined choice as deliberative desire; Aquinas defined the will as the appetite of reason.

7. Sociality (relations possible only between beings of reason and will)—the corresponding good is friendship (we are back in contact with Plato and Aristotle here).

When we ask, "Who are the others?" in a claim that we have ethical responsibilities to others, there are several answers. Correlated with each good there may be a different set of relevant others. If there is a conflict—"my own good or that of others?"—it should occur only at lower levels. If knowledge is the highest good, then it is clearly a good that can be shared indefinitely, with no loss to its original possessor. Augustine has a similar view regarding the vision of God. There is no such thing as a competition for knowledge or for the vision of God. Butchvarov concludes that an adequate ethics is not likely to regard things such as money, offices, fame, power (where we compete) as good in themselves, though they may be means to something that *is* good in itself.

■ SHORT ESSAY QUESTIONS

1. Michael Frayn, in *The Tin Men*, says that scientists developing the Samaritan line of "ethical" computers began by setting up for them the "simplest and purest" form of ethical situation, in which two rational beings are on a raft which will sink if both stay aboard, but will float if only one remains on it. Indicate how each of the following positions discussed would "program" the Samaritan computer to deal with the situation (that is, what general rules would be given to the computer for such situations, and why). Indicate briefly, in each case, how the "program" fits the position. Rank these "solutions" 1 through 7 in order of most satisfactory to least satisfactory from a moral standpoint, and briefly justify the ranking.

   a. Hobbes, the materialist, who says that "laws are the only basis of morality"

   b. Ayn Rand, who says that the achievement of one's own individual happiness is the highest moral purpose (and that certain individuals are more valuable than others because of their creativity)

   c. A cultural relativist

   d. A Utilitarian like John Stuart Mill

   e. Kant (as best you can, based on his general principle(s), recognizing that some extrapolating must be done)

   f. an Epicurean

   g. Butchvarov

2. Indicate and discuss at least three ways in which the ethical views of the Stoics are anticipations of Kant's position.

3. Outline, briefly, the different advice you would get from Jeremy Bentham and Kant on how you should live the next two years of your life.

4. State clearly why Kant says the basis for ethics must lie in a *categorical* (not a *hypothetical*) imperative.

5. Kant argues that suicide is not wrong for the reason that God despises it, but that God despises suicide because it is wrong. Discuss the importance of this distinction.

6. Do you agree with those who say that morality is, like taste, in the "eye of the beholder"? Why or why not? What would Kant say to this claim? Protagoras? Plato?

7. What is the thrust of the Epicurean view on morality? Be careful to distinguish Epicurus himself from what some of his "followers" thought. Is it an adequate theory? Why or why not?

■ LONG ESSAY QUESTIONS

1. Try to write an account of the following: your day, your best friend and why you are close, your ambitions (goals), your favorite way to relax (pick one) using only scientific, deterministic language (getting rid of all references to consciousness, mind, value, choice, etc.). If you have difficulties writing this account, comment on why you have the difficulties and what this tells you about the adequacy of the deterministic account.

2. In the translator's introduction to Kant's *Foundations of the Metaphysics of Morals*, Lewis White Beck raises nine common criticisms of Kant's ethics (as expressed in the *Foundations*), and attempts to assess or answer them briefly. Write a paper that takes on criticisms 1, 2, and 6.*

State the criticisms clearly, assess their relevance to any "good" ethical theory, and then, using the text of the *Foundations*, provide as good a

---

*Criticism 6 raises a broader issue. It is said that a teleological theory like Mill's is concerned only with the consequences of actions, and a deontological theory like Kant's is concerned only with intentions. Can/does Kant ignore the consequences of actions altogether? Look carefully at this question.

defense of Kant to each criticism as possible (go beyond Beck's brief responses). If you find that Kant does not stand up adequately to a criticism, then make it clear how he fails.

[This essay will require you to do a careful reading of Kant with a particular issue (one at a time) in mind; it should also get you thinking about criteria in general that any good ethical theory should meet.]

3. Peter Van Inwagen wrote an excellent book, *An Essay on Free Will*, on the free will issue. Read it, or at least the chapter "What Our Not Having Free Will Would Mean," and write a critical paper expounding and evaluating his argument.

4. Read Thomas Nagel's *The Possibility of Altruism* (1970), and evaluate his argument in a critical paper.

5. In contrast to the previous topic, read Ayn Rand's *The Virtue of Selfishness* (1961), and evaluate her arguments in a critical paper.

6. Examine some congressional debates on a difficult issue, such as censorship of the Internet, or pornography, or wiretapping, or Carnivore, or appropriation of funds for the Ballistic Missile Defense Organization. Much of this is now available on-line as well as in your local library; for instance, the *Congressional Quarterly* is available by online subscription (for a fee), but it also has a free trial period (www.cq.com). You can access the *Congressional Record* online at

www.access.gpo.gov/ u_docs/aces/aces150.html

Another useful source of information, with an index, can be found at

http://thomas.loc.gov/home/textonly.html

See how many instances you can find of approaches we discussed in this chapter to moral decision making, such as utilitarian calculations, Kantian universalizability of maxims, appealing to developing virtuous character, or evaluation of issues based on their contribution to achieving higher-level goods (and minimizing evils). Now compare these cases with any you can find that fit ethical egoism, or any of the views in Chapter 2, such as "there is no truth about these issues," "we can never reach universal agreement," "these 'moral' rules will take away my freedom," "morality is just a matter of feeling, or personal taste," "science has shown people are all incurably selfish," "morality can only be based on a feeling of sympathy," cultural relativism, "law is the only basis for morality," or "don't talk about what is *good* or *right*, talk to me about what is *scientifically* proven fact." Given our analysis and what you read in the proceedings, assess just how satisfactory, effective, or moral these various attitudes are.

7. Write a thoughtful essay on how computers have changed what we value.

■ REFERENCES AND RECOMMENDED READINGS

Abelson, Raziel, and Kai Nielsen. "Ethics, History of." In *Encyclopedia of Philosophy*, vol. 3 (New York: Macmillan, 1967), pp. 81–117.

Aristotle. *Nicomachean Ethics. Eudemian Ethics.*

Augustine. *On the Free Choice of the Will.*

Ayer, A. J. "Freedom and Necessity." In *Philosophical Essays* (New York: Macmillan, 1954), pp. 271–84. Also in Watson, pp. 15–23.

Beauchamp, Tom L. *Philosophical Ethics: An Introduction to Moral Philosophy.* 2nd ed. New York: McGraw-Hill, 1991.

Bentham, Jeremy. *Principles of Morals and Legislation* (1789).

Butchvarov, Panayot. *Skepticism and Ethics.* Bloomington, IN: Indiana University Press, 1989.

Encyclopedia of Philosophy. New York: Macmillan, 1967. See the articles here on the major philosophers and positions discussed, as well the articles on "Freedom" and "Determinism."

Epictetus. *Enchiridion.*

Epicurus. *Letter to Herodotus. Letter to Menoeceus. Fragments.*

Frayn, Michael. *The Tin Men.* London: Collins, 1965.

Hook, Sidney, ed. *Determinism and Freedom in the Age of Modern Science.* New York: Collier, 1961.

Hume, David, *A Treatise of Human Nature* (1739).

Kant, Immanuel. *Critique of Pure Reason* (1781).

Kant, Immanuel. *Foundations of the Metaphysics of Morals* (1785). Trans. Lewis White Beck. New York: Macmillan, 1985.

Leibniz, Gottfried Wilhelm. *Monadology* (1716). *Principles of Nature and Grace* (1714). *Theodicy* (1710).

Lyons, David. *Forms and Limits of Utilitarianism.* Oxford, England: Clarendon Press, 1965.

Lyons, David, ed. *Rights.* Belmont, CA: Wadsworth, 1979.

MacIntyre, Alasdair. *A Short History of Ethics.* New York: Macmillan, 1966.

MacIntyre, Alasdair. *After Virtue.* 2nd ed. Notre Dame, IN: University of Notre Dame Press, 1984.

Mill, John Stuart. *Utilitarianism* (1863).

Moore, G.E. *Principia Ethica* (1903).

Nagel, Thomas. *The Possibility of Altruism.* Oxford, England: Clarendon Press, 1977.

Plato. *Meno. Republic. Gorgias.*

Pojman, Louis P. *Ethical Theory: Classical and Contemporary Readings.* Belmont, CA: Wadsworth, 1989.

Rachels, James. *The Elements of Moral Philosophy.* New York: Random House, 1986.

Rand, Ayn. *The Virtue of Selfishness.*

Robinson, John M. *An Introduction to Early Greek Philosophy.* Boston: Houghton Mifflin, 1968.

Spinoza. *Ethics* (1675).

Van Inwagen, Peter. *An Essay on Free Will.* Oxford, England: Clarendon Press, 1983.

Watson, Gary, ed. *Free Will* (Oxford Readings in Philosophy). Oxford, England: Oxford University Press, 1982.

Part Two

Ethics Applied to a Computerized World

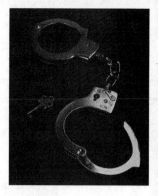

Chapter 4

Software Piracy, Property, and Protection

*I*n order to look into the potential and existing issues connected with computer hardware and software, some distinctions first need to be made. A computer is usually described in terms of its *hardware* (circuits, disks, buttons, metal or plastic casing, and so forth) and *software* (the programs that make it run). A familiar analogy is that the hardware is the body of the machine, the software its "mind."

 ## A BRIEF HISTORY OF HARDWARE

The first calculating device was the abacus, first mentioned in Herodotus around 450 B.C., but probably dating back in China to at least the sixth century B.C. Other early calculating devices were the Aztec calendar stone and the navigator's astrolabe in the Middle Ages. The history of hardware may also be connected to the history of mechanical toys that imitated human behavior. (For a delightful pictorial history of these, see Chapuis and Droz, *Automata*, 1958.) Such toys included statues of gods in ancient Thebes controlled by the priests, flying doves and marionettes in ancient Greece, pictures that move, animated masks, and mechanical clocks dating from the beginning of the fourteenth century (such as those with humanlike figures that come out and strike the hour on a gong).

In 1623, during the Thirty Years War, William Schickard built a device to mechanically add and subtract. A record of his device was found in his letters to Johannes Kepler. In 1643, Blaise Pascal (after whom a programming language would later be named) at age 20 built a mechanical device, which used ratchets to perform addition and subtraction, to aid his father in calculating tax revenues. Gottfried Leibniz built a more efficient calculating device than Pascal's in 1673, one that would also do multiplication and division. His goal was to free humans from the drudgery of doing laborious calculations, in order to give them time to be more creative. In 1805, Joseph Jacquard, a weaver, built a loom that used cards with holes to control the placement of threads (warp and weft) in weaving textiles. Another set of cards would result in a different pattern in the cloth produced, automating the weaving process.

Charles Babbage, a virtual recluse living in England in the early nineteenth century, built a Difference Engine and an Analytical Engine. The latter had (1) a *store* of quantities (variables) to be operated on, and to contain the results of the calculations, and (2) a *mill* to perform the operations. The Analytical Engine took two sets of cards, one to direct operations and the other to provide values to be operated on. Augusta Ada Byron, Lady Lovelace (the only legitimate daughter of the poet Lord Byron), was an accomplished mathematician who studied with the famous mathematician Augustus DeMorgan. She wrote programs for Babbage's Analytical Engine to direct its operations—thus she was considered the first programmer. She wrote articles for the London newspapers to stimulate interest in Babbage's work, and observed that the Analytical Engine wove algebraic patterns in much the same way that the Jacquard loom wove flowers into cloth. In the 1970s, the Department of Defense created a high-level programming language, Ada, named in her honor. Babbage received little support in his own time, and died bitter and frustrated. His work was rediscovered in the twentieth century, when he was widely recognized as the true father of modern computing.

At the end of the nineteenth century, Herman Hollerith and John Billings, working in the U.S. Census Office in Buffalo, New York, were dismayed by the handling of the data for the 1880 census, which was not completed until 1890 (at which point it was time to take a new census!). They developed a system of using cards containing punched holes to represent the data collected, and a mechanical device (a kind of sorter) to sort the data into appropriate categories. Using this system, the data from the next census were completely processed a month after collection was finished. Out of this grew, for Hollerith, a commercial venture, the American Tabulating Machine Company. In 1914, a young man named Thomas J. Watson joined the firm, and by 1924 he had taken over control; he renamed the company the International Business Machines Company. The punched card used to represent data and enter programs remained in use through the 1960s and early 1970s, and was referred to as a *Hollerith card*; the characters coded on the cards were called *Hollerith characters*.

By the late 1930s, Howard Aiken at Harvard and George Stibitz at Bell Labs were building calculating machines, using telephone relays as parts, which were quite similar to Babbage's Analytical Engine. Around 1940, John V. Atanasoff at Iowa State University built a specialized computer to solve linear equations, in which he used vacuum tubes to store information.

Building large calculating devices requires money, and such money can often come from government support, if the project promises a payoff the government is interested in. An interest in ballistics—the paths of projectiles—goes back to Galileo (there is a story of his dropping objects of different weights off the Leaning Tower of Pisa), Newton and his apple, Lagrange, and Laplace (who was Examiner of the Royal Artillery in 1748). World War II created the demand for ballistics tables for artillery pieces and bombing raids. Such tables were very complex and took a long time to calculate by hand, since they had to take into account many variables, such as wind velocity, temperature, angle of the artillery piece (or speed at which a bomber is flying), and weight of shells (or bombs). The calculations for a 60-second trajectory required about 750 multiplications, and took one person roughly 20 hours to complete.

Responding to the need to speed up this process, scientists, through U.S. government support, designed the Electronic Numerical Integrator and Calculator (ENIAC), a calculating machine "hard-wired" to do just one job—calculate trajectories for different projectiles under varying conditions. The information (data) on a particular projectile was "input" to the machine, which always performed the same set of operations on the data it was given. The details of the ballistic trajectory formed the "output." The trajectory that had taken a human 20 hours to calculate was completed by ENIAC in 30 seconds. The ENIAC occupied 1,500 square feet of floor space and weighed 20 tons. Made up of 19,000 vacuum tubes and 1,500 telephone relays, it had a high failure rate. The principal designers of the ENIAC were John Presper Eckert Jr. and John W. Mauchley, both of the Moore School of Electrical Engineering at the University of Pennsylvania. It is interesting to note that Mauchley had visited Atanasoff in 1941, two years before the start of the ENIAC project. Atanasoff later sued Mauchley and Eckert for trying to patent what he claimed were originally his ideas. In 1974, a federal court validated Atanasoff's claims.

Work on similar projects involved the first professors at the Princeton Institute of Advanced Studies—Oswald Veblen (father of economist Thorstein Veblen), Albert Einstein, Hermann Weyl, Eugene Wigner, and John von Neumann. The brilliant mathematician von Neumann (who, with Oskar Morgenstern, developed mathematical game theory) noted the weakness of having a huge and very expensive machine like ENIAC that could perform only one job, a job that would be of little interest when the war was over. Thus von Neumann developed the idea of the "stored program computer," in which the set of operations to be performed (the "program") could be input to the machine as well as the data to be operated on. Thus one computer could be used to do any number of different tasks. This gave rise between 1949 and 1952 to the development of Electronic Discrete Variable Automatic Computer (EDVAC), the first general-purpose stored-program computer.

By 1948, IBM had built the first commercially available computer (Ssec– Selective Sequence Electronic Calculator) and dominated the large computer ("mainframe") market for many years thereafter. The advent of transistors led to a second generation of computers between 1957 and 1959, that were much smaller and faster than those that had used vacuum tubes and relays. The extensive use of integrated circuits ("printed circuits") led to the third generation of computers. A number of transistors, diodes, and other components equivalent to 64 complete circuits could be placed on a silicon chip less that one-eighth of an inch square. Microminiaturization has come a long way since then. Advances in Very Large Scale Integration (VLSI) led to a fourth generation of computers between 1971 and the present. What is being called the "Fifth Generation" of computers is really more of a software notion, the development of "artificially intelligent" machines operating on even faster and smaller hardware.

Of course, mainframes ceased to be the only game in town with the advent of minicomputers in the 1970s and microcomputers in the 1980s. The hardware technology continues to advance, making machines smaller, faster, and cheaper. In addition, supercomputers were developed which were faster and had a great deal of memory, for solving very large-scale problems such as aircraft design, weather prediction, or mapping the human genome. The bigger issue is what can be *done* with these machines, and that is where the software comes in.

 ## A BRIEF HISTORY OF SOFTWARE

The history of software might be construed to be the history of (systematic) thought, or at least the history of logic and mathematics. The scope of these is clearly beyond this brief introduction (see, for example, William and Martha Kneale, *The Development of Logic* (1962), and any of a number of good histories of mathematics); here we will point to only a few highlights that seem particularly relevant to computers.

The history of logic goes back at least to Aristotle, who was the first to formulate laws of argument in the syllogism (in the *Prior Analytics* and *Posterior Analytics*). In an even earlier period in mathematics, a religious group made up of followers of Pythagoras attempted to bring order out of the chaos of the world by asserting that "all is [rational] number." Thus, one would only need to discover the unique numbers of all things, and their relations to each other (which would, of course, follow nice, regular rules), and one would completely understand the world.[1]

Axiomatic systems (which have a set of basic rules or "prime directives") are epitomized in Euclid's *Elements*. If an axiom system is "closed" (that is, *consistent* and *complete*), then given the axioms, definitions, and rules of inference, all of the true theorems of the system are deducible given enough time and effort. A system is said to be *consistent* if no contradictions can be derived within the system (that is, one cannot prove both "X" and "not-X" from the axioms). A system is said to be *complete* if any well-formed-formula (wff) or statement that is expressible in the system and is true can be proved within the system. If all interesting axiomatic systems were consistent and complete, then, given enough time, our modern computers could prove all of the theorems of these systems. But, unfortunately, this is not the case. In 1931, Kurt Gödel proved that any system complex enough to represent simple arithmetic could not be both consistent and complete.

A major step in the development of systematic thought came when Galileo introduced "mathematical physics" around 1600. The rules for understanding the (physical) world evolved as mathematical rules (much like the ideal sought by the Pythagoreans). In 1580, François Vieta introduced the use of letters for unknowns in algebraic equations (a development that would later become important to the use of variables in computer languages). In 1614, John Napier "invented" logarithms, and used "Napier's bones" (two ivory rods with logarithmic markings) to make calculations. Based on this, work by Edmund Gunter in 1620 was the forerunner of the slide rule, which was perfected in 1632 by William Oughtred. In 1637, Descartes discovered analytical (Cartesian) geometry, which the historian Joseph Needham called "the greatest single step ever made in the progress of the exact sciences." In Cartesian geometry, spatial (geometric) points are identified with algebraic coordinates. This showed how concepts in one area (such as a geometric curve) can be taken as represented by concepts in another area (an algebraic formula). Thus the circle of radius r centered at $(0, 0)$ in the two-dimensional x, y plane can be represented by the algebraic equation $x^2 + y^2 = r^2$.

Leibniz (1646–1716) had great faith that logic and mathematics could provide a "universal calculus" by means of which we could *deduce* all the truths about the world: if a question arose (any question, including one in ethics or politics), we could simply, like the mathematicians, sit down and say "let us calculate" to find the answer. Leibniz considered that everything in the world was a mixture of All, or God (1) and Nothing (0), so each thing in the world would have a unique binary number (like 0.1110011... for something high in perfections, or 0.00000101... for something badly flawed, with a large mixture of Nothing in it). Leibniz's "universal characteristic" would manipulate such numbers according to mathematical laws to determine the answers.[2] What better to manipulate such binary values to find answers than a binary digital computer?

Around 1860, George Boole developed an algebra of classes (arising out of his interest in probabilities) based on a 0, 1 notation. This interest in an algebra of classes was picked up in 1861 by John Venn, an admirer of Boole. Venn developed diagrams using overlapping regions to represent the relationships among such classes; these circular diagrams were reminiscent of those drawn by Ramon Lull in 1245 in his *Ars Magna*. Since Boole's attempt to discover the "laws of thought" was easily expressed in simple rules, Jevons was able, in 1869, to see the possibility of mechanizing them. In the next year he exhibited, before the British Royal Society, a "logic machine"–a device looking much like a cash register, with signs representing different combinations made to appear by pressing keys. In 1885, Allan Marquand suggested an electrical analogue of Jevons' machine. Claude Shannon, at Bell Labs, noticed the relationship between Boolean expressions and switching circuits in the late 1930s. In 1945, an electrical computer was constructed at Harvard for the solution of Boolean problems.

The realization that both symbols (numbers and characters) and rules for their manipulation could be represented on a binary machine led to the explosion of computing technology in the past 50 years. Today, software generally refers to any program for manipulating information in a computer, or for using the computer to control the action of some other device.

In the earlier years of digital computers, the programs written were generally done "in-house" to solve particular scientific or engineering problems as part of a larger project. If such software was sold, it was usually done so as part of a larger package, often in fulfillment of a government contract.

Some distinctions should be drawn at this point. A computer is made up of binary (two-state) components, and so everything in it–numbers, natural language, instructions–must take this binary form. Thus base-10 numbers we are familiar with must be transformed into binary before they can be represented internally on the computer. For example, the decimal number 25 is 11001 in binary (base 2), and would be represented internally on the computer by a set of binary (on/off) devices in an "on-on-off-off-on" pattern.

The *instructions* that a computer can execute include mathematical manipulations (beginning with addition, and progressing to subtraction, multiplication, and division by building on this), "shifting" bit (*binary digit*) patterns right or left, storing values, erasing values, testing whether two values are equal or unequal (the first greater than, greater than or equal to, less than, or less than or equal to, the second), branching to another location (either unconditionally, as in JUMP TO X, or conditionally, as in IF A = B, JUMP TO X), and stopping. Each of these instructions is represented as a unique binary string internal to the computer, which causes the appropriate action to be taken. A **software program** is a sequence of such commands, expressed in binary, that are stored in the machine and then executed. The only language the computer understands is binary. This is why it is humorous in *Star Wars* when C3PO tells Luke Skywalker's uncle that of course he can speak the binary language Bocce, that it is "like a second language" to the robot.

Early programmers of computers actually had to program in binary **machine language.** That is, they had to convert all the numerical decimal values into binary before entering them into the computer, and learn the binary strings for each instruction we discussed, and enter those strings to make up the program. This was very difficult to do, and it was hard to think through a complex program to solve a difficult problem; the programmer wanted to think in broader terms such as "sort this list of values into ascending order" but was forced to think in terms of tiny, discrete *load, compare,* and *jump* instructions represented in binary! Such programming was difficult and hard on the nerves of the programmers. So **assembly language** was developed, which allowed programmers to write instructions in short mnemonic codes such as ADD, SUB, STO, JMP, JNG (to stand for the fictitious example instruction "jump on negative [value]"), and the like. This was somewhat easier on the programmers, but the machine did not understand ADD, SUB, or the rest, so a program had to be written (in binary machine language) to translate these humanlike codes into binary; such a program was called an **assembler.**

As the power of the computer became more and more recognized, the desire to apply it to larger and more interesting problems increased. The slowdown in translating what a programmer wanted the machine to do into machine code or even assembly language became intolerable, and so "higher-level languages" were developed. Among the first of these were FORTRAN ("FORmula TRANslator") and LISP (LISt Processing language), then COBOL (Common Business-Oriented Language), and a "tower of Babel" of other languages that did not survive for very long. Other languages came along that did survive the test of time, such as BASIC (Beginner's All-purpose Symbolic Instruction Code), Pascal (named after Blaise), and Ada (named after the first programmer). These languages used commands closer to English or algebraic notation, employed symbols for mathematical operations (+, -, *, /, and ** or ^), and used single instructions in the language (such as DO or FOR, PRINT) to represent *sets* of operations at the machine level. For a program written in such a high-level language, another translator program, called a **compiler**, was needed to transform the programmer's code into machine code.

A program is generally written according to an **algorithm,** a finite structured sequence of instructions that comes to an end in a finite amount of time. It is named after the ninth century Arabic mathematician al-Khôwarizmi; it was through the translation of his work on algebra that Arabic numerals became known in the West. A simple example of an algorithm (though not one usually performed by a computer) is a cooking recipe. A finite set of instructions that violates the algorithmic condition of coming to an end in a finite amount of time is the set of instructions found on most shampoo bottles—Apply, Lather, Rinse, Repeat. This creates what is called in computer parlance an *infinite loop*.

A paradigm example of a mathematical algorithm that can be translated directly into a computer program is the Euclidean algorithm for finding the greatest common divisor of two whole numbers (integers a and b):

Euclidean Algorithm for Greatest Common Divisor

1. Call the larger number M and the smaller N.

2. Divide M by N and determine the remainder R. (The remainder is the whole number left over when N multiples of the quotient Q have been taken away from M. For example, if you divide 35 by 10, the quotient Q is 3 and the remainder is 5.)

3. If R is greater than zero, make M the value of N, and make N the value of R. (You can imagine these values stored on slips of paper with the titles M, N, and R; each time you change a value you erase the old value and write in the new one.) Then repeat from Step 1.

If R is equal to 0, then the current value of N is the greatest common divisor of your original numbers a and b.

THE END[3]

SOFTWARE PIRACY

The biggest change in software development was spurred by the introduction of the personal computer (PC) at the beginning of the 1980s. Small but reasonably powerful desktop computers became available for the general public. However, most people were not programmers and had little desire to become so. This inspired manufacturers who wanted to sell their microcomputers to the general public to provide them with software "packages" that could perform various tasks—from word processing, spreadsheets, and income tax programs to games. Some of these programs were "bundled" with the microcomputer purchased, while others could be bought later. Thus many people (not just those building the PCs) got into the business of creating many and varied software packages for computer users to buy.

These software packages have become a billion-dollar business. Nowadays someone develops a "neat" package to do Z, convinces the general PC public that they desperately *need* Z, and then sells many copies of the package at great profit. Here is the American dream—young entrepreneurs who built small computers in their garages, or who developed a few clever software packages, become today's millionaires and billionaires.

Operating systems for computers—which test memory, keep programs from wiping each other out, handle input and output controls, and so on—are also programs that are needed to communicate with the machine and make it run.

The problem we need to consider in this chapter comes up because not everyone who has access to package Z or an operating system or interface has paid a fair price for it. Software piracy—from small-scale to very large-scale—is rampant today. We will examine the extent of such piracy, why it is so easy, and what is currently being done about it. We also will examine to what extent this is an *ethical* problem. A related problem, that of one software package being *too much like* another existing package, gives rise to accusations of espionage, stealing of ideas, and the like.

What Is Software Piracy?

When Thucydides wrote of the times in Greece prior to the Peloponnesian War, he told of the prevalence of pirates in the area. Many towns were built somewhat inland (as was Athens), with a small seaport (like Piraeus) where ships might dock, so that the town was protected from the attacks of pirates.

Such a profession was "considered quite honourable" at the time, and we find many of the characters in earlier stories asking a newcomer, "Are you a pirate?" with no hint of disapproval.[4] It may be that a similar attitude prevails in our society regarding today's software pirates.

Generally, a software pirate is someone who copies a program that is normally sold for a price, without paying anything for it. Often a friend or acquaintance will ask to borrow a software package that someone has bought, make a copy of the program disk(s), and return the original. There are now software rental stores, and no one asks what those who rent the programs do with them when they get them home, as long as the rented copy is returned intact. A student who is required to use a software package for a class might check it out at the library loan desk, then make a personal copy before returning it to the desk. These are small-scale, individual cases, and most people who do this get away with it. Do they feel guilty? (This is a *psychological* question.) *Should* they? This is an *ethical* question. We need to examine whether what they have done is *morally wrong* (clearly, it is *legally wrong* now).

The law says that copying such material is illegal (analogous to the warnings on videotapes that it is illegal to copy them). If the culprit is caught, there are potential fines and even jail terms. Few if any of these small-scale cases will even be detected, much less go to court. But the software industry knows that they happen; those selling the software know that there are many more copies of their package "out there" than they have received payment for.

Then there are midscale cases. Charlie gets his parents to buy him an expensive word-processing program, then makes copies for everyone he knows (the disks used cost him about $2 for each copy) and charges them $20 for the program; he also photocopies a few essential pages from the manual to give them. (It should be noted that a small publishing industry grew up on the basis of the existence of such copying. There are many books published on how to use various word-processing programs, spreadsheets, database management programs, and the like, that would have no market if everyone was buying the original software that contains its own full documentation and explanations.) Charlie is happy, since he has pocketed a profit; his friends are happy, since they have copies of an expensive program for only $20; the only people who are unhappy are those at the company that markets the software package, since they were paid for only one copy in a case where now many are in use.

On a strict utilitarian analysis, more people would gain pleasure from getting good software inexpensively than the balance of pain to the few people in the company who are not getting their large profits. But it is not as simple as this. There is the matter of *justice*, of fair recompense for creative work done, of how the people now benefitting from the inexpensive software would feel if the positions were reversed. There are other aspects to the question that must be examined as well—the high cost of the software, whether huge profits are justifiable, whether good ideas should be shared with everyone without cost, and so on. We will examine these aspects as the discussion progresses.

The last category is that of large-scale piracy, which has two aspects that are distinct. The first is the large corporation that buys one or a few copies of a useful software item, and then makes illegal copies for all the rest of its employees. "Raids" on large corporations (such as Montedison in Italy, Westinghouse in Brazil, and the Maxwell publishing empire in England) resulted in uncovering large amounts of such illegally copied software in use. This is clearly in violation of the intent of the software license agreement, and breaks the law. Several such corporations have been sued for their violations of the law. Among these are the Davy McKee engineering company and the New York City Council.[5]

The Westinghouse branch in Brazil was threatened with fines of as much as $2 million for their copyright infringement of the Microsoft MS-DOS operating system software.[6] It is interesting to note that only "several" copies of MS-DOS were mentioned in the Westinghouse raid, but in the raid on Italy's Montedison, Ashton-Tate and Lotus claimed that 90 percent of the company's software had been illegally copied.[7] Pirated copies seem to be a way of life in Italy, to the tune of about $500 million worth a year.

The German software company Cadsoft uncovered in 1993 the fact that employees of IBM, Philips, the German federal ministry of the interior, and the federal office for the protection of the [German] constitution were making illegal copies of one of its programs. The companies accepted Cadsoft's offer of a free demonstration program, a program that turned out also to search their hard disks for unauthorized copies of the other program and report back to Cadsoft (through a voucher for a free handbook that the free program printed out and invited the user to return).[8] A large-scale software scam was perpetrated in 1994 in the San Francisco area by a man selling stolen and illegally copied software through the mail; he advertised his amazingly low prices in the *Chronicle* and other newspapers. At the time of the report, he was facing up to $500,000 in fines and up to 10 years in prison.[9] In 1996, Microsoft filed a suit against small Houston computer manufacturer Premium for installing pirated software on the computers it sold.[10] This was part of a wider piracy crackdown in Texas, Silicon Valley, and New York/New Jersey.

Suspects were indicted in 1995 for selling $3 million of pirated software in 1992–93; they allegedly made 200,000 illegal copies of Microsoft programs.[11] The city of Philadelphia had to pay almost $122,000 in fines to the Business Software Alliance in 1997 because two city offices had made illegal copies of hundreds of software programs.[12] Philadelphia made the news again in 2001, when a Philadelphia school district was accused of using bootleg Microsoft computer programs in its classrooms.[13] The school district faces a multimillion dollar suit brought by Microsoft.

The most recent software piracy sweep (December 2001) is being made of college campuses (including Duke, Purdue, MIT, and UCLA), as well as several computer and software companies around the country, looking for copies of illegal software distributed by the DrinkOrDie network, which originated in Russia in 1993 and has a reputed 200 members worldwide. Raids were also carried out in Britain, Australia, Finland, Norway, and Sweden.[14] Some of the "software" they are looking for includes bootleg copies of the movie *Harry Potter and the Sorcerer's Stone.*

One 1999 estimate claimed that software vendors in the United States are losing more than $3.6 billion a year from piracy at home; they may lose up to five times that much from piracy abroad.[15] Recent worldwide losses from software piracy are exceeding $12 billion a year. It is estimated that over 80 percent of all the software programs in the world come from the United States. The Software Publishers Association estimates that 37 percent of all software is pirated, with 95 percent of that occurring at corporate sites.[16]

The second aspect of large-scale piracy involves those who make piracy into a global business. Such piracy has always been greater outside of the United States, with the Far East, the Middle East, Italy, and some Latin American countries being particularly active in this area. Several *Wall Street Journal* articles in 1993 reported claims by Microsoft that piracy was severely damaging its business in Japan, and that software piracy was growing rapidly in China; today the Business Software Alliance (BSA) reports that 94 percent of the software in China is illegally copied, with 97 percent in Vietnam, and 89 percent in Indonesia.[17] These same countries do a large-scale business in copied books as well.

In 1990, BSA initiated a series of spectacular raids in Asia, finding 5,000 copies of MS-DOS and many copied manuals in various languages in Taiwan (valued at $22.5 million if sold legitimately), a multimillion dollar business in illegal business computer manuals in Singapore in 1991, and a mail order business operating out of a hut in Hong Kong in 1989 (over 109,000 copied manuals and 6,600 copied disks), with a legitimate market value of roughly $50 million.[18] In November 2001, pirated copies of Windows XP went on sale in Thailand (at $2.70) almost two weeks before Microsoft's formal launch date there.[19] The litany of such illegal activities goes on and on. When a software package like Lotus can be bought in Thailand for one-tenth its cost in the United States, it is very tempting. Such disks may also be infected with computer viruses, a topic to be discussed in Chapter 6.

There is hope that government action may have an effect on large-scale piracy abroad. In an article appearing in the October 18, 1993 *Washington Post,* Bill Gates wrote in support of approval of NAFTA, indicating how sales of Microsoft products in Mexico had greatly improved since NAFTA negotiations began. He believed that NAFTA would create an improved legal climate in Mexico, through its strong intellectual property provisions. It would codify software protection through copyright, "and turn a large piracy market into a major software market."[20] Gates believes that a legal crackdown on software pirates under NAFTA will mean more exports from the United States and so more jobs, including in the area of Spanish-language programs, training, and support. "Moreover," says Gates, "every new job in the computer industry begets additional jobs for our suppliers." One is reminded of a line from an old "Li'l Abner" sequence: "What's good for General Bullmoose is good for the U.S.A.!" In this line, Al Capp most likely had General Motors in mind, but the software industry has challenged the automobile industry for preeminence in the United States. It is interesting to note, as we discuss property protection for software in upcoming sections, that comparisons to patent protection in the auto industry will often be made.

Some people who may be "soft" on software piracy call it "technology transfer" or "sharing," which has a legitimate ring to it; another term used, however, is "softlifting." Other countries should be encouraged to develop their own software industries, and trade agreements the United States signs with them should include recognition and enforcement of whatever property rights (copyright, patent, or something better) the United States places on their software. These issues should be clarified through GATT (General Agreement of Tariffs and Trades) talks, and in trade negotiations with China. In January 1993, there was congressional discussion of an agreement called TRIPS (Trade Related Aspects of Intellectual Property Rights).[21]

We have seen a wide range of software piracy cases, from the individual who copies an occasional program to the large-scale businesses in illegally copied software. Such a range presents the ethical analyst with a "slippery-slope" problem. Is it all right to copy one program, but immoral to make a big business out of selling copied programs? If it is all right to copy one time, how about two? Or three? Just where do you draw the line? (This is where the slippery slope comes in.)

An analogy might be drawn with plagiarism. Plagiarism is taking someone else's work (usually words) as your own. But at what point does a case constitute plagiarism? One word? Surely not. Two words? No. Three words? No. Well, when? There is no precise number of words that constitutes minimal plagiarism. Let us look at the other extreme—if someone takes a whole book, changes only the author's name (and perhaps the title), and tries to publish it, that is clearly plagiarism. It is both immoral and illegal. The extreme cases are clear, but the in-between cases are not so clear. There is even a "fair use" consideration that allows the use of short quoted sections of a work to appear in another work.

The software pirate is not claiming authorship of the copied program; he just wants to *use* it, so the plagiarism analogy breaks down here. We need to look for better analogies, and if we do not find them, because the issue is unique, we must try to appeal to our fundamental ground for ethics that we were at some pains to lay in the first three chapters.

An easy (but not satisfactory) solution is to just say that all the cases between the extremes are the same, and either condone or condemn all together. There are some, as you will see, who think that all software should be free as air, so piracy should not be an issue. At the other extreme, some might claim that *any* copying, even of one program, that is not authorized by the seller, is wrong. If so, we have to examine *why* it is wrong.

Is it because we are failing to give fair recompense for someone's work? But how much is fair? As we mentioned, a shortsighted utilitarian might approve at least through middle-level piracy, since it makes many more people happy than it makes sad. But the farseeing utilitarian might recognize that it would have bad future consequences, because no one would want to put in the effort to create good software, because they would not be rewarded for it. A Kantian would say that it is not moral unless you could will that everyone would freely copy software (we will see later in this chapter that computer scientist Richard Stallman wills just that), but another Kantian might balk at this, and will that no one would copy software. Virtue ethics would probably say that taking what does not rightfully belong to you will create bad character, and so is wrong. Those who considered the range of goods and evils would ask what long-term, higher-order *goods* and *evils* are involved, for the individual and society.

Clearly, we are going to have trouble determining the precise line between what is fair and what is unfair within the wide spectrum of software copying, complicated by the circumstances of the individual cases along the continuum. Since we tend to be better at making judgments in concrete cases, especially in "gray" areas where it is not obvious whether a general principle applies or not, it is useful to begin our ethical analyses with such specific cases.

Common language contains the notion of a **judgment call**, a decision based on the best estimate of what to do in the case at hand, even though one cannot fully articulate the principles behind the decision. What ought to lie behind such calls are familiarity with the details of the case, a good will, and considerable thought about moral issues. It seems reasonable that we should not attempt, in the longest chapter in this book, to resolve by ethical analysis the entire continuum of cases on the copying problem. Thus we will provide an ethical analysis of a few concrete cases in this chapter as illustrations of such analysis and leave the remainder as exercises for the reader.

One concrete example involving software piracy was provided in 1991 by a *Wall Street Journal* report that software companies were secretly searching electronic bulletin boards in search of "pilfered products."[22] A high-profile result of this monitoring was the first charge of piracy on the Internet, leveled against a 20-year-old MIT student named David LaMacchia. LaMacchia had posted materials on an electronic bulletin board so that others could copy them, and encouraged others to do the same; the estimated worth of the programs was more than $1 million, and LaMacchia was charged with "wire fraud" (a federal offense).

The Software Publishers Association called LaMacchia's actions "flagrant." The *New Scientist* article reporting on this said that U.S. law does not explicitly bar the posting of software programs on electronic bulletin boards, and asked if this does occur with copyrighted material, who is to be held responsible?[23] Should it be the system operator (in this case, LaMacchia)? But would that be like holding the head librarian responsible if someone photocopies a whole book from the library, and then sells bootleg copies of it on the sly? The broader issue of *responsibility* will be taken up in Chapter 10.

The thing to note here is that if LaMacchia did not know that what he was doing was illegal, then there may well be a failure of communication (and clarity) in our current system. The rules regarding software, and what can and cannot be done legally with it, should be clearly spelled out and made widely available to the general public. On December 28, 1994, the Massachusetts District Court dismissed the case against LaMacchia, on the basis that he did not personally profit from the activities. The court said, "It is not clear that making criminals of a large number of consumers of computer software is a result that even the software industry would consider desirable." Judge Stearns called LaMacchia's actions "heedlessly irresponsible," "self-indulgent," and "lacking in any fundamental sense of values."[24] He further suggested that criminal penalties should perhaps attach to such activities, but such a modification of copyright law is up to the legislature, not the courts.

Some economists like to raise the question of whether ethics is relevant to any action that has been judged feasible, legal, and profitable. The answer is, of course, "of course," but the question shows just where ethics enters the LaMacchia case. He did it, so it certainly was feasible. It wasn't obvious that his action was illegal and, in fact, he was acquitted. It wasn't profitable, which is, essentially, why he was acquitted. Thus the remaining question is whether LaMacchia's action was moral.

The facts of the case are known. The rough principle we are using is that an action ought to be done with good intentions (Aristotle and Kant) and it ought to bring about more higher-level goods than evils. It would seem that LaMacchia's intention was to share information, not to damage anyone. As noted, he did not profit from his act, and there seems nothing malevolent in his intentions. The issue is about ends, not means. What is *not* at stake here is whether using an electronic bulletin board was worse or better than sending a large mailing that contained the same information. So the basic question is whether LaMacchia caused more fundamental good than harm.

One need not be a shortsighted utilitarian to agree that many people may have benefitted from LaMacchia's postings. One need not be a rule utilitarian to see that if all software were freely distributed, software companies and a great deal of funded software research and development would cease to exist. Profits aside, there is harm in this. There would be less development, thus less knowledge, and a large number of people would become unemployed. Now if we changed the facts of our society and dispensed with free enterprise (whether we should or not is a much larger question), our analysis would be greatly altered. But it is not clear that LaMacchia's motivation was this grandiose.

Thus we are confronted with judging an act under the social conditions in place. Those conditions involve a free enterprise system that is reasonably tolerant of actions that do not damage the system. The facts of life in this system are that acts like LaMacchia's are not typical, and they constitute little threat to the overall enterprise. Our reading of the case does not generalize easily. It is analogous to Dostovesky's thesis that the punishment should fit the criminal, not the crime.[25] One must decide this on a case-by-case basis. It is difficult to make a strong case that LaMacchia acted immorally.

In more recent legislation, Section 230 of the Communications Decency Act (a part not struck down by the Supreme Court decision) states that providers or users of an Internet Service cannot be considered publishers "of any information provided by another information content provider." This means a BBS provider is not liable for what others publish on the site.[26]

An interesting piracy case is that of *Inslaw Inc. v. U.S. Department of Justice*. In 1982, Inslaw had a contract with the Department of Justice to install its PROMIS (Prosecutors Management Information Systems) case-tracking software in DOJ offices. The software integrates information in disparate databases, such as those of the DOJ, CIA, NSA, the Attorney General's Office, and the IRS; this shared information permits the effective tracking of a lawbreaker, a lawyer's or a judge's actions, political dissidents, or intelligence operations and operators. It can even be used to track troop movements. It is a very powerful tool, one that brought the detailed analysis of such activities or people out of the "dark ages" into the light of modern technology.

Inslaw invested further effort improving the system (at an estimated cost of $8 million), expecting the government to cover this when the contract was renegotiated. But the Justice Department, after it obtained the new source code, refused to renegotiate the contract, withheld $1.8 million in payments to Inslaw, and "astonishingly went on to pirate a further twenty copies of the new PROMIS."[27] Inslaw's president and CEO William Hamilton was able to bring a $30 million suit against the DOJ, only because he was in Chapter 11 bankruptcy as a result of the government's actions. Normally, one is unable to sue the government (it requires a lengthy process to be authorized by the Contract Appeals Board), but this restriction is waived if a company is in bankruptcy proceedings.

In February 1988, after three years of court battle, "Inslaw was awarded $6.8 million in damages, not including legal fees and 'consequential damages' for lost business opportunities," both of which will be the subjects of upcoming trials.[28] And the saga of PROMIS continues. An investigative journalist, Danny Casolaro, was working on a book about the case as part of a wider picture he called "The Octopus," in which he thought the DOJ, the intelligence agencies, and even the mob were manipulating government activities for profit. Casolaro was discovered dead in a West Virginia motel in 1991 under mysterious circumstances, both wrists slashed. The body was embalmed before the family was notified, and the room was cleaned immediately. The West Virginia authorities ruled it a suicide, but the family still does not believe that it was. Casolaro had told his friends that if anything happened to him, it would not be an accident.

From 1989 to 1992 the House Judiciary Committee investigated the Inslaw affair, and concluded that high government officials, including Edwin Meese, Attorney General under Ronald Reagan, conspired to steal PROMIS from Hamilton. The report said that the DOJ "acted wilfully and fraudulently" and took PROMIS by "trickery, fraud and deceit." They recommended that Inslaw's claims be settled immediately and fairly. Hamilton could receive from $25 million to $50 million or more in damages for his mistreatment by the DOJ. The *ABA Journal* reported in November 1994 that a bill introduced in the House in late July by Charlie Rose (D-S.C.) would send the case to the U.S. Court of Federal Claims. Rose said, "After years of wrongs and numerous acts of coverup and denial, the Department of Justice now stands unrepentant in the face of compelling evidence that it has dealt with citizens of this country in the most egregious way." [29] Unfortunately, Rose's House Resolution 4862 was killed.[30]

There is evidence that the DOJ sold PROMIS to Israel and perhaps to other nations as well. Though the CIA denied having any copies of PROMIS, it may have been in use in that office, and perhaps also by Oliver North to track political activists.[31] It is also speculated that Osama bin Laden may have gotten PROMIS software from the Russians, who got it from spy Robert Hanssen. Britain, Germany, and the U.S. all indicate they have recently stopped using PROMIS.[32] All in all, it seems that in the Inslaw case we see piracy of very sophisticated software at high government levels that has serious implications regarding government investigative techniques, the full impact of which will be examined in Chapter 7 on privacy.

The most blatant cases of piracy are those of people who go into business illegally copying and selling software products. This goes on all over the world, but seems particularly rampant in the Far East, especially in Hong Kong. The ethical question is more clear here. The rights of the software developer and manufacturer to sell the product for profit are being infringed upon by someone who had no part in the development. The original developer or company is the only one with the right to profit from the product *as developed*, and just copying it and selling it is both illegal and immoral. It boils down to a matter of theft. This undermines trust and the principles upon which business is constructed in society. The practice, if generalized, would lead to a complete breakdown of the system. Once the thieves start stealing from one another, the picture becomes even more clear. Thief A, whose goods are stolen by thief B, will want reparation; to get this, thief A would have to go to the law (which he cannot), or engage in a small war with thief B, which will damage both of their operations. Not only is legitimate society harmed by this practice, but the "society" of thieves self-destructs.

The question gets more complex when we ask, "what about those who develop another product based on a similar idea?"

 # HOW CAN SOFTWARE RIGHTS BE PROTECTED?

This question has no easy answer, at least at the present time. Traditionally, there have been three methods of protecting rights to products: patents, copyrights, and trade secret legislation. Yet none of these is a perfect fit for software, for various reasons we will examine. First of all, most *products* under legal protection are basically physical *things*, such as drugs, or automobile engines, or *processes*, such as a method for curing rubber, or a technique for creating a petroleum-product substitute. But the physical part of a software product is the few magnetic disks on which it resides, an inexpensive medium; the essential part of the product is the *idea* it embodies, the program that some clever person or group of people developed to do a common job in an elegant way. An example would be a tax-return software program, which is based on the governmental forms for filing, and then has step-by-step instructions for the person filing to enter the relevant information, and get the greatest possible tax benefit given the current tax laws.

Much of what we will discuss here reflects the current *legal* status of intellectual property, but that should not be our only consideration. Laws change as conditions change and human sensibilities evolve. If there are some problems with the way things are now, and if the current legal measures are inadequate to deal with intellectual property (specifically, software), then an educated public and legislature must make improvements. Moral education and a familiarity with the issues and the technical aspects of the problem are required to do this. The issues must be clarified, and the moral implications examined. We attempt to do this in what follows, in the context of the current legal situation. We do not expect a perfect solution to emerge full-blown from these considerations, but we do hope to lay a groundwork upon which rational progress can be made.

Arguments for Private Property

Not too many thinkers have paid attention to arguments to justify private property, but such arguments are essential as a basis for any reasonable position to be reached with regard to the ownership of computer software. We must therefore begin by examining the various positions related to this topic. The first writer to put forward a coherent argument for private property was John Locke, in his *Second Treatise on Government*. Locke argued that a person *owns* his or her *own* body, so we must begin there (this of course rules out slavery as a legitimate practice). If you own your body and your mind, then you also own the products of your labor (physical *and* mental). Your labor is an extension of yourself.

Locke's primary concern was with the ownership of land and its products. He argued that the earth was given to humankind in common, citing Genesis. To take something (like an apple) out of the common and make it your own, you must mix your labor (part of yourself) with it, by picking it up. He meets the objection that you would have to have everyone's permission to take it out of the common wealth by arguing that universal agreement and permission would be impossible to obtain, yet God would not have given the world to us and yet made it impossible for us to use it. We would starve if we had to obtain everyone's agreement, so obviously (to the "light of reason") it is sufficient for us to make the land or the apple ours by mixing our work with it (as long as it does not already belong to someone else). The only considerations of reason, according to Locke, that should guide such taking are that, in doing so, we leave "as much and as good" for others, and that we should not allow what we take to spoil (go to waste). Note that this whole argument can be made just as reasonably without need for reference to God or the Bible.

Locke's argument is a *moral* one, appealing to a natural *right*[33] to one's own body (we have added "and mind"). But, as we have discussed, rights are not basic; goods are basic. One has a natural *right* to one's body because of the basic *good* of freedom. Freedom should be preserved and nurtured for its own sake. One should be free to use one's body and mind *and their products*; if someone takes them away, this freedom is abrogated. However, as we will point out, knowledge (and intellectual "property" in general) is unique in the sense that if someone else has your knowledge, you have not lost it, in the way that they can take away your land or the pot you made. One might also question whether ownership properly extends to the *products* of body and mind; perhaps these should be shared.

Some have objected to Locke's argument by saying that it is self-defeating if one looks at the case of children. Clearly a child is the product of the parents' labor, and thus according to Locke should belong to the parent as property. However, all humans are supposed to own themselves for the theory to work. Locke would have rejected this argument, since human life and freedom was taken as basic, with the rest of the conditions for property derived from that. The private property Locke is concerned with is land, food, and other natural resources, and how a person may legitimately lay claim to any such property.

Another problem with Locke's theory (for physical goods) is that of scarcity. He relies on being able to lay claim to property and still leave as much and as good for others but, in a world of rapidly increasing population and shrinking resources, this is not always an easy condition to meet. However, as scarce as knowledge may be, its sharing does not make it more scarce.

A different basis for property rights might lie in what have been referred to as "squatter's rights"—whoever gets to the property first (be it land, gold, or the like) has the legitimate claim to it. This is a sort of "first come, first served" or "possession is nine-tenths of the law" theory. However, such a theory has difficulties that lie primarily in various ambiguities—what counts as "being there first" (is it like a race, as was the case in the development of some parts of the American Midwest?), what counts as "occupying" the property, and how much can be occupied? If a man comes to a lake heretofore unpopulated, can he claim the whole lake? What about land? Where are the boundaries?

David Hume, in Book III of the *Treatise*, observes that humans have been created especially *needy*, but with "slender means" for satisfying these multiple needs. He argues that only society allows humans to fulfill these needs adequately. A lone individual dissipates energy in mere survival, without having enough "force" to "execute any considerable work." Society provides a remedy for the *inconveniences* of isolated effort:

> By the conjunction of forces, our power is augmented: By the partition of employments, our ability increases: And by mutual succour we are less expos'd to fortune and accidents. 'Tis by this additional *force*, *ability*, and *security*, that society becomes advantageous.
>
> (Hume, *Treatise*, III, II, iii, p. 485)

Humans are productive and creative, but they can produce and create much more by working together. The question then arises about who will have ownership or control of the products.

Humans wish to enjoy the fruits of their "industry and good fortune," and it is the function of society both to secure these rights to the creative individuals and to reduce the general scarcity of goods by augmenting productivity. This is therefore a kind of utilitarian position, in which the necessity of social institutions for human survival is the justification for the right to individual property. Humans whose basic needs are met and who have a security (provided by society) in their rightful possessions are more likely to be benevolent to others. If one's own survival is protected, the *sympathy* for others has opportunity to develop. However, sympathy for others is simply a *means* toward more fundamental ends.

A careful, contemporary analysis of property rights is given by Lawrence C. Becker, in *Property Rights: Philosophic Foundations*. Becker suggests two other possible bases for property rights: *desert* and *political liberty*. The argument from *desert* is simply that some individuals, because of particular properties they exhibit, may be especially deserving of having property. Someone might lavish property on another because of the latter's great beauty (there are many instances of this to be found in history as well as in our own time). Other characteristics that might be deemed deserving of special consideration regarding property might be outstanding virtue, unusual power, great skill (we see our modern athletes reap great rewards for their skill), or intelligence of a particularly high level.

One problem here is that, in some of these cases, no effort or labor is involved (as with the person who is naturally a striking beauty), and that one must carefully look at the disproportionate rewards given to those considered deserving in some cases (for example, the multimillion-dollar athlete). Such considerations may well be relevant when examining the case of profits for those who sell software. A more serious problem is that too much emphasis is put on a rather trivial good—property—when there are much more important and valuable goods that should be given priority, such as knowledge and friendship. Is the prize (property) of more value than the good of knowledge?

The second basis suggested by Becker is that of **political liberty**. The argument is that people are naturally going to try to acquire things and keep them for themselves, and any restriction on this sort of activity is a violation of their liberty. Therefore, property rights to protect the results of these activities are necessary to preserve individual liberty. It is basically a *noninterference rule*, not to interfere with what another is doing. Obviously (as Becker notes) this is too broad, because among the things that another person might be doing, many are immoral and/or illegal. If any limitations are to be put on the noninterference principle (and it is clear there must be), then presumably they will be something like this: Don't interfere with another's actions *as long as what the person is doing is moral*. Of course, the question then shifts to defining what is moral, and how we will meet this rule. Political liberty becomes one issue, but liberty to do *what* is seen as a more fundamental issue. So we must retreat, in the property case, to a more basic justification of property rights, such as Locke's or Hume's.

Arguments Against Private Property

It can be argued that most conflict in human societies arises over issues of possession. Machiavelli thought that it all came down to property and women (and he had in mind possession in both cases). If there were no private property, and no *possession* of spouse or children, these conflicts would not arise, and perhaps humans could get down to the more serious business of being creative, free, and happy. In Plato's *Republic*, the guardians of the ideal state were not allowed to have any private possessions, and women and men were to be held "in common." If the precepts were followed in such an "ideal state," the conflicts would dissolve, and justice (each doing his or her own business *for the good of all*) would reign.

Karl Marx also thought that the ideal communist state would be one in which all property was common. He advocated the abandonment of traditional marriages, because they had made wives and children into slaves. He argued (in the *Communist Manifesto, 1844 Manuscripts*, and elsewhere) that (bourgeoise) private property has been the source of alienated labor: human beings alienated from themselves and unable to fulfill the promise of their *species being*—creative work. In Marx's ideal society, one would indulge one's creative urges in any direction that beckoned. (Of course, everyone must do a share of the "drudge" work, but that share would be small, and machinery would help carry it out.) Work would be done not for the sake of possessions, but for the sake of fulfillment.

Can those of us living in the world's most materialistic society imagine a life such as the one characterized by Marx as satisfying? This requires us to take a hard look at what it is that we find valuable in possessions, and whether we would value them highly as long as everyone had enough of everything from the common store to be comfortable. The hard look should begin by asking, Are not friendship, knowledge, and the appreciation of beauty really more valuable than the acquisition of material things? I am reminded of a student who, when asked what was the great goal or aspiration of his life, said it was to own a really fancy, expensive car. Is that really all there is to human happiness?

In a later section, we will look at the ideas of several people who believe that all software should be free and be shared with everyone. Such a view fits into anti-private property views such as those in the *Republic* and in Marx.

Intellectual Property

So far, most of our discussion about private property rights has been about physical things, such as land, crops, and artifacts made by humans (such as tables, cars, computers). But there is another kind of property that people have: *intellectual property*—their ideas and the working of their minds. Perhaps the rules and the justifications with regard to physical property carry over easily into the intellectual domain; then again, perhaps it is not so simple. There certainly is a definite difference between an idea and a thing (such as a chair)—if someone takes away the thing, I no longer have it or the use of it; however, if someone shares my idea, I still have it.

Mental entities such as ideas are uniquely private; no one else can know what I am thinking unless I say it or write it. If I speak or write the idea, then it is in the mind of the hearer or reader, but it is still mine as well. Knowledge can be shared without the person who originally had it losing it. Aristotle, at the end of the *Nicomachean Ethics*, advocates the life of true happiness for a human being as the life of contemplation, understanding. All other contenders for happiness—wealth, beauty, power, honor—can be lost, or depend on others. No one can take away your understanding (at least while you live). Furthermore, the rational faculty is what is unique to human beings; true human happiness should be linked to what is unique in humans. A life of pleasure would be a good life for a pig as well; the fulfillment of the human potential in reason is what will be the best life for a human being. In addition, it is the most "godlike" life. A god would have no need of wealth or power, so a godlike life would be one of contemplation.

Augustine, in *The City of God*, says that true human happiness will come only in the vision of God. Clearly, this is not something to be hoarded, since, like knowledge, one person having it does not prevent others from attaining it.

Some people do very hard physical labor, or have various physical skills (as athletes do), and get paid for this. Others may not be as good at such physical endeavors, but they are very intelligent; they are good at using their minds to solve problems or to design things. They put just as much effort into their work as the physical laborer, and they also deserve reward. They produce *ideas*, instead of *things*. A manual laborer can make a chair, and then sell it, and earn a reward. Someone might copy the chair, but a lot of work must go into making the copy. If someone sells an idea, the idea is very easily copied and transmitted from one person to another. It is harder to protect an investment in intellectual effort.

The English Lord Upjohn said that "in general, information is not property at all; it is normally open to all who have eyes to read and ears to hear."[34] This is one position that can be taken, in which case we should not be worrying about the protection of software at all. The issue then becomes whether anyone would develop good software without the incentive of a monetary reward for doing so.

A careful examination of motives is in order here. The desire to inquire and to solve problems is not satisfied by money and fame, but the need to eat (to preserve the good of *health*) and eat well (for *pleasure*) requires some money. But how much money is enough? Money is not an end in itself, it is only a means. The drive to acquire a great deal of money (to what end?) often gets in the way of acquiring the real goods of human life.[35]

Software Protection

It has been recognized for hundreds of years that intellectual property requires protection, just as physical property (such as lands and goods) does. There are three usual ways at present that various kinds of intellectual property are protected under the law—trade secrets, copyrights, and patents. We will examine each of these categories, and see how none of them fits perfectly the unique characteristics of software.

Trade Secrets   Many companies owe their success to a marvelous idea that they have implemented and sold. A few examples would be recipes for a unique product, such as Coca-Cola, or Colonel Sanders' fried chicken, or Twinkies. The continued success of such products depends on having something the competition does not have, and so the recipe must be kept a *secret*. It is reported that the formula for Coca-Cola is kept in a vault to which access is closely guarded,[36] and other such recipes are carefully protected as well. The product is what is sold, and the way to make it is kept a secret.

Similarly, the design specifications for many products may be kept as trade secrets, in order to stay ahead of competitors. This is an effective method, barring successful espionage where the secret may be stolen, because one can sell the product to many satisfied consumers without having to reveal the formula or design. (Of course, packaged food products must display a list of their ingredients, in order of amount used, but, as any good cook knows, there is a great gap between a list of ingredients, especially without specific amounts, and a successful recipe.) But what happens if employees with knowledge of the secret leave such a company? Generally, an employee who will work closely with the company secret must sign a nondisclosure clause as part of the initial employment contract, promising not to reveal the secret. Even if the employee leaves the company to join another, the promise is binding not to reveal proprietary information, on penalty of serious legal action.

Trade secret laws vary from state to state and country to country, but generally they enforce strict penalties for violation of trade secrecy agreements. The problem with using trade secret laws to cover software is that the product (the program) *is* the idea itself. When someone buys the software package, what is purchased is a working copy of the program itself, on a disk, along with instructions on how to use it. The program on the disk may be in machine code (binary), but the idea of *what* it does and *how* at least some of it is accomplished is revealed in the program operation and documentation. Another problem lies in the fact that trade secret laws differ from one state to another, and in other countries they may be based on common law (set by custom and precedents). Thus a company that sells a product worldwide may have to deal with a whole array of different trade secret legal coverage in various locations. Whereas the product may be well protected in one country against trade secret violation, in another the law may not help.

A trade secret is not protected against "reverse engineering," which means that, for example, some sophisticated chemists might be able to, after analyzing samples, figure out the formula for Coca-Cola and thus market another cola with the same taste without ever having to steal the secret from the vault. In the software area, some sophisticated programmers might be able to work with a program enough to figure out what it does and how, without ever seeing the source code. They might even be able to "read" some of the binary code of the object program and work back to what instructions had been translated into that code.

Once a trade secret is "out," it is considered in the public domain and available to anyone. So even though the initial violator may be prosecuted, the secret is no longer a secret, and the company has lost any protection against others benefitting from its knowledge. Such protection would only be afforded by additional coverage—say, under patent.

When a software package is sold to a business to do a specific job for them, it is often necessary to make modifications in the package to suit the particular business. An example of this would be software marketed to colleges and universities to keep track of all their academic bookkeeping—student records, class schedules, course registrations, and the like. The company may sell this software to many colleges, but each installation probably has its own peculiarities that must be accommodated. In order to make the software viable, the company must make some of the original program code available to the college to allow for its appropriate modification. Once this is done, the secret is out of the bag. And yet the software could not be sold without this capability to change it as the need arises.

Steven Frank observes that trade secrecy might well be the best method of protection for many artificial intelligence (AI) programs, since such programs are generally produced for a single user or a small group of users, which would make it practical to issue licenses and identify any violators. "Perhaps most importantly," Frank adds, "the haphazard and largely uncertain scope of federal protection under the copyright and patent laws can leave AI researchers without any realistic alternative" (Frank, 1988, p. 73).

Trademarks   A trademark is just a name or logo used to uniquely identify a product; it has little or nothing to do with how the product is made. A trademark is defined as "any word, name, symbol, or device or any combination thereof adopted and used by a manufacturer or merchant to identify his goods . . . and distinguish them from those sold or manufactured by others."[37] So a trademark is obviously not a secret—far from it, it is spread abroad as much as possible to encourage sales of the product. What is protected by law is the *use* of this trademark to identify a product. Thus, if *Lotus 1-2-3* is the trademark of an integrated software package, other software packages may not use this name. A legal issue might arise if another company wanted to market similar software and call it *Lily 1-2-3*.

The trademark itself does not protect a product, or prevent others from marketing a similar or identical product; they just must not use the same trademark on it. Other kinds of protection (such as trade secrets or patents) must be used to keep the product itself protected. In choosing a trademark name, *generic* terms such as 'software' or 'computer' are not protected. A *descriptive* term, however, like 'spellchecker', may be too general to be protected against use by others. So *suggestive* or *arbitrary* terms are those most likely to receive trademark protection. A combination of generic and suggestive terms can be seen in the names of the Word and WordPerfect word-processing programs.[38]

Some software manufacturers may get some mileage out of another company's trademark by using it on their packaging to say that their product is *compatible with* the other product. They may do this as long as (1) they do not do it to disparage the other product, (2) the other trademark is not likely to become a part of the name of the new product, (3) the use of both marks on the product is not likely to cause confusion to the purchaser as to the source, and (4) the product manufacturer clearly identifies the other trademark as belonging to the other company in any advertising.[39] One can thus imagine some clever ways that developers of new software might use to get considerable mileage out of saying their product is compatible with some very famous brand.

Apple Corporation ended up paying $30 million to use the trademark name "Apple" on its products. The apple had already been used as a trademark by the Beatles, who had recorded their music on their own label, Apple Records. When Apple Computer Corporation was founded in 1976, the originators agreed that they would not use the "Apple" name in the music business. When the MacIntosh computers included a capability to play music, the Beatles sued Apple for violating the original agreement. Apple Computer settled by paying the Beatles roughly $30 million for the right to continue using the Apple trademark (Heckel, 1992, p. 134).

Copyrights Copyright and patent law in the United States arises from a provision in the Constitution (Article I, Section 8.8) which states that the Congress shall have the power "to promote the progress of science and the useful arts, by securing for limited times to authors and inventors the exclusive right to their respective writings and discoveries." We should keep in mind the basic intent of this provision as we go on: the purpose of these rights is to promote scientific progress, for the good of the nation as a whole. The underlying presumption in providing the authors and inventors limited rights is that they will be more inspired to come up with new ideas if they may benefit (financially) from them. In an ideal society, perhaps people would do such work for the joy of discovery and of helping others, and would share their knowledge freely; but in today's acquisitive society the incentive of reward may be necessary.

Thomas Jefferson had some insight into intellectual property and the importance of its dissemination:

> If nature has made any one thing less susceptible than all others of exclusive property, it is the action of the thinking power called an idea, which an individual may exclusively possess as long as he keeps it to himself; but the moment it is divulged, it forces itself into the possession of everyone, and the receiver cannot dispossess himself of it. . . . He who receives an idea from me, receives instruction himself without lessening mine; and he who lights a taper at mine, receives light without darkening me. That ideas should be spread from one to another over the globe, for the moral and mutual instruction of man and improvement of his condition, seems to have been peculiarly and benevolently designed by nature.[40]

Again, the idea is that everyone should benefit from knowledge.

A copyright protects the *form of expression* of a work, but not the idea behind it. Thus we have seen, in literature, many cases of works with much the same "plot" as older works, but where the words and perhaps the characters differ, and so they do not violate copyright coverage. (Consider, as just one example, the many reworkings of the ideas in Shakespeare's *Tempest*, including a 1956 science-fiction movie, *Forbidden Planet*, which introduced us to "Robbie the Robot.") Since a computer program is a string of symbols in a language, its form of expression could be covered by copyright.

The Software Copyright Act of 1980 explicitly extended copyright coverage to computer programs as "literary works." It also defined a computer program as "a set of statements or instructions to be used directly or indirectly in a computer in order to bring about a certain result" (17 U.S.C. Section 101). For some time, it was not clear whether only the higher-level language program (the *source code*) was coverable by copyright, but not the machine language, binary code (the *object code*), presumably since the latter was not "human-readable"—at least by *most* humans! But by 1983, the courts came to a ruling in two cases—*Williams Electronics, Inc. v. Artic International, Inc.* and *Apple Computer, Inc. v. Franklin Computer Corporation*—determining that object code embedded in ROM (read-only memory) is also suitable for copyright protection.

The Discussion published for the *Apple* decision cites the copyright statute itself, which indicates that copyright covers works in any tangible means of expression "*from which they can be perceived,* reproduced, or otherwise communicated, either directly or *with the aid of a machine or device*" (17 U.S.C. Sec. 102 (a), emphasis added). This only makes sense since, in effect, the object code is just a *translation* of the source code. If *Crime and Punishment*, originally written in Russian, is translated into English, and if the original version is covered by copyright, the translation should be covered by copyright as well. The Discussion also mentions that the defendant in *Williams* had argued that a copyrightable work "must be intelligible to human beings and must be intended as a medium of communication to human beings" (685.F.2D at 876-7). The decision, however, indicated that the words of the statute itself defeat this argument.[41]

The case of *Apple v. Franklin* also established that operating systems are copyrightable. This makes sense, since an operating system is also a program; if the object code of an applications program is copyrightable, that of an operating system should be so as well. Franklin had attempted to build "Apple-compatible" personal computers, such that software that had been developed to run on Apples would run on their ACE 100s too. Franklin admitted copying Apple's operating system (some of the code still contained the trademark name Apple), but claimed that it was necessary to have that operating system in order to ensure compatibility with software programs written for the Apple. Franklin's contention, then, was that Apple's operating system did not contain copyrightable material.

Franklin appealed to the Copyright Act, Section 102(b), which states explicitly that:

> In no case does copyright protection of an original work of authorship extend to any idea, procedure, process, system, method of operation, concept, principle, or discovery, regardless of the form in which it is described, explained, illustrated, or embodied in such work.[42]

Franklin tried to claim that an operating system is a "process," a "system," or a "method of operation," and thus does not fall in the class of what is copyrightable. Apple's claim was that it was not trying to copyright the *method* (which would be a more suitable entity for patent), but precisely the *mode of expression*, and that is what Franklin had blatantly copied. Franklin also hoped to win its case on the basis of the many unresolved aspects of copyright law as applied to computers.

Judge Sloviter granted the injunction, denied by a lower district court, preventing Franklin from using the programs at issue, and left the remainder of Franklin's challenges to be dealt with in the final resolution of the case. Franklin, however, settled out of court, so no final court decision was required. One speculates that the reason was that Franklin saw the "writing on the wall" (or on the computer terminal). The judge had determined that the language of the statute—that a computer program (which is coverable by copyright) is a set of instructions to be used in a computer to bring about a certain result—"makes no distinction between applications programs and operating programs."[43] One cannot help but suspect that the lower district court, whose ruling was reversed in this action, was influenced by sympathy for the small company going up against the giant Apple.

Just what does a copyright on a software program protect? It does not protect the *idea*, or the algorithm, on which the program is based, but only the *mode of expression*. Thus there can be many different programs that implement the same algorithm but will not be considered to infringe on one another. The question then arises, just *how different* must one program be from the next not to represent copyright infringement. Michael Gemignani (1985) points out that the plaintiff in a copyright suit must prove that the offender had copied the work (so it must be shown that said offender had *access*) and that the copying constituted an "improper appropriation."

In a time when programs are routinely transmitted electronically and so leave no "paper trail," and a person does not need to be physically in the vicinity of the original program, *access* may be very hard to show. Further, "improper appropriation" is rather vague; Gemignani says that the courts speak in terms of two programs having "striking similarities," but again this is vague. Just *how* similar must two programs be for the resemblance to be "striking"? One line in common? (Surely not.) Two lines? (Nah.) Just where does this "slippery slope" have its cutoff? Gemignani comments that "most courts do not possess significant technical background to determine whether striking similarities exist between seemingly dissimilar works" (1985, pp. 312–13). Expert witnesses can be called to testify on either side of such a case. Furthermore, programs may be written in different languages and may not look very similar at all to an untrained eye. A copyright does not protect the program (say, the object code) from being "reverse engineered" and the user figuring out how to do the same job with slightly different instructions, perhaps using a different language to write new source code.

The "striking similarities" condition may be disregarded in cases where there are only a few options as to how the idea or algorithm might have been implemented effectively. For example, if you have written a copyrighted program to do taxes, and I write one independently, I should not be penalized for the fact that my output fits the federal tax form, since for the program to be useful, I am constrained to that form of output. This is related to the "merger of expression and idea" consideration, which "holds that if an idea is inseparable from its expression, then only one or a few options exist for accomplishing a specific function" (National Research Council [NRC], 1991, p. 26). In such a case, the expression is not protected, since it would grant a monopoly on an idea.

The Software Copyright Act of 1980 states that a program may be protected as soon as it is "fixed in any tangible medium of expression." The problem of when a program becomes "fixed" is a difficult one. Programmers are always tinkering with their programs, trying to improve them or to remove unwanted "bugs." Which version is protected by copyright?

The problem of "fixation" of the form of the program is particularly vexing with respect to artificial intelligence programs that "learn" by experience. Some AI programs (such as some that play chess) are designed to modify their own programming based on real-world interactions. Programs using nonmonotonic logic can have a dynamic nature such that executions of the program in various contexts will result in a change in the basic program code. Programs that were sufficiently altered by such executions ("experience") might not be comparable enough to the original (copyrighted) program to be covered by that copyright (Frank, 1988, p. 66).

This raises some very interesting issues. There might well be two versions of the original program that were executed under different conditions (had "different experiences"), perhaps several executions each, that would end up not only being very different from the original program but also very different from each other as well. This not only raises problems as to whether the new program(s) in operation would be covered by copyright; it raises problems of responsibility for the action of the program, since it is no longer the same code written originally by the programmer, and there is no way the programmer could have predicted that this exact code would result. A program with learning capabilities is thus *unpredictable*, whereas the results of an algorithmic, nonlearning program are predictable, and always the same under the same conditions.

A copyright is relatively easy to get, and there is no demand for novelty. Only the "mode of expression" must be unique, even if it embodies a totally non-novel idea. The cost of a copyright is quite low (a small filing fee), so this form of protection is quite attractive to many authors. The period of protection of a copyright is the life of the author plus 50 years (or, in some cases, 75 years). The main problem with a copyright for software is that it provides *no* protection of the idea behind the program, and so someone can take the idea and write it in a different way and profit. A copy of the program must be filed for copyright (though this may be waived on request), which would preclude any secrecy as to its content. In some cases, a flowchart (which is much less revealing) may be filed instead.

Damages and attorneys' fees may be collected on proof of copyright infringement, and any illegal copies must be destroyed. But before this can occur, the plaintiff must prove access and "improper appropriation"; this may be difficult and expensive. As we saw in the LaMacchia case, access on the Net is easy and would be very difficult to prove; this is discussed further in Chapter 6.

Information on copyrights can be obtained from:

U.S. Copyright Office
Library of Congress
101 Independence Ave., S.E.
Washington, DC 20559-6000
Tel. (202) 707-3000
Website: www.loc.gov/copyright

Digital Millennium Copyright Act   A new law (Public Law 105-304) was signed into law on October 28, 1998, that attempts to clarify some of these issues. The text of the law can be found online, and excerpts have been published in Spinello and Tavani (2001, pp. 215–25). The law begins with this statement: "No person shall circumvent a technological measure that effectively controls access to a work protected under this title." Traffic in any technology designed to circumvent such measures is forbidden. This includes descrambling or uncrypting said work or avoiding or deactivating the protective measure. "Reverse engineering" is allowed under certain limited circumstances "to achieve interoperability . . . with other programs." It is yet to be seen, through the application of this addition to copyright law to many actual cases, how successful it is in protecting the intellectual property of the digital age.

Dmitry Sklyarov is the first real test case for the DMCA. He wrote a decrypting program that gets around the security for Adobe e-books. Adobe squawked, and Dmitry was thrown in jail. Members of the Electronic Frontier Foundation persuaded Adobe to see that he was released from jail, but the charge is still unresolved. This case could bring about a change in the law.[44]

Licensing and Copyprotection   For a time in the 1980s, software vendors attempted to protect their products from illegal copying by installing forms of "copy-protection" that would (presumably) prevent copying of the programs, and in some cases actually do damage to the computer system of the person attempting the illegal copy. A similar method was tried in the earlier days of videotaped movies. Both methods failed. First, the use of copyprotection spawned a new industry of devices to "beat" copyprotection, from actual boxes that were sold to "break" copyprotection on video tapes to software programs that claimed they would defeat any software copyprotection. Second, in the case of computer software, manufacturers soon found that the consumers were much less likely to buy products that were copyprotected. (Savvy users, in particular, who wanted to be sure of having a "backup" copy in case of disaster, found a condition preventing the making of such a backup was very unattractive.) The software manufacturers soon got the message, and grudgingly removed forms of copyprotection. However, the new Microsoft Windows XP release requires the user to "activate" it (online or over the phone) to gain full use of all its features, a process that lets Microsoft extract information about the user's computer, and makes it impossible to activate XP on another computer. (In other words, if you own two computers, you have to buy *two* copies of Windows XP.)

Obviously, we are dealing here with the issue of directly pirated exact copies of an original program, either by individuals, large corporations, or true pirates who will sell large quantities of the copy for profit. We are not talking about competing software from different companies where an infringement of one program by another is claimed. Yet copyright protection is also invoked by software manufacturers for the case of program pirates. The technique that has been adopted by the software manufacturers is to say that they own the program and the copyright rights to it, and that when someone purchases their software, all that has been bought is a license to *use* the software, under specifications set by the manufacturer. This usually includes the right to make only *one* archival copy, and limits the number of machines on which the software may be used.

The user generally does not find out about this licensing agreement until the software has been purchased and opened. The license agreement is in the box containing the software, a box that has been "shrink-wrapped." The user is required to sign and return the license agreement, on pain of having no support, remedy for a flawed product, or access to updates if the license is not signed. John Weld, a Washington, DC attorney with the Computer Law Center, wrote a very clever article in the September and November 1986 issues of *Monitor,* entitled "Would You Buy a Shrink Wrapped Automobile?" This article exposes clearly the enormity of what the software vendors are putting forward through these license agreements.

When you buy a software package (let us make up an imaginary package called Wordy), you have not really bought the program at all. Even though you have a copy of Wordy in your hand, on several computer disks, and extensive documentation on how to use it, you do not *own* the program. What you have purchased (according to the Wordy Corporation) is only the "right to use" this software. You may make "an" (i.e., one) "archival copy" of the program disks, but that is all. You may not rent or lease the software. You may use it only in the quantity (one) indicated on the agreement.

Initially, such agreements generally said that you could only use the software on the one machine for which it was purchased, which did not take into consideration your buying a new machine later, having one machine at work and one at home, and so on. Now such agreements often "generously" say that you *may* use the software on a home or portable computer *as long as the extra copy is never loaded at the same time as the copy on your primary computer*! So the program you thought you bought you have only leased, with rather severe restrictions on how you may use it.

Even if you do not sign and return the registration and license agreement, the software manufacturer considers you bound by the details of the agreement, and would try to enforce them if the issue arose. The reasonable question arises whether you can be legally (or morally) bound by an agreement that was not visible when you purchased the product, but is hidden in the shrink-wrapped package. Weld points out that the Second Restatement of Contracts says that users "are not bound to unknown terms which are beyond the range of reasonable expectation." Terms hidden inside a shrink-wrapped package that do not come to light until the purchase is made and the package opened are surely "unknown," and the stated limitations on your use are definitely beyond reasonable expectation.

Weld compares the shrink-wrap restrictions to your buying an automobile, then finding when you unwrap it that you do not own it but are only leasing it, that you are forbidden to let anyone else drive it, or to sell or lease it, and that you cannot use it as a trade-in or give it as a gift. You are also restricted as to where you can drive it. Furthermore, the car is sold "as is," with the manufacturer assuming no responsibility as to its continued performance or freedom from design faults. This clever analogy points up rather clearly that software license agreements are well beyond "reasonable expectation."[45]

The Software Publishers Association (SPA) has sponsored ads and billboards that picture a pair of handcuffs with the following caption: "This is the hardware you can get free if you copy software illegally." SPA and the Association of Data Processing Service Organizations (ADAPSO), now the Computer Software and Services Industry, are both associations of software manufacturers who want to discourage software copying to increase their profits. In practice, currently anyone who is caught making ten or more illegal copies of copyrighted software valued (in total) at $2500 or more, over a six-month period, is subject to criminal prosecution. The result of such prosecution could be (for a first-time offender) a jail term of up to five years and a significant fine. A lesser offense would be considered a misdemeanor, if the copying is for commercial advantage or personal gain, and punishable with up to a year in jail and a smaller fine.

The February 15, 1993, issue of *Research Recommendations*, published by the National Institute of Business Management, reports that the war on software piracy is spreading, and that in 1992 $3 million in fines were levied against U.S. firms found using unauthorized programs. According to this article, the SIIA and the Business Software Alliance (BSA) "urge workers to inform on employees who are breaking copyright law." This "tattletale" system seems to be working (as we saw in some of the piracy "busts" we discussed), but we must be wary of actions that are reminiscent of the informants encouraged in Nazi Germany.

Let's look again at your Wordy agreement. It might also say (as some other products do) that "you may not decompile, disassemble, reverse engineer, copy, create a derivative work, or otherwise use" the software except as the agreement allows. Of course, the Wordy people may write what they like, but one has to wonder on what basis they can legally forbid you to reverse engineer the product. From what we have seen, neither trade secrecy legislation nor copyright law provides protection from reverse engineering. How about patents? What happens if the manufacturer has obtained a patent on the program? Is there a statement that Wordy is operating under patent number such-and-such on the package or the license? We will examine the nature of patent protection for software next.

Anne Branscomb says that it is the principle of trade secrecy that underlies the "shrink-wrap" license (Branscomb, 1988, p. 40). But it is a very strange secret that a company sells in great quantity on the open market. In the case of Coca-Cola, the trade secret is the formula, but the product sold is the drink made according to the formula. In the case of a software package, it is the program itself that would be the trade secret *and* it is the program (compiled into ROM on disk) that is sold. Frank (1988), Browning (1986), and others have questioned the legal standing of such licenses on mass-produced software. Branscomb says that "to consider a computer program used by millions of people a trade secret offends common sense."

Patents Section 101 of the U.S. Patent Code (35 U.S.C.) states that "whoever invents or discovers any new and useful process, machine, manufacture, or composition of matter, or any new and useful improvement thereof, may obtain a patent therefore, subject to the conditions and requirements of this title." A patent, when granted, has a duration of 17 years. The cost of obtaining a patent can be high (Frank states that application fees and maintenance fees over the time covered by the patent can be more than $3000 at the time of his writing in 1988),[46] and the time it takes for one to be granted can be "interminable"; "two to five years can elapse between the filing of an application with the Patent and Trademark Office (PTO) and the date the patent is finally issued" (Frank 1988, p. 69). Since software generally has a rather short lifespan, it can easily become obsolete while waiting for patent protection.

There are five *substantive requirements* that must be met by an invention to qualify for a patent: (1) patentable subject matter, (2) novelty, (3) utility, (4) originality, and (5) nonobviousness (Patent Code, 35 U.S.C., Sections 101–103).

Patentable Subject Matter. The categories stated in the patent code, quoted at the beginning of this section, include "process," "machine," "manufacture," and "composition of matter." Susan H. Nycum explains: "These categorical labels are legal 'words of art'; that is, their meaning can only be understood by reference to the court decisions which have added or subtracted phenomena from these categories over the history of patent adjudication" (1978, p. 5). Some rules have been developed to cover which phenomena will be included or excluded; one of these is that "mental processes" are not included. Another rule is that a patentable process "act upon or change materials to a different state or thing" (Nycum, 1978, p. 5).

Novelty. It must be shown that the invention has not been anticipated by "prior art." The Patent Office requires a thorough search of all prior patents in the area to determine that the proposed invention does not infringe on any of these cases of "prior art." This can be a very time-consuming process. Once this has been canvassed, a strong case must be made as to how the invention proposed for patent coverage differs significantly from this prior art. Note that no such prior art search is required for the issuing of a copyright.

Utility. This requirement stipulates that the invention have a practical, useful application. This ties in with the rule that the process, machine, or other composition must alter something in the physical world. This points out that certainly some things (such as some works of literature) that would be the object of copyright would not be suitable for patent. An idea itself is not patentable; the Supreme Court decided this in 1863 (Nycum, 1978, p. 21). What can be granted a patent is some process or device that will be *useful* to humankind. This ties in with the Constitutional intent of promoting the useful arts.

Originality. According to Nycum (1978, p. 6), this requirement merely means that the patent applicant must be the inventor. She says that this condition has not been of importance in the software patent context. It would seem that much of what one might think of as coming under *originality* is covered under the *novelty* condition.

Nonobviousness. Section 103 of the Patent Code states that a patent may not be obtained "if the differences between the subject matter sought to be patented and the prior art are such that the subject matter as a whole would have been obvious at the time the invention was made to a person having ordinary skill in the art to which the said subject matter pertains." This is a difficult criterion to apply, but Nycum points out that there is a complex legal history behind the proper use in this context of the words 'obvious', 'ordinary skill', etc. Ultimately, the application of this criterion is "a subjective decision based on the overall impressions of a judge" (Nycum, 1978, p. 5).

Thus an invention may be novel but also obvious, and so not qualify for a patent. The novelty may just be due to the fact that no one thought the product was worth designing before, though the way of doing it would have been obvious.

A patent grants the recipient the right to exclude others from making, selling, or using the invention during the period of the patent. It gives the inventor essentially a *limited* monopoly for that period. The right for the inventor to exploit the monopoly by making and selling the product is covered by other legal constraints, particularly antitrust laws (Nycum, 1978, p. 7). In addition to the five substantial requirements listed, certain kinds of processes are explicitly excluded from patent coverage.

The "Mental Steps" Doctrine. "Mental processes" and "abstract intellectual concepts" have been deemed unpatentable by the courts. One cannot obtain a patent on a mathematical formula or a "law of nature." In *Gottschalk v. Benson* (409 U.S. 63 [1972]), the Supreme Court denied a patent to a computer program whose purpose was to solve a mathematical problem—in this case, to convert binary coded decimal numbers into binary. The Court ruled that the process was an algorithm, and thus not amenable to patent. To grant a patent would have given Benson a monopoly on a general mathematical technique and all of its applications. The Court would not allow anyone to *own* the basic tools for scientific research.

In *Parker v. Flook* (1978), the patent was sought for a catalytic conversion process in which a computer program was used to calculate an "alarm limit" signal to indicate the need to stop or change the process. The Court decided that the basis of the process was the mathematical calculation of a *number,* the alarm limit, and so was not a proper subject matter for patent.[47]

Nycum reports that early "mental steps" cases deemed unpatentable any process claiming steps that could be performed mentally, at least "established that '[a] method is not *per se* unpatentable because its practice requires that the operator must think' (*ex parte Bond*, 135 U.S.P.Q. 160, 162 [Pat. Off. Bd. App. 1961]), an observation perhaps too obvious to mention" (Nycum, 1978, p. 20).

Ownership of Mathematical or Scientific Laws. To allow one person to *own* a thought or idea would then mean, if carried to its logical conclusion, that no one else would be allowed to think it. A patent excludes the selling and *use* of the entity patented. This could then put a restriction on freedom of thought, a basic right of human beings, recognized in the U.S. Bill of Rights, particularly in Amendments I and IX. For someone to *own* a mathematical formula or a law of nature would mean that no one else could make use of the formula or law. Newton did not have a monopoly on Newton's Laws of Motion (nor did he apparently desire to); for him to have had such ownership would have greatly impeded scientific advance.

Private ownership of such general mathematical ideas or scientific laws would not only be grossly unjust, but it certainly would not contribute to the overall progress of the arts and sciences (which is the whole intent of Article I, Section 8.8, of the Constitution, on which protection of intellectual property in the form of "writings and discoveries" is based).

Some questioned whether mathematics should be considered non-patentable just because there has been "no immediate correlation between the discovery of a mathematical relationship and the implementation of that relationship in the physical, tangible world of machines."[48] The writer here wants coverage for *all* processes, mental or physical, and so is challenging the designation of mental processes as not "statutory" (i.e., meeting the substantive requirement of patentable subject matter). The key word here is 'discovery'. If mathematical truths and scientific laws are facts independent of human thought, but discoverable by human thought, then they cannot be owned by an individual.

Regular relationships in nature that obey certain natural laws (such as the law of gravity) are clearly external to us and exist independent of whether we notice them. Nature *is* as it is, and our thought does not change that. We may learn to operate within the natural regularities to make some changes in the natural world (such as building bridges, or blasting away mountains), but we do not change natural laws. Anyone may discover these relationships, and no one can own them.

The status of mathematical objects and relationships is a bit more controversial, but a large majority of mathematicians are Platonists, which means that they believe that mathematical truths are expressions of the eternal relations among eternal mathematical entities, and that these relationships can be discovered by humans but not changed by them. A second, less common, view of the nature of mathematics is that of Kant and various schools following from his thought. Kant argues that we, as human beings, structure the data of experience in certain ways due to our nature; the laws of mathematics are simply the ways in which this structuring occurs. If this is the case, one person still cannot be said to own a mathematical theorem, because any human being has the potential to recognize the way in which our thought is structured.

John Stuart Mill said that mathematics is just a matter of induction, that we have become conditioned by our experience to believe in certain mathematical relations because they have held up over time. This does not mean that these relations exist necessarily; they might change tomorrow. But mathematics represents our current set of beliefs in this area. If this were the case (setting aside the basic difficulties with this position for our discussion here), one person still could not be said to uniquely own a mathematical belief. What you believe or do not believe should place no restrictions on what I may believe. My beliefs, as much as anything, are my own property, and just because you come to have a particular belief *earlier* than I do does not prohibit my coming to believe the same thing, and to act on that belief (for example, by applying it in my work).

The Formalist view is that mathematics is just a system of games for manipulating symbols (marks on paper, etc.). The Formalist position makes no claim that this set of games has any correspondence to physical reality, and so it should be of little interest to the hungry patent-seeker, who wants to profit from an idea for a process or device that will alter the world (even if only slightly). As for ownership of mathematics on this view, it would seem that any of us can always make up a new game. As for the existing games, the appropriate analogy would seem to be that no one owns the game of chess, and that we may all play chess and even construct our own boards and carve our own playing pieces, without infringing on anyone else's property rights.

Ludwig Wittgenstein had a view of mathematics as a set of games and rules that we have found to be useful—no more, no less. He believed that this position avoided any difficulties attendant on talking about eternal mathematical objects, necessary truths, and the like. According to his view, could someone be said to *own* a useful rule? Couldn't someone else make up a game that happened to have the same or similar rules? Think about the world of games you are familiar with, and the fact that there is no proprietary ownership of these games. Anyone can play basketball if there are a few players, a ball, and a hoop; no one is restricted from using the game for pleasure. If our useful mathematical games also bring us innocent pleasure, who has the right to stop us?

We have seen that *no* account of the nature of mathematics could be used as the basis for a coherent argument in favor of the private ownership of mathematical principles.

Diamond v. Diehr Sets a Precedent   In the early 1960s, the Patent Office specifically excluded computer programs from patent because of their relation to ideas. In 1965, the President's Commission on the Patent System was established to look into the issue further, and recommended that computer programs be considered unpatentable. In 1968, the Patent Office stated that "computer programs . . . shall not be patentable," although the Court of Customs and Patent Appeals rejected this the next year (Gemignani, 1981, p. 317). Until 1981, the Patent Office continued to reject computer programs as patentable and the Court of Customs and Patent Appeals continued to question many of the PTO's rulings.

In 1981, the case of *Diamond, Commissioner of Patents and Trademarks v. Diehr et al.* was brought before the Supreme Court. In 1975 Diehr had requested a patent on a process for curing synthetic rubber. The unique contribution claimed for the process was the ability to constantly measure the temperature inside of a rubber curing mold and then feed the data to a computer that calculated the appropriate curing time using the Arrhenius equation; the computer would then prompt the opening of the mold when the calculated time had elapsed. The Commissioner of PTO rejected the patent application on the grounds that the steps in the process carried out by a computer program were nonstatutory. The Commissioner's view was that the patent was being sought on the computer program, which was not an appropriate subject matter for patent.

The Court of Customs and Patent Appeals reversed the PTO's decision, and the case went to the Supreme Court for review. The Court decided 5-4 in favor of the patent for Diehr. Judge Rehnquist delivered the holding of the Court:

(1) although by itself a mathematical formula is not subject to patent protection, when a claim containing such formula implements or applies it in a structure or process which considered as a whole is performing a function designed to be protected by the patent laws the claim constitutes patentable subject matter; (2) subject process constituted patentable subject matter notwithstanding that in several of its steps it included the use of a mathematical formula and a programmed digital computer, as process involved transformation of uncured synthetic rubber into a different state or thing and solved an industry problem of "undercure" and "overcure"; and (3) [the] fact that one or more steps might not be novel or independently eligible for patent protection was irrelevant to [the] issue of whether the claims as a whole recited subject matter eligible for patent protection. (*Diamond v. Diehr*, in Johnson and Snapper, p. 326)

In the details of the opinion, Rehnquist admitted the similarity of this case to *Benson* and *Flook*, in that all involved computer programs and mathematical formulas. But the distinctive difference in *Diehr* was said to be that the *process*—that of curing rubber—was appropriate for patent, and "a subject matter otherwise statutory does not become nonstatutory simply because it uses a mathematical formula, computer program, or digital computer" (*Diamond v. Diehr*, in Johnson and Snapper, p. 330). Judge Rehnquist appealed to Justice Stone's explanation in 1939, which stated "When a scientific truth, or the mathematical expression of it, is not a patentable invention, a novel and useful structure created with the aid of scientific knowledge may be" (*Mackay Radio & Telegraph v. Radio of America*, 360 U.S. 86, 94, 59; S. Ct. 427, 431, 83 L. Ed. 506 [1939]).

The dissenting opinion argued that the Diehr case was not significantly different from *Benson* or *Flook*, both of which had been rejected on the grounds that they requested patents on mathematical formulas. It was argued that the inventive claim in the process was the use of the computer program to calculate the curing time, since no evidence was provided that the method of measuring the temperature in the mold or controlling the mold heater or opening the mold are novel. Thus if the mathematical formula part of the method is considered a part of prior art, as it should be, there remains nothing in the application justifying patentable invention (*Diamond v. Diehr*, in Johnson and Snapper, pp. 336-38).

Yet the decision of the Court stands, and it has prompted a flood of patent applications involving computer programs since 1981. Our careful look at the decisions and rationales in this arena has been carried out in the hope that it will provide a clear-eyed basis for intelligent future decision making.

Patents to Protect Intellectual Property   The courts have to work all of this out, but it is obvious from the cases and decisions we have looked at that the lines are not clearly drawn as to what may be patented and what may not. An idea *per se* is said not to be patentable, but the *use* of a novel idea in a physical process is. This seems to be a very fine and difficult distinction to draw. We have already discussed the justifiable reasons why no one should be able to own an idea, under the section on copyrights. If one is to be allowed 17 years' control over the implementation of an idea in a process (or machine), then it must be made very clear what the limits of that control should be. For example, Samuel Morse, in seeking a patent for the telegraph, wanted the patent to cover *all* types of communication using electromagnetic transmission. In 1863, the Supreme Court (*O'Reilly v. Morse*, 56 U.S. 62) denied approval of this broad patent coverage on the grounds that "permitting a single individual to obtain control over an entire phenomenon of nature would constrict, rather than promote, the progress of science" (Frank, 1988, p. 70). Clearly a patent right should not be so broad as to exclude other useful development in an area.

A computer program itself was not considered patentable but, as *Diamond v. Diehr* shows, a process utilizing a computer program *might* be patentable. Since the appropriate subject of a patent may be a process or a *machine*, then presumably a computer (which is a machine) which embodies a computer program that has a novel effect in the physical world may be patentable as well.

What of the increasingly sophisticated expert systems that are being developed through artificial intelligence (AI) research? (These will be discussed in more detail in Chapter 12.) The aim of an expert system is to replace a human decision maker in doing a humanlike intellectual task (such as diagnosing a disease or finding oil deposits). Yet the "mental steps" prohibition in current patent litigation should exclude such programs from gaining patents. If they are excluded, then what sort of coverage, that is fair to its creator, would be appropriate for the AI program?

The current position is that a mathematical formula may not be the subject of a patent. Yet a computer program in binary form can be considered as a number, a (long) string of 1s and 0s that defines the program in memory. Surely if mathematical formulas are not patentable, numbers should not be either. It seems that none of the current legislation fits computer software well, and perhaps the old laws should not be bent and reinterpreted to fit the new phenomenon. Perhaps new legislation unique to computer software is required to do it justice.

There is a heated disagreement in the computer world about the appropriateness of patent coverage for computer programs. Paul Heckel, responding to an article in the *Communications of the ACM* (January 1992) by the League for Programming Freedom titled "Against Software Patents," wrote "Debunking the Software Patent Myths" in the June 1992 issue of the same journal. In this article, Heckel, himself a holder of a software patent, says that "most patent lawyers conversant with software are virtually unanimous that it should be patentable" (Heckel, 1992, p. 125). This is not surprising, given all the business that patent suits on software will bring them!

Heckel cites D. Chisum who said that the *Benson* decision "is not supported by the authorities on which it relied, that the court misunderstood the nature of the subject matter before it, and that the court failed to offer any viable policy justification for excluding by judicial fiat mathematical algorithms from the patent system" (Heckel, 1992, p. 130). Heckel discusses nine patents covered in the League article to show that they were unfairly criticized. He says that "To discard the patent system because some bad patents exist would be the same as suppressing free speech to stamp out lies" (p. 131). The analogy is very poor here. Free speech is a fundamental right, not an arbitrarily constructed set of rules that may have flaws.

Heckel makes a number of recommendations to strengthen the patent system of coverage for software, urging that this will further strengthen a competitive marketplace.[49] Pamela Samuelson, a lawyer specializing in intellectual property law, responded to Heckel's article in the October 1992 *CACM*. She begins by objecting to Heckel's innuendo that anyone who objects to software patents does so out of jealousy, and his claiming that only a "knee-jerk intuitivist" ignorant of intellectual property law or a Marxist would question patenting software. She points out that Chisum's concerns over *Benson* are misunderstood by Heckel, and that Chisum is arguing that unless the *Benson* decision is overturned by the Supreme Court or Congress, "the legal basis for patenting algorithms and many other software innovations is shaky" (Samuelson, 1992, p. 16).

Samuelson showed in an article in the *Emory Law Journal* 39 (1990), "Benson Revisited," that the Court's decisions in this area up to that time were consistent with existing law. She argues that the established laws for copyrights and patents have been designed to cover different subjects. Copyrights are applicable to writings and patents to machines (or processes). "Never have copyright and patent rights been applied to the same innovation. Nor should they be because it would distort the economic effects that these two different laws are intended to bring about" (Samuelson, 1992, p. 16).

Yet we have seen a shift in software manufacturers from seeking copyrights to asking for patents. The problem is "that software is both a writing and a machine at the same time," and so far there is "no consensus even within the legal community about the boundaries of patent or copyright law as applied to software" (Samuelson, 1992, p. 16). She suggests that perhaps new *sui generis* legislation is needed for software, since, although patent law has caused the manufacturing industry to flourish, there is no guarantee that it will be appropriate for the information industry. She reminds Heckel and her readers that if Congress does consider new or revised legislation regarding software, its primary purpose should *not* be to secure the rights of innovators, but to promote progress in the software area, for the general good of the population.

It is of considerable interest to note that in June 1995 the U.S. Patent and Trademark Office gave the official "green light" for software patents and, apparently, the agency was preparing to hire computer science majors.[50] We will discuss the opposition to software patents, by experts such as Stallman and Garfinkle, in an upcoming section.

Since knowledge is a fundamental higher good, it should be maximized as much as possible. The general good of the society would be best served by increased knowledge and progress in the "useful arts and sciences," as Samuelson points out. Thus future legislation should attempt to enhance such progress; whether this is best done by protecting the property rights of innovators or by disseminating information is a *practical* problem.

Information on patents and trademarks may be obtained from the following:

General Information Services Division
U. S. Patents and Trademark Office
Crystal Plaza 3, Room 2C02
Washington, DC 20231
Tel. (703) 308-HELP or 1-800-PTO-9199
Website: www.uspto.gov

Look-and-Feel Legislation In 1986, the Third Circuit Court of Appeals decided in favor of the plaintiff in *Whelan Associates v. Jaslow Dental Laboratory*, a case that was to have considerable impact on the software industry.

Elaine Whelan had written a dental office management program for Rand Jaslow; Jaslow paid the development costs and kept the program for his use, but Whelan was allowed to retain rights to the program. Finding the program a useful idea, Jaslow decided to create a new version of a similar program that would run on IBM PCs. Jaslow wrote his version in BASIC, whereas Whelan had written hers in EDL (a now-defunct Event Driven Language) for an IBM mainframe, and he apparently did not copy from her code. However, Jaslow had helped design the user interface (the screen displays and command structure for the user), and both programs came out looking quite similar. Whelan sued Jaslow for copyright infringement.

The Circuit Court decided in favor of Whelan, not on the basis of copied or "significantly similar" code, but because the appearance (the "total concept-and-feel") of the two programs was strikingly similar. Samuelson suggests that there was a certain naiveté on the part of the judge, who assumed that because the two user interfaces were so similar, the programs running them must be similar in structure (Samuelson, 1989, p. 567). Thus the case was decided on certain "nonliteral" features of the program, similar function, and inferred similarities in structure, sequence, and organization. The decision was appealed to the Supreme Court, but the appeal was denied the next year.

There are similar cases that painted a background for this decision. One was a suit by one greeting-card company against another in 1970, which was decided in favor of the plaintiff because the cards in question "conveyed the same mood and character" (Rosch, 1987, p. 293). The first significant computer case involving the "total concept-and-feel" was a suit brought by Atari in 1982 against a company whose K. C. Munchkin game was said to infringe the copyright for Atari's PAC-MAN. "Although the layout of the mazes, the number of gobbled-up dots on the screen, their arrangement, and the sounds and colors used by the two games were different, the court found that Atari's copyright had been infringed on" (Rosch, 1987, p. 293).

However, in an earlier case in 1979, *Synercom Technology, Inc. v. University Computing Co.*, Synercom had developed, for use by engineers, a structural analysis program with a particular way of entering the data to be analyzed; a defendant had designed a similar analysis program that used the same data input format as Synercom's program. However, in this case the court decided that there was no infringement; the defense lawyers convinced the court that granting the claim would be like allowing the first automobile manufacturer that used the H-pattern shift in its car to have exclusive rights to that pattern (Samuelson, 1989, p. 566). What is seen here is the beginning of a defense of certain program similarities on behalf of **standardization**. Imagine if each standard-shift car model had a different gear pattern! Surely accidents would have increased, and driver education would have been most difficult.

In *Broderbund Software, Inc. v. Unison World, Inc.*, a case that arose a few months after the circuit court decision in *Whelan*, design choices such as similar screen displays and the choice of commands were the basis of the infringement suit, which was awarded to the plaintiff (Samuelson, 1989, pp. 567–68). In the *Whelan* case, the suit had been brought claiming copying of the program *structure*, and the judge had decided that this was evidenced by the similarity of the interfaces. In *Broderbund*, the judge, "relying on the Whelan case, . . . said that the menu screens displayed by the programs were protectable by copyright" (Samuelson, 1989, p. 568). The decision emphasized the fact that there were many different displays available that could have been used as evidence of infringement, and talked a lot about the aesthetics of the displays. Thus this case was decided on the basis of the overall way the two programs look and feel to the user when they are executed.

In 1987, in *Digital Communications Associates, Inc. v. Softklone Distributing Corp.*, the plaintiff won the infringement suit based on similarities in the main menu screens of the two programs. The judge decided the case on the basis that the two programs had similar commands *and* that for the shortened forms of the commands both programs capitalized and highlighted the first two letters of the command (Samuelson, 1989, p. 568). Thus if Softklone (perhaps an unfortunate choice of name for a company that is facing a copying charge) had used the same command word (let us suppose the command is "Send") and then allowed the capitalized first two letters, "SE," to invoke the command, the judge held them liable for this and other similarities. First of all, there is not a wide variety of choices of meaningful and obvious commands in this instance, and "send" is the most effective. Furthermore, "the judge seemed to think that the capitalization of the first two letters was simply a stylistic expression of the author" (Samuelson, 1989, p. 568). The judge's position implied that "EN" or "ND" would have been just as effective a short command as "SE." But anyone who has spent much time using a computer program would recognize that the abbreviated "SE" is the *only* sensible choice.

This group of decisions set the stage for two much larger-scale copyright infringement suits. In the first, on January 12, 1987, Lotus Development Corporation brought suit against Paperback Software (for their *VP-Planner*) and Mosaic Software (for their *Twin*—again, perhaps an unfortunate name choice) for infringing on their *Lotus 1-2-3* program. *Twin* had advertised a "work-alike" spreadsheet, and *VP-Planner* had advertised that it is a "feature-by-feature work alike for 1-2-3" and "designed to work like Lotus . . .

keystroke for keystroke" (Branscomb, 1988, p. 38). These companies, perhaps unaware of the current court actions, had blatantly advertised publicly that they had copied the "look-and-feel" of *Lotus 1-2-3*.

From a teacher's point of view, it would be desirable to have standardization in the software industry. One could then teach students how to use a particular word-processing program, or spreadsheet, or database, and be confident that they could readily carry that knowledge to other software programs that do the same jobs. But if copyright infringement claims as to "look-and-feel" are successful, it will make the whole software enterprise very chaotic. Of course, this may well be what the giant companies want— "you'd better teach your students Lotus, and have them buy Lotus." But people (students and employees) often do not have a choice over the software they are provided. Standardization is of great value in the software industry, and there is an overseeing group—the American National Standards Institute (ANSI)—that sees to it that there is a basic standard set of instructions and operations in any programming language.

This "look-and-feel" legislation will harm much of the software industry, and turn the large, powerful companies into monopolies (we have certainly seen the trend with Microsoft). Until recently, as Winn L. Rosch puts it, we were operating under the "freedom-to-clone" policy. In hardware, a whole industry grew up in IBM personal computer clones. Until the court decisions we discussed, manufacturers and their lawyers had the understanding that one should not copy code, but anything else was fair game. "If you could duplicate the operation of a program without copying the underlying code, you could clone anything you wanted" (Rosch, 1987, p. 289). It is competition that drives innovators to *improve* their products. If competition is stifled by one company having a monopoly on a certain kind of software program, there will be no incentive for them to improve it. "Buy us! We're the only game in town."

On June 28, 1990, a federal court judge in Boston handed down a decision in favor of Lotus against Paperback Software; they were deemed liable for copyright infringement because they copied the whole menu setup of *Lotus 1-2-3*, which the judge decided was a protectable "expression" of the *Lotus* program (Samuelson, 1990, p. 29). Terms used in the wording of the decision referred to Lotus' "creativity," "organization," and "insight." Does this decision have a narrow impact of saying that you can't directly copy another program's interface, or a much broader impact (Samuelson, 1990)? After all, if the "organization" and "insight" of a program are protected under copyright, any program just trying to accomplish a similar job may be vulnerable.

Lotus was not "squeaky clean" itself. Lotus had built its *1-2-3* program on the ideas of the earlier *VisiCalc*. Three months after Lotus brought suit against Paperback and Mosaic, the company that created VisiCalc sued Lotus for copyright infringement.

On a larger scale, Apple Corporation sued Microsoft and Hewlett-Packard, claiming that their "windowing" software is a violation of Apple's copyrighted software on the Macintosh. (It should be noted that Apple was accused of copying the idea of icons and using a mouse from Xerox Corporation.) The judge's opinion in this case stated that the arrangement of the principal elements of the Macintosh interface "serves a functional purpose in the same way as the visual displays and user commands of the dashboard, steering wheel, gear shift, brakes, clutch and accelerator serve as the user interface of an automobile. Purely functional items or an arrangement of them for functional purposes is wholly beyond the realm of copyright" (law library, p. 1006, Vol. 799 of the Federal Supplement books). This seems a sensible conclusion, but it is not at all clear why the Lotus user interface should not also have been considered functional.

Again the automobile is being used as an analogy (as in the case where the H-pattern of the gear shift was mentioned); yet that is a physical device, and the software is for the manipulation of information that might be considered nonphysical. Is the difficulty here that courts are trying to fit existing law, Procrustean-bed style, to a new category that the original law never anticipated? It is difficult to see how the Lotus look-and-feel can have been judged to be violated and the Macintosh not to have been. Such blatant inconsistency simply points to the inadequacy of current law to cover software.

What is the main ethical issue here? It seems to be to determine what will be in the overall good for society. Software is *useful*; it helps people working on difficult problems—from an individual doing a tax return to a scientist trying to estimate the impact of certain changes on the environment. Certain innovations in software, such as the use of "windows," make the programs run more effectively. Such general improvements *do* seem analogous to innovations in the auto industry that generally made driving more safe, and so should not be kept as the exclusive domain of one manufacturer. Allowing the broader use of such innovations will improve software in general, and thus foster *progress*, which is of benefit to all. A true "free enterprise" system would not put artificial restrictions on what developers could do. Adam Smith's idea of **unrestricted competition** was that the *best* products will win out, and everyone will benefit.

In February 1994, a federal jury in Los Angeles found that Microsoft's MS-DOS 6.0 software infringed on a patent for data compression held by Stac Electronics. Stac was awarded $120 million in damages from Microsoft.[51] Thus around and around we go, and it seems that in the end just about everyone will get penalized for copying something from someone else.

Samuelson points out that "look and feel" is a phrase coined by two lawyers who wrote an article in 1985 about the possibility of user interfaces being covered by copyright. The phrase has no legal meaning, at least so far, but it is clear that this is the major criterion on which these last cases have been decided. Samuelson argues that these considerations are more about the *functional* nature of programs than about their expression, and so they are pushing software protection closer to patents than to copyrights. She blames these problems, of not having the right category for software protection, on a Congress that put software (a technology) under copyright coverage, when copyright precedent had no experience with technologies (Samuelson, 1989, p. 569).

It would be nice if there were some logical basis for the software protection decisions, but it seems that they are often being made under inapplicable laws by courts that have little knowledge about what they are dealing with. The direction of the "look and feel" decisions has serious implications regarding intellectual property and progress.

The Opposition to Legal Protection of Software

Richard Stallman used to work for the MIT Artificial Intelligence Laboratory, and was referred to by some as the "last true hacker"—intended as a term of praise in this case, referring to a very imaginative, inquisitive programmer. He left MIT in the early 1980s, apparently because he felt that they restricted his freedom to create and share his ideas. Stallman believes that all software should be free and available to anyone, and has tried to make his belief into reality by writing and making available valuable software for general use. In "The GNU Manifesto," Stallman describes GNU (which stands for GNU's Not Unix), a Unix-compatible software system he has written to "give it away free to everyone who can use it" (Stallman, p. 308). (Unix is a sophisticated operating system developed by Bell Labs, a research subsidiary of AT&T.)

Stallman describes why he "must write GNU":

> I consider that the golden rule requires that if I like a program I must share it with other people who like it. Software sellers want to divide the users and conquer them, making each user agree not to share with others. I refuse to break solidarity with other users in this way. I cannot in good conscience sign a nondisclosure agreement or a software license agreement. . . So that I can continue to use computers without dishonor, I have decided to put together a sufficient body of free software so that I will be able to get along without any software that is not free. I have resigned from the AI lab to deny MIT any legal excuse to prevent me from giving GNU away. (Stallman, 1987, p. 309)

Stallman then proceeds to describe how users can get this free software (and documentation). They may change it in any way they like, as long as any improvements are also made available as *freeware* like GNU. Stallman continues to look for contributions of money, hardware, and programmer time to advance his project. He argues that good system software should be free "like air" and that making it so will avoid wasteful duplication of programming effort that "can go instead into advancing the state of the art" (Stallman, 1987, p. 311).

In the GNU Manifesto, Stallman argues for a Kantian ethics view, saying that extracting money from users is destructive because it limits the ways the program can be used, and this "reduces the amount of wealth that humanity derives from the program." (A few get wealthy instead of the "wealth" of knowledge being shared by all.) He continues, "since I do not like the consequences that result if everyone hoards information, I am required to consider that it is wrong for me to do so." (Kant would talk in terms of the rule to hoard not being universalizable; Locke would also disapprove of hoarding.)

Stallman and his associates founded the Free Software Foundation in 1985.[52] The Foundation proceeded to boycott Apple for its suit against Microsoft and Hewlett-Packard, claiming that it was an attempt to keep people from writing programs that are even remotely like those on Macintosh computers, and creativity was being stifled. The Foundation recommended that people considering buying Macintosh computers should wait for a Mac-clone, so they "don't feed the lawyers!"

A copy of Stallman's "Free Software Sing" can be found at

www.gnu. org/music/free-software-song.html

It begins "Join us now and share the software / You'll be free, hackers, you'll be free," and goes on to compare the hackers (favorably) with the (presumably evil) hoarders.

In a 1994 article in the *Communications of the ACM*, Richard Stallman and Simson Garfinkle spoke out "against software patents" (1994, p. 17). They began by observing that the Patent Office had refused to hire computer scientists as examiners,[53] and that it did not offer competitive salaries. Without someone trained in the area, how can the PTO judge whether software that comes before them is novel or nonobvious? They describe several software patents that write a cursor on a screen and erase it, scroll multiple subwindows, or do a recalculation in a spreadsheet, and point out that these common techniques are now off limits because of their patents. "Nothing protects a programmer from accidentally using a technique that is patented, and then being sued for it" (Stallman and Garfinkle,

1994, p. 18). MIT had used a technique on its LISP machines but did not apply for coverage since it seemed obvious. AT&T subsequently applied for a patent on the same technique, and so MIT may be forbidden to use a method they had initiated and had distributed free. The authors remark that "obvious patents are like land mines" (p. 20); one could trip over one at any time and be harmed.

By January 1992, the Patent Office had granted more than 2,000 software patents. If this keeps up, the software giants like Apple, Microsoft, and IBM will have patent control of many software techniques and be able to force others to pay a high price to use them in their programs. Note that IBM acquired Lotus in 1995 in a $3.3 billion takeover.[54] The Refac Technical Development Corporation (New York) owns the "natural order recalc" patent, and demands 5 percent of the sales of all major spreadsheet programs (Stallman and Garfinkle, 1994, p. 21).[55]

One can imagine a crazy scenario in which you wrote a program that used techniques from more than 20 such patents (not because you have no new ideas, but because certain techniques are essential to effective programs). If each patent-holder demanded 5 percent (or more) of your sales, you would be paying all of your "profits" out to such patent-holders and still going into debt. It would not pay to be a small innovative programmer, and the big companies would control all of the software. In *The Producers*—Mel Brooks' first screen feature, now transformed into a hit Broadway musical—the producers sell investors interest in well over 100 percent of a show. The only way they can make a profit (keep back some of the investments) is for the play to be a flop. This is not a promising analogy for the software industry.

Susan Nycum, writing in 1978, long before any of these more recent decisions, and even before *Diamond v. Diehr* extended patents to software, referred to the following imagined specter raised in a brief for the *Benson* case: "Patent protection in the United States might induce the transmission of data abroad for processing in countries without such protection" (Nycum, 1978, p. 63). This is not beyond the realm of possibility. One can also imagine talented programmers emigrating to countries where their creativity would not be so stifled by patents.

What *Is* Reasonable and Fair?

Clearly it is immoral to steal something that does not belong to you. And just as clearly it seems that espionage with regard to secret hardware or software and large-scale piracy for profit are certainly not questionable issues. Stealing someone else's ideas to create a competitive product would be wrong, but the matter gets less clear when the ideas may be based in mathe-matical truths that anyone might come to discover. We have seen through-out this chapter that the distinctions between what can be owned and what should be free to everyone in intellectual property are very murky, especially in the software arena. Clarification is needed of words like 'own' and phrases like 'belongs to you' before we can come up with general ethical principles to apply here.

A just system of protecting copyrighted material allows for what is called "fair use." Several factors are taken into account in determining fair use: the purpose of the use (use for purposes of scholarship, comment and criticism, teaching, and news reporting are allowed); the type of work under copyright (is it out of print? is it published or unpublished? is the material used strictly factual material, and so presumably accessible to all?); what proportion of the work is used; and whether the use will negatively affect the market value of the original work.

There are certainly many cases in scholarly work where the ideas of an earlier work form the basis of a new one that generally criticizes and tries to improve on the earlier work, or might be only a commentary on it. The work may be quoted in part (with credit always given), and the world benefits from the new discussion. If software is to be covered by copyright, then per-haps some clear guidelines should be drawn for "fair use" of software in new programs, that will allow improvement to occur. After all, the byword from the Constitution is 'progress'.

If software is to be protected by copyright, does that justify the software license agreement restrictions put on users? Generally, copyrights are given on books, pieces of music, and other "literary works." If I buy a book, it is mine to do with what I like, except that I may not make copies of the whole book or substantial segments of it to sell or give away. If I were to do this, it would cut into the author's right to profit from honest effort and talent. As a matter of fact, not a large part of the profits from a book go back to the author; most of them revert to the publishing company. But in any case, it is the author and the publishing company who have put in the time and money to make the book available, and they are the only ones who have a legiti-mate right to profit from it.

I have other rights with regard to any book I buy, which apparently the software manufacturers do not want me to have with regard to any software I buy: I may lend my book to a friend, or give it away, and I can even sell my own copy if I like. I can use it (read it) wherever I please. I have title to the book, in the way I have title to a car I buy (not a shrink-wrapped one!), and it is part of my property—it will be part of my estate when I die, and be passed on to my beneficiaries. This raises an issue that I have not seen discussed in the software literature—if the software license is (according to the manufacturer) issued to me and me alone, no one else is supposed to use it, and I am not to transfer it to anyone else, what happens to the right to use the software when I die? Does my death signal the expiration of my temporary license? All of this seems a bit bizarre, and if it is, perhaps the rules should be changed.

In her insightful article, "Who Owns Creativity?" Anne Branscomb points out that any "realistic legal rules depend on a social consensus about what kind of behavior is acceptable and what is not." She points out that "some degree of unauthorized copying has become accepted social practice" (Branscomb, 1988, p. 40); this occurs with journal articles, pieces of music (think of a number of Charles Ives' compositions), and other originals, quite often. In addition, there is the practice of "fair use" copying, as long as it is not too extensive. I would not want to say that the law (or morality) is merely social consensus, and I do not really think Branscomb is suggesting that. Laws and morality should (as we have discussed) have a basis in fundamental principles. But she is pointing out that laws should also be *enforceable* and *realistic. Is* it realistic to have a law that says that a person may not make a copy of a software program or a videotape for a friend when the law is effectively not enforced on the small scale? It would certainly do a great deal toward solving the job shortage problem if the authorities had to employ enough personnel to effectively enforce noncopying legislation against the average person in this country!

Another problem that ties into the small-scale copying of software is the exorbitant cost of some software. A scan of the Amazon.com website recently revealed the following "low" prices for popular software: Lotus 1-2-3 Millennium Edition, $319.99; Microsoft Excel X for Mac, $349.99; Microsoft Excel 2002, $289.99; Lotus 1-2-3 5.0, $324.99; FileMaker Pro 5.5, $249.99; Microsoft Access 2002, $289.99; QuickBooks Pro 2001, $249.99; Adobe Acrobat 5.0, $249.99; WordPerfect Office 2002, $359.99; MS Word for Mac, $379.99; MS Word 2002, $289.99; Report Writer, $549.99. It should be noted that most of these programs do not involve more than four to six computer disks, which have a raw value *as disks* of under $5; occasionally there is extensive documentation as well.

Initially, software manufacturers justified the high cost of their software by the programmer-years of research and development (R&D) that had gone into it; they wanted to recoup their investment and make a profit. At the outset, they have no way of knowing how many copies of a program will sell; so the higher they can set the price (short of ridiculously high), the sooner the investment will pay off. Today, large companies with fabulously successful software packages that have been selling for years justify keeping their prices high because of the high rate of piracy. Not all copies of their software (probably less than 30 percent) in use are ones for which they received payment. Thus they are in effect charging the legitimate buyer for the pirated copies.

Does software need to be so expensive? If a company estimates that they have lost $200 million in potential revenues to piracy, and have made only $75 million, are they in financial difficulty? They are also assuming that all of the pirated copies in use would have been purchased if somehow the piracy could be prevented; this is not necessarily the case at all. If inexpensive pirated versions of a "high-priced spread" spreadsheet program were not available, these potential customers might well not pay the big bucks for it, but would probably look for more reasonably priced spreadsheets, or to freeware, public domain software, and the like.

Richard Stallman and the Free Software Foundation advocate that good software should be free to everyone to use, modify, and improve; it would then be their moral duty to put their improved versions of existing programs and their innovative new programs into the public pool. Stallman wanted this software to be *freeware*, rather than *public domain software*, so that everyone could be allowed to modify and redistribute the freeware, with no restrictions. There is a great deal of public domain software, some of it good, but a distributor can place restrictions on its modification and redistribution, thus inhibiting what Stallman hopes for in a totally free exchange of ideas.[56]

Another concept is that of *shareware*, in which software is made available, and if users find it helpful they can send some money to the program creator in thanks. It seems to be a sort of "honor system" that is becoming popular, but the quality of the software and support may not be as high as one would hope. Linux is an operating system available as shareware that could come to challenge Microsoft.

The 1992 Code of Ethics issued by the Association for Computing Machinery (ACM), the main professional group in the field, states (Clause 1.5) that it is a "moral imperative" to "honor property rights including copyrights and patents." But a July 1993 *Communications of the ACM* "Forum" article points out that the "scope and meaning of copyrights in software is uncertain and controversial; most members [of ACM] disapprove of having patents in software at all." This article was signed by some of the most respected people in the computer field, including Guy L. Steele Jr., Danny Hillis, Richard Stallman, Gerald J. Sussman, Marvin Minsky, John McCarthy, John Backus, and Fernando Corbato.

There is certainly a critical need for the computer community and the legal community to come to some logical and fair consensus regarding how software innovation should be treated. As it is, we have the two extremes: at one end, those who say that all software should be free and freely shared, and, at the other end, the large software manufacturers who want every protection—to treat their software as trade secret (with the software license agreements), and as copyrighted material, and as falling under patent protection (as the situation calls for). There is also a continuum of positions in between, all of which are tolerated under the current conditions. We also have apparently inconsistent court rulings about the protectability of entities like user interfaces. It is time to straighten things out.

We need to clarify concepts of ownership, especially in relation to intellectual property. We need to examine just how viable Locke's argument for personal property is, particularly whether it extends to mental as well as physical labor. To say that someone *owns* an idea would seem to infringe on the freedom of thought of others. We also need to take a close look at utilitarian considerations; many have claimed that if there is no reward, software production will degenerate, but this might not be so. The consequences for all just might be better with no proprietary software. The future consequences are always difficult to judge, but we still must try.

We must make a clear distinction between means and ends. Profit (money) is not a good in itself, it is only a means. Thus we should look closely at the higher-level goods that should be our ends, and then ask which means best accomplish them. If our goal is a society in which human happiness in general can flourish, how can this best be accomplished? What role should software play in this, as a means, and what will contribute most to fruitful progress in the development of software and its significant contribution to society?

The National Research Council's report on *Intellectual Property Issues in Software* includes a set of general goals for the intellectual property system, developed by Robert Spinrad of Xerox Corporation. He refers to these as the "Five Cs":

- **Coverage** (or protection) of the "brilliant idea" in a software product, and the "hard work" that went into it.
- **Continuity**, "the ability to build on existing standards and conventions at reasonable cost" (so the emphasis, he says, should be on *access* and not *appropriation*, so programs can build on existing standards, and not be forced to use different interfaces, etc., which would be detrimental to the user).

- **Consistency** in the scope and application of intellectual property protections, so there are no "surprises," and companies can make reasonable marketing and development decisions.
- **Cognizance,** "the timely awareness of other intellectual property rights claims," which involves improvement of the current means of dissemination of information about what is under copyright, protected by patent (or "in the pipeline") in a particular area that would restrict other work in that area.
- **Convenience,** a "straightforward system" that "minimizes the need for litigation" (National Research Council, 1991, p. 85).

Though these goals may be very difficult, if not impossible, to achieve at the same time, they certainly make clear the major concerns. As we have seen, some proposals satisfy some but not all of the goals. One of the most difficult to achieve may be that of *convenience* (which Spinrad fears may be "asking for the moon"), but freeware would accomplish that and essentially all of the other conditions *except* coverage. We should ask whether we might replace "coverage" (implying protection of some imagined right) with "recognition" (though it spoils the 5-Cs pattern). Is profit (due to "coverage") the highest goal, or might appreciation of the value of one's work by others be more satisfying? This recognition is closer to the fundamental goods of friendship and knowledge (in the best sense, when it is shared without loss to anyone).

NEW ISSUES RAISED BY THE INTERNET

The rapid expansion of the Internet has complicated difficult issues even more. To begin with, *plagiarism* is much easier than it ever was before, since so much material is available on the Net, and it is sinfully easy to download it intact right into one's paper. (One doesn't even have to retype it!) Furthermore, a number of services are available online where students can buy a paper on just about any subject (a striking change from the past, when the student in search of a paper had to find and make a deal with the expatriate student living in "collegetown" and making spare change writing papers for others). There was a recent plagiarism scandal at the University of Virginia, a school dedicated to the "honor system." Plagiarism was discovered in a number of papers, and degrees that had been awarded were actually withdrawn. One thing the student who does plagiarize large sections of a paper from sources online should know is that it is also extremely easy for a professor to type in a phrase from a suspect paper and quickly get back the source reference from a search engine such as Google.

Another problem arises with hypertext, the capability in a web-based text to highlight certain words or names such that, if the user clicks on a highlighted entry, a **link** is made to the actual source. This can be very helpful to the user, and it makes research much easier and more rapid. However, those who create the links generally do not ask permission of the owner of the web page to which the link is made. The general assumption seems to be that if anything is put up on a web page for all to see, it is also fair game to link to it. Certainly the potential for linking to sections of text out of context always exists, no matter what the form. One could, for example, claim in the home web site that Socrates believed that "might is right" and link to a section of the *Republic*, Book I, where that is said, without noting that it is in the mouth of Thrasymachus, a sophist, whose views Socrates decisively defeats. However, a bad writer could also do this in print (though it is not very likely such a work would get published, whereas on the Net, anyone can "publish" anything there).

The real problem seems to arise with *deep linking*, which involves linking directly to a segment of a web page without going through the home page, on which there may be proprietary information, advertising, and the like. For example, in 1997, Ticketmaster brought a lawsuit against Microsoft for trademark infringement and unfair competitive practices (see Spinello, "An Ethical Evaluation," 2001; Wagner, 1997). Microsoft linked to a subpage of the Ticketmaster site, bypassing their home page with related advertising and a special promotion for using MasterCard; Ticketmaster claimed "foul!" and the loss of revenues. The case was settled out of court, but Microsoft did modify its link to go through Ticketmaster's home page.

One more problem worth mentioning is that there is absolutely no editorial scrutiny and little or no censorship on the Internet. This has the virtue of encouraging open communication, which is presumably a good. The problem is that, in an era of such tremendous information explosion, it is good to have some way of sorting out the good from the "junk" and the downright subversive. If someone looks up information on some topic such as abortion, many reputable sites will be listed along with some that merely express personal opinion without any justification and others that advocate the murder of doctors who perform abortions, along with their names and addresses. Internet users need a way to sort through mountains of information and misinformation to find the truth, which can be difficult. The advantage of printed matter is that, at least in most cases, what is published must first undergo the scrutiny of those who are knowledgeable in a field.

Those using the Internet as a reference source should thus think about the old Roman adage "Let the buyer beware!" Today the new caution should be adapted to "Let the reader beware!"

■ ENDNOTES

1. The first crisis in mathematics arose when one of the Pythagoreans discovered that even within their own geometry there was something that was demonstrably not representable as a rational number—that is, as an integer or the ratio of two integers. In a simple right-angled triangle of unit sides, the length of the hypotenuse—the square root of 2, according to the Pythagorean theorem—can be shown not to be a rational number. It is said that the Pythagoreans threw the discoverer of this awful truth into the ocean. This may be only symbolic, since the Ocean in Greek thought of the time was taken to be representative of Chaos, and this member of their group had destroyed the order they thought they had discovered for the world and thrown them back into chaos.

2. For Leibniz, a **contingent truth** (true only in a particular world) would have a representative, *infinite*, nonrepeating fraction (a *surd* or *irrational* value, like pi or the square root of two) and be completely knowable only by God, whereas a **necessary truth** (one true in all possible worlds) would have a *finite* or a *rational* representation, and thus be knowable by human beings.

3. You can try this algorithm on any two positive integers—say, 26 and 15, 69 and 24, or 19 and 5 (it works on primes, too; the GCD of any two primes will turn out to be 1). This algorithm can easily be written as a computer program in a high-level language, and it is often a functional part of a much larger program to do some interesting job.

4. Thucydides, *The Peloponnesian War*, Book One, Introduction, trans. Rex Warner (Harmondsworth, England: Penguin, 1979), 5, pp. 37–38.

5. Tom Forester and Perry Morrison, *Computer Ethics: Cautionary Tales* (Cambridge, MA: MIT Press, 1994), p. 54.

6. Patrick G. Marshall, "Software Piracy: Can the Government Help Stop the Drain on Profits?" *CQ Researcher* 3, no. 19 (May 21, 1993), 443–48.

7. "Microsoft Corp.: Raid at Westinghouse Unit Yields Unauthorized Copies," *Wall Street Journal*, 7 May 1991, sec. B, p. 4.

8. "Antipiracy Tactics: 'Computer Cheats Take Cadsoft's Bait'," *Software Engineering Notes* 18, no. 2 (April 1993), 14.

9. Jon Swartz, "Software Scam in Bay Area/Piracy Case Called Biggest in Region," *San Francisco Chronicle*, 12 April 1996, p. B1.

10. Dwight Silverman, "Microsoft charges Piracy in Suit Against Premium," *Houston Chronicle*, 9 July 1996, p. 1.

11. "South Bay/Arrest of Suspect in Software Piracy Case," *San Francisco Chronicle*, 18 September 1996, p. A16.

12. Julia King, "Philadelphia Fined in Software Piracy Case," *Computerworld*, 7 July 1997, p. 3.

13. *Times Education Supplement*, 3 August 2001, p. 10.

14. Philip Shenon, "Internet Piracy Is Suspected as U.S. Agents Raid Campuses," *New York Times*, 12 December 2001; and "U.S. Expands Investigation into Piracy of Software," *New York Times*, 19 December 2001, p. 5.

15. Edward Iwata, "Increase in Software Piracy Could Blight Financial Future," *USA Today*, 1 August 2001, p. B01.

16. William Brandel, "Licensing Stymies Users," *Computerworld* 28, no. 16 (April 28, 1994), 1, 12. See also Iwata (2001), previous note.

17. David P. Hamilton and Jacob M. Schlesinger, "Microsoft Targets Software Piracy by Japan PC Users," *Wall Street Journal*, 4 March 1993, sec. A, p. 10; "World Wire: Software Piracy in China," *Wall Street Journal*, 14 October 1993, sec. A, p. 13. See also "Coalition to Combat Software Piracy," *Info World* (December 7, 1987), 5. For newest statistics, see Iwata (2001), footnote 15.

18. Forester and Morrison, 1994, pp. 69–70.

19. "Bangkok Buccaneers," *Client Server News*, 19 November 2001.

20. William H. Gates III, "Protection from Pirates," *Washington Post*, 18 October 1993, p. 19.

21. Suzanne P. Weisband and Seymour E. Goodman, "Subduing Software Pirates," *Technology Review* (October 1993), 32–33.

22. G. Pascal Zachary, "Technology: Software Firms Keep Eye on Bulletin Boards," *Wall Street Journal*, 11 November 1991, sec. B, p. 1.

23. Jeff Hecht, "Internet 'Pirate' Charged in US," *New Scientist* 142, no. 1922 (April 23, 1994), 7.

24. EPIC (Electronic Privacy Distribution Center) Alert (January 18, 1995), sec. 5. See also David L. Wilson, "Ruling on Software Piracy Prompts Debate," *Chronicle of Higher Education* 41, no. 18 (January 13, 1995), A20.

Two more convictions in similar cases raise questions as to just where the line should be drawn. Microsoft and Novell received a court settlement that a New Jersey teenager operating the Deadbeat Bulletin Board that distributed free copies of their copyrighted software should pay them $25,000 ("New Jersey Teenager Agrees to Pay $25,000 to Microsoft, Novell," *Wall Street Journal*, 6 February 1995, p. B4). Richard D. Kenadek, the operator of the Davey Jones Locker bulletin board, was sentenced to six months home confinement and two years probation for selling copyrighted software ("Bulletin-board Owner Sentenced for Selling Illegal Software Copies," *Wall Street Journal*, 13 March 1995, p. B6).

25. Perhaps LaMacchia should be sentenced to a virtual reality multiuser dungeon, where he imagines that he is serving a sentence in jail. See Tom Dworetzky, "Crime and Punishment: Raskolnikov Does MUD Time," *Omni* 16, no. 11 (August 1994), 16.

26. Jonathan A. Friedman and Francis M. Buono, "Limiting Tort Liability for Online Third-party Content under Section 230 of the Communications Act," *Federal Communications Law Journal*, 52, 3 (May 2000), 647–65.

27. Forester and Morrison, 1994, p. 55.

28. Mary Jo Foley, "A Small Software Firm Takes on Uncle Sam—and Wins," *Datamation* (April 15, 1988), 26.

29. Henry J. Reske, "12 Inslaw Sponsors," *ABA Journal* 80 (November 1994), 22. The article adds that a Justice Department report in September indicated that its own investigation showed "no credible evidence that its employees stole the software," adding that no more payments should be made, and that the case should be closed.

30. Anthony Kimery, "The Inslaw Octopus Lives On," *Wired* 3, no. 4 (April 1994), 76. The Attorney General Janet Reno led the attack.

31. For much greater detail on this interesting case, see Richard L. Fricker's "The INSLAW Octopus," Wired Ventures, Ltd., 1993/4 (info@wired.com). My thanks to Bob Gonsalves ("pinknoiz") for making this article available for my reference.

32. David Farber, "Bin Laden/Hanssen: Excerpt of Fox News Special Report," 17 October 2001 (www.interesting-people.org/archives/interesting-people/200110/msg00237.html).

33. Locke argues that each person's natural right is to "life, liberty, and property." It is Locke's work on which the thought in the American Declaration of Independence is based, which states that it is a self-evident truth

that all humans are created equal and have "certain unalienable Rights, that among these are Life, Liberty, and the Pursuit of Happiness." Locke would probably agree with the rephrasing, only pointing out that property (on his view) is necessary to the pursuit of happiness.

However, it is not self-evident that property *is* essential to happiness, as Plato and Marx, among others, pointed out. It is important to maintain life and health, and to have time to pursue higher goods such as friendship and knowledge. The means to such ends do not necessarily involve property (except, of course, the property in and freedom of one's own mind and body).

34. *Boardman v. Phipps* (1967) 2 AC 46, 127; quoted in Martin Wasik, *Crime and the Computer* (Oxford, England: Clarendon Press, 1991).

35. In 1832, Alexis de Tocqueville wrote the following about rich American businessmen: "most of those who now enjoy leisure were absorbed in business during their youth; the consequence of which is, that, when they might have had a taste for study, they had no time for it, and when the time is at their disposal, they have no longer the inclination" (*Democracy in America*, ed. Richard D. Heffner [New York: Mentor/NAL, 1956], p. 53).

36. Stanley M. Lieberstein, *Who Owns What Is in Your Head?* (New York: Hawthorn Books, Inc., 1979), p. 124.

37. Sec. 45 (U.S.C. 1127) of the Trademark Statute.

38. Saul Lefkowitz and E. Robert Yoches, "The Role of Trademarks in the Protection of Computer Software," *Communications of the ACM* 32, no. 12 (December 1989), 1392.

39. Lefkowitz and Yoches, p. 1391.

40. Thomas Jefferson, *Writings of Thomas Jefferson*, Vol. 6, ed. H. A. Washington (1854), pp. 180–81.

41. *Apple Computer, Inc. v. Franklin Computer Corporation*, in *Ethical Issues in the Use of Computers*, eds. Deborah G. Johnson and John W. Snapper (Belmont, CA: Wadsworth, 1985), p. 345.

42. *Apple v. Franklin*, in Johnson and Snapper (1985), p. 347.

43. *Apple v. Franklin*, in Johnson and Snapper (1985), p. 348.

44. Scott Harris, "Digital Martyr," *The Industry Standard* 4, 31 (August 20, 2001), 68.

45. David Browning presents an interesting way to challenge the shrink-wrap licenses in an article called "Warranties and Vendor Relations" in the June 1986 issue of *Monitor*. In the article, Browning drafts a letter to a software vendor in which he returns the license agreement, unsigned, along with specific objections to aspects of the license agreement (such as its statement that the licensee may only use the software on a single computer, that he is responsible for taking precautions against any unauthorized copying of the program, and the hidden condition that execution of the software constitutes acceptance of the agreement, which he refers to as deceptive business practice).

46. A basic filing for a utility patent is $370, and for a design patent (for an article of manufacture) is $165; if the patent is granted, another fee is required before the patent is issued. These fees are for "small entities" and fees are double for corporations. Furthermore, "maintenance fees" are required at specified intervals during the life of the patent (**www.uspto.gov**).

47. *Diamond, Commissioner of Patents and Trademarks v. Diehr et al.* 450 U.S. 1048–1073 (in Johnson and Snapper eds., *Ethical Issues in the Uses of Computers* (Belmont, CA: Wadsworth, 1985), pp. 329 and 336–37).

48. Popper, *Current Status of Patent Protection for Programmable Processes,* 7 Pat. L. Ann. 37, 42–3 (1969). Quoted in Nycum, p. 22.

49. Heckel urged those who "want to correct the misinformation about software" to join or contact ALPHA (the Abraham Lincoln Patent Holders Association), 146 Main Street, Suite 404, Los Altos, CA 94022 (an association he founded).

50. Robert P. Bill, "Viewpoint," *Computerworld,* 26 June 1995, p. 37.

51. *Software Engineering Notes* 19, 3 (July 1994), 8.

52. See also Stallman's article, "Why Software Should Be Free," in Johnson and Nissenbaum, pp. 190–200.

53. Note that the statement by the Office of Patents and Trademarks that they *will* hire computer scientists shows a change in this policy. One has to wonder whether criticisms such as those of Stallman and Garfinkle prompted this change. If so, there is hope that other rational criticisms may have an effect.

54. Michael Fitzgerald, "Lotus on the Block," *Computerworld* 12 June 1995, p. 1.

55. Stallman and Garfinkle urge others concerned about the violations of intellectual freedom that are threatened by the current legal cases to contact the League for Programming Freedom, 1 Kendall Square # 143, P.O. Box 9171, Cambridge, MA 02139 (e-mail: league@prep.ai.mit.edu).

56. See also Deborah Johnson's essay, "Should Computer Programs Be Owned?", in Bynum, ed., *Computers and Ethics* (Oxford, England: Blackwell, 1985), pp. 276–88.

■ SHORT ESSAY QUESTIONS

1. Carefully analyze and compare the copyright coverage on a literary work (for which the copyright system was intended) and that expected on a software program. What latitude with respect to a literary work is allowed under copyright that software developers may want restricted for their products? Is the difference sufficient to conclude that copyrights are an inappropriate method of coverage for software?

2. Try to briefly but clearly explain the software licensing system to someone not familiar with it. Does it have any parallels with any other products that one buys? Can you (or can the manufacturers) justify this as a *fair* practice?

3. Pamela Samuelson (1992) argues that patent and copyright coverage has never been granted to the same "invention," and that it is appropriate that they should not be. Yet software comes very close to breaking this precedent, since some software has been copyrighted and other software has been patented (though no one software item has obtained both coverages). However, it is quite conceivable that someone will soon ask for both, to cover all their bases. Outline Samuelson's position on this and assess its validity.

4. If the purpose of patents is primarily to encourage development in an area, and they have caused manufacturing to flourish, why might they *not* have the same sort of effect on the "information industry," as Samuelson suggests?

5. If a computer program is a number (it can be represented as a long string of 0s and 1s), and numbers (like mathematics) cannot be the subject of patent coverage, discuss whether all of the software patents that have been granted thus far should be rescinded.

■ LONG ESSAY QUESTIONS

1. Elaborate on the various moral considerations (utilitarian, justice, role-switching, and any others you feel are relevant) to the question of the midscale software piracy discussed in this chapter. Base this essay on your appreciation of various ethical positions developed in Part One of this book.

2. Examine carefully David Hume's distinctions regarding the acquisition and right to property in the *Treatise*, Book III, Part II, Sections iii-iv,

making the distinctions clear and then applying them to current issues in software property rights.

3. If you work for a large corporation, and in your spare time you invent something, or write a winner software package, your employer may well try to claim the rights to your creation (this happened to the man who invented Gatorade). Does this seem right? Apply some of the discussions from this chapter on the right to private property to this case. What do you conclude?

4. Try to develop utilitarian arguments both *for* and *against* the legal protection of software. If you can find strong arguments on both sides, where does this leave you? Does it point out some weaknesses in utilitarianism? If Kantian and virtue ethics both lead to support for no-ownership of software, what does that suggest to you? What does the position on maximizing higher-level goods suggest on this issue?

5. Philosopher Sir David Ross, in *The Right and The Good* (Oxford, England: Clarendon Press, 1930), bothered by Kant's strict requirement to universalize any moral duty, suggested that there are a number of *prima facie* duties, duties that seem obvious. The duties he lists are: (1) of **fidelity** (to keep promises and tell the truth); (2) of **reparation** (to "make good" any harm we have done); (3) of **gratitude** (to return favors); (4) of **justice** (*distributive* justice); (5) of **beneficence** (to improve the conditions of others); (6) of **self-improvement** (with respect to virtue and knowledge); (7) of **nonmaleficence** (to avoid harming others). Now perhaps one Kantian (like Stallman of the Free Software Foundation) might will that everyone should contribute software to society, and another "Kantian" (like Bill Gates of Microsoft) might consistently will that everyone should be rewarded for their software and have their rights to their rewards protected. This suggests a weakness in the Kantian approach. Is Ross' view any better? How many of his *prima facie* duties are relevant to the issue of software protection? What does one do if the duties conflict? (This is a problem for Ross' view.)

■ REFERENCES AND RECOMMENDED READINGS

Anthes, Gary H. "Piracy on the Rise; Companies Fear Liability." *Computerworld* 28, 16 (April 28, 1994), 12.

"Apple Computer, Inc. v. Franklin Computer Corporation." U.S. Court of Appeals, Third Circuit, No. 82-1582. In Deborah G. Johnson and John W.

Snapper, eds., *Ethical Issues in the Use of Computers* (Belmont, CA: Wadsworth, 1985), pp. 339–52.

Becker, Lawrence C. *Property Rights: Philosophic Foundations.* London: Routledge & Kegan Paul, l977.

Brandel, William. "Licensing Stymies Users." *Computerworld* 28, 16 (April 28, 1994), 12.

Branscomb, Anne W. *Who Owns Information? From Privacy to Public Access.* New York: Basic Books, 1994.

Branscomb, Anne W. "Who Owns Creativity?" *Technology Review* (May-June 1988), 38–45.

Chapuis, Alfred, and Edmond Droz. *Automata: A Historical and Technical Study.* Trans. Alec Reid. Neuchatel, France: Editions du Griffon, 1958.

Cohen, Julie E., Mark A. Lemley. "Patent Scope and Innovation in the Software Industry." *California Law Review* 89, 1 (January 2001), 1–58.

Cohen, Morris Raphael. "Property and Sovereignty." In Johnson and Snapper, 298–304. From *Cornell Law Quarterly* 13 (1927).

Diamond, Commissioner of Patents and Trademarks v. Diehr et al. 450 U.S. 1048–1073. In Johnson and Snapper, pp. 326–39.

Einstein, David. "Additional XP Copy Needed for Each PC." *San Francisco Chronicle*, 11 October 2001, p. D10.

Fisher, Lawrence M. "Xerox Sues Apple Computer Over Macintosh Copyright." *New York Times*, 15 December 1989, sec. D, p. 1.

Foley, Mary Jo. "A Small Software Firm Takes on Uncle Sam—and Wins." *Datamation* (April 15, 1988), 26.

Forester, Tom, and Perry Morrison. *Computer Ethics: Cautionary Tales and Ethical Dilemmas in Computing.* 2nd ed. Cambridge, MA: MIT Press, 1994, ch. 3.

Frank, Steven J. "What AI Practitioners Should Know About the Law (Part One)." *AI Magazine* 9, 1 (Spring 1988), 63–75.

Friedman, Jonathan A., and Francis M. Buono. "Limiting Tort Liability for Online Third-party Content under Section 230 of the Communications Act." *Federal Communications Law Journal*, May 2000, pp. 647–65.

Gemignani, Michael C. "Legal Protection for Computer Software: The View from '79." In Johnson and Snapper, pp. 305–25.

Gould, Carol C., ed. *The Information Web: Ethical and Social Implications of Computer Networking.* Boulder, CO: Westview Press, 1989, ch. 6.

Graham, Robert L. "The Legal Protection of Computer Software." *Communications of the ACM* 27, 5 (May 1984), 422–26.

Grant, Daniel. "Computer Copycats Blur Rights: Electronic Manipulation of Images Has Made Copyright Infringement Hard To Combat." *Computer Science Monitor* (October 3, 1991), 12.

Guzman, Rafer. "AOL Case Will Test ISP Liability." *Wall Street Journal*, 18 August 1999, p. F1.

Gwynne, Peter. "Stalking Asian Software Pirates." *Technology Review* 95, 2 (February–March 1992), 15–16.

Harris, Ron. "Technology Leaders Oppose Copyright Law Exemptions." *St. Louis Post-Dispatch*, 20 May 2000, p. 9.

Harris, Scott. "Digital Martyr: Digital Millennium Copyright Act Ensnares Dmitry Sklyarov." *The Industry Standard* 4, 31 (August 20, 2001), 68.

Heckel, Paul. "Debunking the Software Patent Myths." *Communications of the ACM* 35, 6 (June 1992), 121–140.

Hollander, Patricia A. *Computers in Education: Legal Liabilities and Ethical Issues Concerning their Use and Misuse.* Asheville, NC: College Administration Publications, 1986.

Honore, A. M. "Ownership." In A. G. Guest, ed., *Oxford Essays in Jurisprudence.* Oxford, England: Clarendon Press, 1961, 107–47.

Hume, David. *A Treatise of Human Nature* (Book III, Part II, iii). Ed. L. A. Selby-Bigge. Oxford, England: Clarendon Press, 1960 [1888].

Jakes, J. Michael, and E. Robert Yoches. "Basic Principles of Patent Protection for Computer Software." *Communications of the ACM* 32, 8 (August 1989), 922–24.

Johnson, Deborah G. *Computer Ethics.* 2nd ed. Englewood Cliffs, NJ: Prentice-Hall, 1994, ch. 4. Or see ch. 6 in 3rd ed. (2001).

Johnson, Deborah G., and Helen Nissenbaum, eds. *Computers, Ethics, and Social Values.* Englewood Cliffs, NJ: Prentice-Hall, 1995, ch. 3.

Johnson, Deborah G. "Should Computer Programs Be Owned?" *Metaphilosophy* 16, 4 (October 1985), 276–88.

Kneale, William and Martha. *The Development of Logic.* Oxford, England: Clarendon Press, 1962.

Lawrence, John. "Intellectual Property Futures: The Paper Club and the Digital Commons." In Charles Ess, ed., *Philosophical Perspectives on Computer-Mediated Communication.* Albany, NY: SUNY Press, 1996, 95–114.

Lefkowitz, Saul, and E. Robert Yoches. "The Role of Trademarks in the Protection of Computer Software." *Communications of the ACM* 32, 12 (December 1989), 1391–96.

Lieberstein, Stanley H. *Who Owns What Is in Your Head? Trade Secrets and the Mobile Employee.* New York: Hawthorn Books, 1979.

Locke, John. *Second Treatise of Government* (1698). Arlington Heights, IL: Harlan Davidson, 1982.

Machrone, Bill. "The Look-and-Feel Issue: The Evolution of Innovation." From "Taking the Stand: The Look-and-Feel Issue Examined," *PC Magazine* (May 26, 1987), 166, 168, 174. In M. David Ermann, Mary B. Williams, and Claudio Gutierrez, eds., *Computers, Ethics, and Society.* New York: Oxford University Press, 1990.

Martin, Janette. "Pursuing Pirates." *Datamation* (August 1, 1992), 41–42.

Mungo, Paul, and Bryan Clough. *Approaching Zero: The Extraordinary World of Hackers, Phreakers, Virus Writers, and Keyboard Criminals.* New York: Random House, 1992.

National Research Council (NRC). *Intellectual Property Issues in Software.* Washington, DC: National Academy Press, 1991.

Nichols, Kenneth. "The Age of Software Patents." *Computer* 32, 4 (April 1999), 25–31.

Nissenbaum, Helen. "Should I Copy My Neighbor's Software?" In Johnson and Nissenbaum, eds., 201–13.

Nycum, Susan H. "Legal Protection for Computer Programs." *Computer/Law Journal* 1 (1978), 1–83.

O'Reilly, Tim. "The Internet Patent Land Grab." *Communications of the ACM* 43, 6 (June 2000), 29–31.

Perrolle, Judith. *Computers and Social Change: Information, Property, and Power.* Belmont, CA: Wadsworth, 1987.

Rosch, Winn L. "The Look-and-Feel Issue: The Copyright Law on Trial." From *PC Magazine* (May 26, 1987), 157–8, 160, 164. In Ermann, Williams, and Gutierrez, eds., 288–95.

Samborn, Hope Viner. "May I See Your License?" *ABA Journal* 87 (April 2001), 74–5.

Samuelson, Pamela. "ACM Forum: Once Again, Patents." *Communications of the ACM* 35, 10 (October 1992), 15–17.

Samuelson, Pamela. "Benson Revisited." *Emory Law Journal,* Fall 1990, 39 Emory L. J. 1025.

Samuelson, Pamela. "A Case Study on Computer Programs." In *Global Dimensions of Intellectual Property Rights in Science and Technology.* Washington, DC: National Academy Press, 1993, pp. 284–318.

Samuelson, Pamela. "The Copyright Grab." *Wired* 4, 1 (1996), 134.

Samuelson, Pamela. "How to Interpret the Lotus Decision (And How Not To)." *Communications of the ACM* 35, 11 (November 1990), 27–33.

Samuelson, Pamela. "Why the Look and Feel of Software User Interfaces Should Not Be Protected by Copyright Law." *Communications of the ACM* 32, 5 (May 1989), 563–72.

Scafetta, Joseph, Jr. "Computer Software and Unfair Methods of Competition." *Marshall Journal of Practice and Procedure* 10 (1977), 447–64. In Johnson and Snapper, pp. 353–63.

Snapper, John W. "On the Web, Plagiarism Matters More than Copyright Piracy." In Spinello and Tavani, pp. 280–94.

Spinello, Richard A. "An Ethical Evaluation of Web Site Linking." In Spinello and Tavani, pp. 295–308.

Spinello, Richard A. *Ethical Aspects of Information Technology.* Englewood Cliffs, NJ: Prentice-Hall, 1995, ch. 6.

Spinello, Richard A., and Herman T. Tavani, eds. *Readings in Cyberethics.* Sudbury, MA: Jones and Bartlett, 2001.

Stallman, Richard M. "The GNU Manifesto." (From *GNU Emacs Manual* (1987), 175–84.) In Ermann, Williams, and Gutierrez, eds. 308–17.

Stallman, Richard, and Simson Garfinkle. "Viewpoint: Against Software Patents." *Communications of the ACM* 35, 1 (January 1994), 17–22, 121.

Wagner, M. "Suits Attack Web Fundamentals." *Computerworld* (May 5, 1997), 125.

Wagner, Suzanne C. "Considerations in Ethical Decision-making and Software Piracy." *Journal of Business Ethics* 29, 1/2 (January 2001), 161–67.

Warwick, Shelly. "Is Copyright Ethical?" In Spinello and Tavani, pp. 263–79.

Weisband, Suzanne P., and Seymour E. Goodman. "Subduing Software Pirates." *Technology Review* (October 1993), 30–33.

Weld, John. "Would You Buy a Shrink Wrapped Automobile?" *Monitor* (Capital PC Users Group). September and November 1986.

Zachary, G. Pascal. "Gates's Bid to Acquire Art Images for Computers Is Coolly Received." *Wall Street Journal*, 11 February 1992, sec. B, p. 1.

Chapter 5

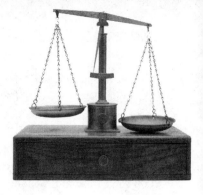

Computer Crime

*T*he development of computer technology has created a vast new potential for crime. We will consider one type of computer abuse, that of computer break-ins and planting destructive software, in the next chapter. We will consider the rest of what may be called computer crimes here. Some of these are just new spins on old-fashioned crimes such as embezzlement, extortion, counterfeiting, and espionage created by the existence of computers; others are new kinds of crimes that would not have existed without computers (such as destructive software and taking advantage of computer roundoff errors to steal money).

A report from the National Institute of Justice on "Dedicated Computer Crime Units" defines computer crime as "*any illegal act for which knowledge of computer technology is used to commit the offense*" (McEwen, 1989, p. 1). A computer may be either actively or passively involved in the crime. It is actively involved if the computer is used to break into files, steal money, or the like; it is passively involved in cases like narcotics dealing, where a computer is used to keep track of clients and goods.

McEwen classifies computer crimes into five categories: (1) internal computer crimes (viruses, logic bombs, etc.), which we deal with in Chapter 6; (2) telecommunications crimes ("phreaking" and illegal bulletin boards, considered in the next chapter, and misuse and theft of telephone communications); (3) computer manipulation crimes (embezzlement, fraud); (4) support of criminal enterprises (databases for criminal activities, or illegal sale of client information); and (5) hardware/software thefts (McEwen, 1989, p. 2). To his list, we should add cyberterrorism.

Federal authority to handle computer crimes comes primarily from the U.S. Code–Section 1029 ("Fraud and Related Activity in Connection with Access Devices") and Section 1030 ("Fraud and Related Activity in Connection with Computers") of Title 18. The FBI, the Internal Revenue Service (IRS), and the U.S. Secret Service are the primary federal units with trained investigators in computer crime (McEwen, 1989, p. 7). On December 15, 2000 the House and Senate passed the Computer Crime Enforcement Act (H. R. 2816) creating a fund of $25 million to help state and local agencies fight cybercrime. All fifty states have computer crime statutes on the books to deal with state violations.

A number of local police authorities have developed dedicated computer crime units; among them are several in California (Alameda and Santa Clara counties, and Los Angeles), Baltimore, the Illinois State Police, Maricopa County (Arizona), and Tarrant County (Texas). The Federal Law Enforcement Training Center in Glynco, Georgia offers training in computer crime investigations for personnel at federal, state, and local levels (McEwen, 1989, pp. 11–12). International computer crime fighting is carried on by Interpol; check out their web site

www.interpol.int/Public/TechnologyCrime/ default.asp

 # KINDS OF COMPUTER CRIME

Computer crimes can be divided into two basic categories: crimes *against* computers, and crimes committed *using* computers. The first category is fairly simple and will be considered briefly. The second category is much more complex, and so will be subdivided into a number of subareas.

Crimes Against Computers

Crimes against computers can involve damage to computers' hardware or software, or theft of computer technology. Damage to software through illegal break-ins will be considered in Chapter 6. Theft of software, which was covered in the discussion of piracy in Chapter 4, will also be considered in Chapter 6. Other instances of crimes *against* computers follow.

Damage to Computers People get angry at computers for a variety of reasons, from being issued an incorrect phone bill for thousands of dollars to being issued a pink slip by the computer. In Olympia, Washington, in 1968, shots were fired at an IBM 1401 computer. In Johannesburg, South Africa in 1972, an "assailant" (who probably received an incorrect bill) fired four shots at a computer, which was dented but kept turning out bills. In Charlotte, North Carolina, in 1974, a computer operator fired a handgun at a computer (presumably it had done something, or failed to do something, that frustrated him) (Whiteside, I, 1977).

In New York, an employee of the Irving Trust Company took a sharp instrument and destroyed all the data on tapes containing information on G.E. accounts. An unhappy employee at Girl Scout Headquarters erased information on magnetic tapes by running a magnet over the tapes. An overworked computer employee of a New York trucking firm destroyed billing records he was unable to enter into the computer by the close of the work day; the records represented about $2 million in billings (Whiteside, I, 1977, p. 63).

Volkswagen apparently lost over $259 million due to foreign-exchange contract fraud in 1987. This involved, according to the report, "erasure of computer data and tampering with computer programs."[1] An "insider scam" created "phony currency-exchange transactions and then covered them with real transactions a few days later, pocketing the float as the exchange rate was changing."[2] The "float" is the interest gained on large amounts of money that can be held for a short period of time before being turned over.

Students at the exclusive Dalton School in Manhattan used their classroom computers to break into a Canadian data communications network and destroy files of two of the network's corporate customers (one was Pepsi-Cola) in 1980.[3] Clearly it was done on a lark, and they probably had no real sense of the value of what they had destroyed.

In September 1987, a man in Somerset County, New Jersey, was arrested for firing eight shots (four hit) from a .44 Magnum handgun, using dum-dum bullets, at his IBM PC. He didn't think he was doing anything wrong, since he was only destroying his own property (presumably out of frustration). But he was arrested for "recklessly creating a risk and using a firearm against the property of another" (since the house, which belonged to a relative, took four hits). He was also charged for not having a permit for the gun, and for discharging a weapon in a restricted area (presumably a residential neighborhood).[4]

In the past, some organizations that were against computing recommended different ways to damage computers, which included pouring a salt solution or a caustic fluid into the operating console, blowing smoke into the computer or spraying it with hair spray, putting an open container of hydrochloric acid in front of the air conditioner, or putting mice under the computer floor to gnaw on the electric wires (Wasik, 1991, p. 57). Some advised recipients of bills that said "Do Not Fold, Spindle, or Mutilate" *to* fold, spindle, and mutilate the bills, or to take the punched-out card pieces from computer punched cards and stick them into the holes on bills or other information cards to mess up the computer when it tried to read them. They also recommended wearing cheap, heavy perfume in the computer room, since it seemed to have an adverse effect on the big machines.

There have been terrorist attacks on computer complexes, and that may be only the beginning of such activity, since taking out key computers can severely damage the communications, military control, or financial infra-structure of an area. August Bequai (1987, ch. 9) offers this report: "During an Easter weekend, members of a mysterious group calling itself the Com-mittee for the Liquidation or Deterrence of Computers (CLODO) broke into the computer centers of Philips Data Systems and CII-Honeywell-Bull, in Toulouse, France, and set them on fire. In a statement justifying their attack, CLODO declared: 'Computers are the favorite instrument of the powerful. They are used to classify, control, and repress.'" Bequai then goes on to spec-ulate about the damage terrorists could do to nuclear facilities or energy storage tanks (a GAO report estimates that the energy in one such tank is 100 times that of the bombs dropped in a raid on Tokyo, Japan, that killed 83,000 people).

Winn Schwartau (1994) hypothesizes an attack that might be carried out by an organization malevolent to the United States. He imagines that on "Day One" they would hit, and take out of operation, the Federal Reserve System, the IRS, and Wall Street. This would cause widespread panic, "an instant decline in confidence in the financial underpinnings of our society"; there would be runs on banks, creating a situation that would put the crash of 1929 to shame. The organization could have implanted computer chips in popular brands of cars that they could cause to fail at the flip of a switch; they could turn all street lights green; they could easily disrupt airport com-munications. Having sabotaged the financial and transportation areas of society, they could turn their expertise on our energy sources—power plants, nuclear plants—and then, to add insult to injury, jam satellite transmissions, so that a frightened public would not only be without money, transportation, and power, but also without information.[5]

The possibilities of terrorist attacks in many guises have become all too real since the September 11, 2001, attacks on the World Trace Center and the Pentagon. Attacks on computer systems would not have to physically harm the computers themselves; there are many ways (as will be discussed in the next chapter) to destroy the *information* on a computer without ever coming physically near it or damaging its hardware. Damaging viruses or worms are propagated routinely today, and the ubiquity of the computer and the inter-connectedness of the Net makes this all the easier. The major arteries of the economy are heavily computerized, as are the power grids, air traffic control, and the mechanisms of government. Can there be enough "firewalls" to protect systems like these from a malevolent attack?

During the Vietnam War, antiwar demonstrators bombed a number of university computer centers (such as the University of Wisconsin, New York University, and Fresno State University), where Defense Department research was being carried out. A double-barrelled shotgun was used to shoot a computer in an American company in Melbourne, Australia, in an antiwar demonstration that caused extensive damage. In June 1976, three armed women gained access to a university computer facility in Rome and set the computer on fire, causing roughly $2 million in damage (Whiteside, I, 1977, pp. 36–37).

In 1988, a woman attacked a computer system (at Vandenberg Air Force Base, north of Lompoc, California) that she believed was designed to launch a nuclear attack. Her tools were a bolt cutter, drill, crowbar, and fire extin-guisher (which she directed into the computer). She was sent to jail for five years and fined $500,000 (Wasik, 1991, p. 57). It is interesting to note the efforts of peace activists which are directed at computers; we will examine the relations between computers and military defense and offense in Chapter 11.

Theft of software or trade secrets, topics covered in Chapter 4, is big business. One notable example that occurred in the early 1980s was IBM working with the FBI to "sting" Hitachi, which was trying to steal trade secrets from IBM. The FBI used hidden cameras and recorders to obtain 100 hours of damaging tapes against Hitachi. A plea bargain was struck in January 1983, where Hitachi pleaded guilty to conspiring to transport stolen IBM property out of the country, but no one went to jail. According to Tinnin (1990, pp. 331–42), among the main items in contention were the "Adiron-dak workbooks: which contained top-secret designs for IBM's new 308X series of computers."

The theft of computers themselves is common, since they are valuable items. For example, about $70,000 worth of computers from the Persian Gulf War theater showed up for sale in Ventura County, California. "Welcome to Saudi Arabia" showed up on some of the screens, and there were maps, information on the deployment of military units, and other leftover military data on the computers.[6] This is an instance of a simple theft that could also represent a military intelligence leak. Today, laptops make a tempting target for theft.

However, the computer theft of choice is that of computer microprocessor chips, especially new designs. In "Your Chips or Your Life!", John Greenwald reports the following recent thefts: In Grenock, Scotland, three men wearing masks and carrying knives overpowered a security guard and stole $3.7 million worth of computer chips and other components. In California, burglars stole $1.8 million worth of computer chips and equipment from a warehouse in January 1994. Five gunmen tied up twelve workers at a semiconductor plant near Portland, Oregon, and made off with $2 million worth of chips.[7] In 1995, thefts of computer chips exceeded $8 billion.

Crimes Using Computers

The computer has become an amazing new tool that can act like an extension of the human mind. It can (like any tool) be used for good or evil. The positive uses are applauded, and should be encouraged to augment human development. Some of the negative uses involve systems that make killing in war more efficient, and the expanding growth of industries supported by computer use that endanger the environment. Other negative applications are in the area of crime, where the computer creates new possibilities for criminal activity *and* can be used as the criminal's tool to carry them out.

Embezzlement by Computer One of the most famous cases of embezzlement using the computer was the Equity Funding Scandal. It inspired an excellent two-part article by Thomas Whiteside in the *New Yorker* in 1977, called "Dead Souls in the Computer." The Equity Funding life insurance company, which was headquartered in Los Angeles, created bogus policies on nonexistent people that it then sold to other insurance companies in a re-insurance arrangement. Whiteside compares this to a novel by the Russian writer Nikolai Gogol called *Dead Souls*, which tells of a man who put the names of dead people (which he obtained from gravestones) on the rolls of his serfs, which he then used as collateral to obtain government loans. Equity created similar "dead souls" in the computer, also to profit from them (Whiteside, I, 1977, pp. 38, 40).

The Equity scandal broke in 1973, when it came out that 64,000 of Equity's 97,000 policies were fake. Equity claimed that the policies recorded up through 1972 were worth $3.2 billion, but apparently $2.1 billion of that was in bogus policies. The scam was discovered when a former employee of Equity reported the goings-on to the New York State Insurance Department and to a Wall Street analyst. Several Equity officers were arrested, tried, and sent to prison for fraud (Whiteside, I, 1977, pp. 40, 42).

A $4 billion class action suit was brought against IBM because Equity had used IBM computers in the fraud. The charge against IBM was that it had failed to inform customers of the susceptibility of computer products to fraud and for failing to provide safeguards. The suit was brought against those who "manufactured said data processing equipment such that it could be used for any business for the purpose of defrauding the public."[8] Incredible as this sounds, IBM had to pay damages in the suit. I still have an ad IBM ran a few years later, which also appeared in the *New Yorker*, in which there is a picture of a line-up with four men in business suits and a computer terminal on a stand. The caption reads, "The computer didn't do it." The ad goes on to say, "Computers don't commit crimes. But they can be misused. That concerns us at IBM, and it should concern anyone involved with computers today. Because keeping computers secure is the responsibility of everyone who uses and manages them. At IBM, we continue to develop security measures that can help keep information safe."

In 1979, Stanley Mark Rifkin, working as a computer consultant for a Los Angeles bank, visited the wire transfer room and learned the EFT code (which was left out in plain view). Then, posing as a branch manager, he called the bank from a public telephone and had $10.2 million transferred to a New York bank, and from there to a Swiss bank. By the time the bank found the fraud, he had flown to Switzerland, converted the money to diamonds, and flown back to the United States. He probably would have gotten away with it if he had not bragged about his accomplishment. He was convicted of wire fraud and served three years in a California Federal Prison Camp.[9]

A chief teller at New York's Union Dime Bank embezzled $1.5 million by skimming money from new accounts and making a simple computer entry to cover it. He probably would also have gotten away with it except for his penchant for gambling. Police investigated a local gambling establishment he frequented, and checked into how a mere teller could afford to lose so much. He felt no guilt about taking from the impersonal bank, and he was careful never to take more from an individual's account than was covered by F.D.I.C. insurance.[10]

This is reminiscent of the 1955 British movie *The Ladykillers*, in which the character played by Alec Guinness tries to convince Mrs. Wilburforce (who has been the unwitting landlady to a gang of thieves) that it would do no good to return the money she has discovered, that nobody wants the money back. He tells her that this particular shipment of money was insured, so the insurance company will pay the loss, and then, to make up for it, it will raise everyone's premiums one farthing for the next year. "So what real harm have we done? Just a farthing's worth. I don't suppose you ever looked at it that way, Mrs. Wilburforce."

Is the argument put here to Mrs. Wilburforce a good moral justification? It has a utilitarian ring to it; the thieves would greatly enjoy their loot, and the insurance policyholders would not even notice the extra farthing on their policies! The act does not generalize well; if everyone carried out such thefts, on the same utilitarian grounds, the insurance companies and banks would either go out of business, or charge exorbitant rates. This would undermine useful services on which society relies. Furthermore, if the thieves are basically dishonest, this will carry over to their dealings with each other; this is dramatically demonstrated in the movie, where they end up killing each other off.

An operations officer for the Wells Fargo bank used the bank's computerized branch accounts to withdraw funds from one branch and deposit them in a bogus account at another, creating bogus credits to cover the withdrawals. He supposedly kept this "rollover" scam going for two years, to the tune of $21.3 million.[11]

The First Interstate Bank of California nearly lost $70 million in an EFT scheme in 1992. A request to transfer funds from one set of accounts to another came on a computer tape, along with an authorization form and signature, and was approved without it being checked (which apparently is not unusual). It was only caught because the transfers created an overdraft.[12]

The National Institute of Justice reported a case in which a manager at a financial institution that insures loans against the eventuality of the death of the borrower figured out a way to make the system work for him. In the event of death, the institution would submit a claim to the insuring company for the unpaid balance of the loan. If a customer having a line of credit with the financial institution died, the manager would generate a fraudulent loan for the difference between the deceased client's line of credit and the current unpaid balance; he would then get a check from the insurance company for the amount, deposit it in an account under a fictitious name, and later transfer it to another bank for withdrawal. The scheme was working well until he accidentally submitted a fraudulent insured loan for a customer over 70 who had died. The insurance company, which had the rule of not insuring anyone over 70 years old, caught the discrepancy and refused to pay. An administrator then submitted the loan to the estate, which paid it, but in the process the fraud was discovered (McEwen, 1989, pp. 47–48).

A British clerk carried on a very successful embezzlement fraud for six years, netting her 193,781 pounds before she was caught. She had the sole charge of a branch bank computer that was linked to a central computer where statements were produced. She systematically debited large amounts from business accounts and diverted them to an account of her own. She was able to cover this up by intercepting the legitimate bank statements that showed the debit, and typing up new ones on appropriate stationery that omitted the debits. She was finally caught when one business customer questioned his account statement, and the account was found to be 15,000 pounds short (Wasik, 1991, pp. 29–30).

Justin Tanner Peterson, who called himself "Agent Steal," used his computer skills to create a $150,000 wire transfer that he used to buy Porsches.[13] It may well be that his taste for Porsches was the tip that led investigators to him.

The switch from communism in the Czech Republic led to a growth of the economy *and* a 75 percent growth of economic crimes in just nine months. One example of such crimes was a 23-year-old employee of the Republic's biggest bank, who transferred "35 million crowns ($1.9 million) from various corporate accounts to his personal account over a period of eight months."[14] He claims to have done this to test the bank's security, and wrote the software to tamper with the corporate accounts himself. He was only discovered when he withdrew about half a million dollars and was caught trying to stuff it into his briefcase. The moral to the computer criminal here is presumably to be cool, and don't take out obscene amounts in bills at one time.

The Belgium branch of the Banque Nationale du Paris was bilked of BFr 245 million (on the order of $7 million) in 1993, by two men who used direct computer access to take funds from other accounts and transfer them into their own accounts at other banks. Apparently, the auditors picked up on the illegal transfers during a routine check of accounts. The money was put back into the original accounts.[15] The point is that these embezzlements keep happening, and we only hear about those few who get caught.

A pay supervisor at Fort Myer in Arlington, Virginia, had regular military paychecks deposited to a fake military officer's account (which he of course controlled), and accumulated $169,000 over three years (1994–1997). A guilty plea earned him a sentence of up to ten years in jail and a $250,000 fine.[16]

In 1999, the comptroller for Halifax Corporation stole roughly $15 million and covered it up with creative accounting. The theft was discovered when a "company doctor" was brought in to try to rev up a slow business. "The money was gone, but Mary Adams Collins, who made $50,000 a year working in the company's Richmond office, had a fleet of cars, a batch of jewelry, and an ostrich farm."[17] The State of Virginia is a prominent new client of the firm. In 2001, two former Cisco Systems accountants illegally issued $8 million in stock to themselves (www.cybercrime.gov/Osowski_TangSent.htm). A former bank vault manager at Bank One gradually stole $663,000 from the bank over a 10-year period. He would take cash from the bank vault, and then adjust the books on the bank's computers to cover the loss. He lived modestly, but lost most of the money at blackjack. But his embezzlement was not discovered; his conscience forced him to confess.[18]

An elegantly simple scheme I heard about was the man who placed his own deposit slips, imprinted with his MICR (Magnetic Ink Character Recognition) account number, in the bins at the bank that hold blank deposit slips for people who forget their own. People would just pick up a slip, fill it out, and deposit their money—but it would go into *his* account. This was because if the deposit slip has an MICR account code, the computerized system would read that automatically instead of any hand-printed account number, and use that account.

Theft of Services   Telephone fraud is rapidly increasing, with people stealing phone credit card numbers, tapping into lines, and using computers to break into switches and private branch exchanges (PBXs). Large companies like Mitsubishi and Proctor & Gamble report losing hundreds of thousands of dollars per year to illicit calls.[19]

In 1987, eighteen New Yorkers were arrested "on charges of illegally altering the memory chips in their mobile telephones so they could make calls without being charged for them."[20] Also arrested were seven others who were said to have actually done the reprogramming of the chips. The assistant director of the FBI in charge of the New York office said it was the first time anyone in the country had been arrested for this kind of crime involving cellular telephones. This fraud had cost the cellular phone company about $40,000 a month. It seems that other people got billed for the calls these people made.

The following is sort of a reverse on theft of services, since it is an example of damaging a system to ensure that you will be called in to service it. A computer consultant to a law firm in Manhattan put a logic bomb in the firm's computer system, such that when claim 56789 was filed, the system would shut down. He was then called in to fix it, and paid an additional $7,000 (besides the $5,000 he estimated to upgrade the old system, and an additional $16,000 in overrun) for the job. He was fined $25,000 by the court.[21] The lesson here may be that the uneducated consumer is often at the mercy of an unscrupulous computer specialist, since the consumer really has no idea what is required to make the system work, or how much time and effort it should take.

Hackers (discussed in Chapter 6) created major denials of service (DOS) by taking down eBay, Yahoo!, amazon, CNN (by Mafiaboy), and Lloyds of London web sites in 2000–2001.

Theft of Information   The General Accounting Office has indicated that data from the FBI's National Crime Information Center is being misused and often sold to outside parties. In one case, a former law enforcement officer from Arizona used data from three different law enforcement agencies "to track down his estranged girl friend and murder her." [22]

A package of computer disks holding crucial telemetry data from an America's Cup syndicate was stolen and "held for ransom" of $10,000 in 1986. Eventually, the stolen disks were recovered without any money being paid. [23]

In November 1993, the computerized records of at least 6,000 people diagnosed with AIDS or who were HIV-positive were reported stolen from Miami's Jackson Memorial Hospital. The danger from such theft is that the records might be used to blackmail patients who would want to keep their condition private. [24] It is the fact that the records were on the computer that made them so easy to steal, since someone walking out with 6,000 paper patient records under one arm would surely have been noticed.

Fifteen car sales personnel in Newark, New Jersey, were charged with using fake credit records of 450 customers to steal millions of dollars. They used the dealership computer to tap into the customers' credit reports, changed the addresses, ordered new credit cards, and ran up big bills in purchases and loans. The average theft per victim was $7,500. The victims did not have to pay, after the theft was discovered, but it took time and was a big inconvenience to correct their credit records. The considerable additional activity on Autoland's computers alerted the dealership managers to what was going on. [25] It should be noted that these last two cases are serious invasions of privacy as well as computer crimes.

"Call the Credit Doctor!" is a slogan used by a business that accesses computerized credit records to alter bad reports for customers, or sells someone's good credit history to another who needs one. The "pioneer" of credit doctoring is Walter P. Hilton, an entrepreneur and sometimes Baptist preacher who, when in his seventies, with partner James Lawson (another Baptist preacher) used a $600 computer to gain access to the Credit Bureau of Greater Houston (Texas). There they would find information on people with good credit records with names similar to those of their customers, and sell the information to their customers for filling out credit applications. They also sold customers a credit history item of having worked for "Hilton & Lawson" for high salaries.[26] On the Internet, one can find the Canadian **thecreditdoctor.com**, or **creditdoctoronline.com**, or **creditfixer.net**, or many others.

Another trick used by credit doctors is to send an avalanche of letters (easy to do by computer) to credit bureaus contesting items in clients' records. Federal law precludes a credit bureau issuing credit information while it is under investigation due to a complaint, and this gives the doctors' clients a "window" of time during which to obtain credit and borrow lots of money while their bad credit record is being checked out by the credit bureau. The credit bureaus say they have made unauthorized access more difficult by requiring more information, but that information is relatively easy to get. They usually ask for name, address (and how long at that address), Social Security number, and date of birth.

Clearly anyone who can access computerized records may be able to change them. Thus, for a fee, someone could fix your bad credit record, your record of unpaid traffic tickets, your arrest and conviction record, or your grades on your school transcript. Or, as we have seen, they can create a whole fictitious person and give him or her a birthdate, birthplace, job, school record, military record, and Social Security number. (This was played out in a 1971 movie called *Paper Man*, in which college students and a computer center worker create an identity in the computer, primarily to get credit cards. Of course, the plan goes awry when an evil person stumbles onto what they are doing, and the college students start getting killed.)

Fraud Of course, embezzlement is a kind of fraud, but we gave the interesting cases their own section earlier in this chapter. Here we will discuss other activities that constitute computer-based fraud.

Three men working at a travel agency in Woodland Hills, California, used a computerized reservation terminal to create fictitious "frequent-flyer" accounts and credit them with miles flown by passengers who were not in frequent-flyer programs. They then used these accounts to obtain free flights, which they sold or gave away to friends. The estimate was that they defrauded American Airlines of $1.3 million in 1986 and 1987.[27]

Four college students who went on a $100,000 spending spree using stolen credit card numbers they accessed using computers were apprehended by Long Island police on March 16, 1995. They were charged with grand larceny, forgery, and scheming to defraud.[28]

A computer program known as Credit Master, which created credit card numbers that could be valid, was available on several major online services.

Though credit card companies say they suffered no significant losses as a result of this program, it has the potential to instigate larceny on a large scale, since it is available to anyone using these services.[29]

Three students from Rutgers University advertised a "New Jersey Scholarship and Grant Search Services" operation, in which they had applicants send their social security numbers, bank account numbers, and credit card data to get help in obtaining scholarships. They apparently intended to use the data to apply for duplicate birth certificates, and to use credit card accounts and withdraw money from bank accounts.[30]

A dairy and produce store owner removed records of $17.1 million in sales so as not to have to pay taxes on them. (He also apparently indicated higher weights—and thus costs—on store items.) This "data diddling" (massaging computer data to make it come out the way you want) "saved" him $6.7 million in taxes, but he now must pay $15 million in back taxes and fines.

This story makes one wonder about markets in which the price is no longer marked on the item but is instead read from the Universal Product Code by a scanner at checkout. This makes it much easier for markets to overprice items without the consumer being aware of it, a practice that Rob Kling (1991, p. 676) indicates is becoming more common. It is very difficult for a shopper to remember each item price that was posted on the shelves to check it against what is charged at the register, and unscrupulous stores can take advantage of this.

Computers have made the doctoring of photographs much easier than it ever was before. Anyone who has seen the movie *Rising Sun* has seen a dramatic example of such photo fraud. Photography is inherently susceptible to manipulation (there are many old examples of famous photographic hoaxes), but computers have made it a snap. Some examples done with computers were a *National Geographic* magazine picture with the Giza pyramids moved together, and a picture of Donald Trump with a homeless man. Newspaper editors are supposedly tough in regulating manipulation of news photos, but tolerant with photos for features.[31] The point is, how would we (the readers) know? Photo manipulation is getting easier, cheaper, and much harder to detect. It seems we are at the mercy of the sense of professional responsibility of news editors. Of course, television footage can be doctored as well.

Anyone with a computer can buy software specially designed to doctor photos—such as PhotoShop, from Adobe Systems in Mountain View, California. There are other similar packages as well, from simple to expensive and complex. Such software could be used, for instance, to create a fake UFO photograph.[32]

Computerized election results present a great opportunity for tampering and outright fraud. Peter Neumann reported on several cases: uncounted votes in Toronto and doubly counted votes in Virginia and North Carolina in 1989; an election in Yonkers, New York, reversed because of the presence of leftover test data in the totals; and other irregularities in Alabama and Georgia. He writes, "Even the U.S. Congress had difficulties when 435 representatives tallied 595 votes on a Strategic Defense Initiative measure."[33] Though the computers were not the major problem, there certainly were serious difficulties with the 2000 Presidential election. He tells further of a computer reporting the wrong winner in an election in Rome, Italy. In Toronto, computerized elections have been abandoned altogether because of the problems. As Neumann points out, if errors can occur accidentally, they can also be created on purpose, through the many ways of tampering with a computerized system.

The *Wall Street Journal* reported in 1990 on a federal review of computerized vote-counting systems that raised concerns over the difficulty of verifying results, the possibility of undetectable fraud, and the lack of technical knowledge among the election administrators. Roy Saltman, a computer scientist at the National Bureau of Standards, recommended a system of "internal controls" such as those used in businesses to improve the accuracy and security of vote-counting computers. "It doesn't matter whether you are counting dollars or votes," said Saltman.[34] A friend of mine who has studied accounting found this suggestion disturbing. He said that in auditing accounting systems ("counting dollars"), auditors set what they call "materiality levels," where they are concerned only about auditing transactions that have a significant effect ("material" effect) on the financial statements. The materiality level is usually based on statistics, and is used to avoid wasteful auditing (say, on petty-cash transactions in a billion-dollar business). But what sort of materiality levels would an auditor set for a vote-tallying system? Aren't *all* votes "material" (that is, shouldn't every single one count)?[35]

Saltman also is especially wary about direct recording electronic systems (DREs), since they have no ballot and thus no independent means of checking the results. There is no redundancy outside the machines, and even if they have internal redundancy, we have to trust implicitly the machine, its invulnerability to tampering, and the vendor.[36]

A report on computerized vote-tallying by Computer Professionals for Social Responsibility (CPSR) in 1991 says that 31 percent of American counties that represent 55 percent of the voters were using computerized systems to tally votes, that these came from a monopoly of private companies, and that lawsuits alleging fraud in elections all involved vote-counting computer systems from the same company (CPSR, 1991, p. 155). They point out obvious weaknesses in the punched-card ballots being used in many systems, and the many ways in which computer programs can be sabotaged to turn out results that are inaccurate and biased toward one side. They begin the report with the statement: "The advent of computerized vote counting over the past two decades has created a potential for election fraud and error on a scale previously unimagined."

CPSR advocates the adoption of a secure system for computerized vote-counting (designed by Princeton computer scientists Howard Strauss and Jon Edwards) that would have the following features: independent reviews of the software by impartial computer scientists; separation of powers (software distribution, ballot creation, precinct elections, election analysis, and determination of final results all kept separate); user-friendly voting software to allow citizen election officials to be in control; no human interaction with the system on election day; ballots that clearly represent the candidates and issues; systems that run on generic hardware; and a system that "never forgets" (by keeping an audit trail that can't be turned off). A Citizens Election Commission of impartial citizens, to include reputable computer scientists, should be established to set system specifications and oversee elections (CPSR, 1991, pp. 160–163). For more recent perspective from CPSR on voting, see the Winter 2001 *CPSR Newsletter* (also available online at cpsr.org) and Roy G. Saltman's article (see References). Perhaps attention to such details might have averted the difficulties and ambiguities involved in the presidential election of 2000. After all, voting is one of our most precious freedoms, and we should not allow it to be subverted.

The president of Quik Tax Dollars, Inc., a major nationwide tax-preparation service, was indicted on charges of bilking the IRS out of more than $1.1 million in a tax fraud. He apparently created 145 false tax returns, complete with names and Social Security numbers (shades of "dead souls in the computer"!) and used an intermediary company to forward the bogus returns electronically to the IRS.[37] It is noteworthy that 12 million tax returns were filed electronically in 1992, and more than 35 million were filed in 2000 (www.irs.gov). The potential for computerized tax fraud in such an environment boggles the mind!

A massive tax fraud began in New York City in 1992, in which some tax records were erased and other tax bills were paid using the money from legitimate taxpayers, all by making use of "computer glitches." Records for $13 million in taxes were erased, and $7 million in interest was lost.[38]

Clerks in the California Department of Motor Vehicles were in a scheme accepting bribes to issue driver's licenses to people who had not qualified to receive them (they pocketed between $200 and $1,000 for each illegal license). They were caught in an ongoing investigation called Operation Clean Sweep.[39]

Carlos Salgado Jr. was arrested in 1997 for selling personal data from more than 100,000 credit card accounts, obtained by hacking into company databases on the Internet. Unfortunately for him, he sold the information (on an encrypted diskette) to FBI agents operating a "sting." His penalty was up to 15 years in prison and a $500,000 fine (roughly twice what he was "paid" for the data).[40]

A relatively new kind of fraud by computer has arisen in manipulating the stock market, and a number of young perpetrators have been caught. "At 27, Nick Leeson brought down Barings Bank with $1.4 million in fraudulent trades. At 25, Gary Hoke faked a Bloomberg news report linked to a Yahoo bulletin board in a stock scam that cost investors $93,000. At 24, Rafael Shaoulian littered financial bulletin boards with unfounded hype that enabled him to sell a stock and pocket $173,000." Mark Jakob (age 23) drove down Emulex stock using a phony Internet report, bought large amounts, and made $241,000 when the hoax was discovered and the stock went back up. And the most recent, and youngest, is Jonathan Lebed, a 15-year-old from New Jersey, who controlled stocks with chat-room hype to the tune of $272,826 in illegal profits for himself.[41] These frauds have been discovered; one has to wonder how many have *not* been discovered (and what role, if any, computer manipulation played in the Enron debacle).

A recent issue of *Computerworld* reported on a 32-year-old Brooklyn, New York, busboy, Abraham Abdallah, who in March 2001 "pulled off the biggest Internet identity heist in history by stealing the online identities of 200 of the richest people in America."[42] There is a rising tide of stealing credit-card numbers from the Internet.

Organized ("Mob") Computer Crime   In Philadelphia, public computer bulletin boards were being used to post requests for child pornography. Child pornographers in that city are known to send pornographic pictures from computer to computer. In Massachusetts, adults used computer networks and bulletin boards to develop relationships with young boys for purposes of sexual abuse. The networks were occasionally used to transmit threats to boys who might have threatened to tell about the abuse (Conly, 1989, pp. 10–11).

In San Francisco, a couple was convicted on July 28, 1994, of eleven counts of transmitting obscenity through interstate telephone lines, with each count carrying up to five years in prison and a $250,000 fine. The couple had been "sending images of bestiality and sexual fetishes" over the

Internet. They charged users $99 a year to connect to their bulletin board. Some Internet bulletin board users are concerned that this represents a government move to censor any material with sexual content sent over the Internet.[43] The differences between this case and the home satellite channels like Spice, TV Erotica, and Canadian EXXXtasy, which transmit pornographic movies, need to be clearly spelled out for the average consumer and entrepreneur.

Concern was greatly heightened by a cover story in *Time* (July 3, 1995) with "CYBERPORN: Exclusive" and the face of a shocked child at a keyboard on the cover.[44] Since there *is* pornography on-line (including sex with animals and "kiddie-porn"), there is no telling what a child might stumble upon while surfing the Net. The article overplays the danger of this, since most such services are complex to access, and carry a charge. Debates in Congress resulted in 1996 in the passage of Jim Exon's (D-Neb.) Communications Decency Act, by a vote of 84 to 16, which prescribes fines of $100,000 or more or two-year prison terms to anyone who "knowingly . . . makes available any indecent communications . . . to any person under 18 years of age." The bill also proposed penalties on anyone who uses "obscene, lewd, lascivious, filthy, or indecent" communications with intent to "annoy, abuse, threaten, or harass" another.

In an article entitled "Cheap Speech," Jeffrey Rosen wrote: "A citizen offended by the Exon bill who sent an obscene E-mail message to annoy Senator Exon could thus be harshly punished, although the same message shouted at Senator Exon on the street would be constitutionally protected. At the end of June, Newt Gingrich, to his great credit, pronounced the Exon bill clearly unconstitutional" (1995, p. 78). A great uprising of negative sentiment led to the bill actually being declared unconstitutional by the Supreme Court.

All of this raises great First Amendment controversies with respect to cyberspace. Child pornography is clearly both immoral and illegal, so the only problems here are the greater facility with which it can be transmitted and sold over the Net. Other pornography and obscene language, versus freedom of speech, is still up for discussion and controversy.

Classical Utilitarians object to harm (pain), as would those who want to minimize evils. But John Stuart Mill might today be soft on pornography, due to his strong libertarian feelings about free speech. Such a utilitarian would object to child pornography, on the grounds of physical harm done, but there are other harms as well—restriction of freedom, damaged development—which can diminish a child's likelihood of inquiring, possessing fortitude, developing friendships, and even of living a sane, full adult life. Aside from religious pronouncements and puritan sexual hangups, where *should* the line be drawn on pornography? Utilitarian calculations fail to assess future harm adequately.

Many argue that pornography does real harm to women, not just by stimulating sexual attacks, but by degrading women.[45] In trying to assess this difficult issue, it may again be helpful to look at extreme cases. Many claim that there is no harm done in simply looking at a *Playboy* centerfold, or in using frank sexual language, sprinkled liberally with four-letter words. If this is the most innocent case (at one extreme), and if child pornography or "snuff" films (where the participants in making the film are actually harmed) are at the other end, at what point in the spectrum is the line to be drawn? At *Playboy* or at a magazine (or a computer service) showing still pictures of explicit sexual acts? What about X-rated movies? And so on. A careful look at the spectrum, and just what it is that makes almost everyone agree that cases on the far end of the spectrum are evil, may clarify how the intermediate cases (and the "innocent" end) of the range should be assessed.

Computer crime investigation units have reported cases that include "the use of computers in connection with organized prostitution, pornography, fencing, money laundering and loansharking" (Conly, 1989, p. 12; cf. McEwen, 1989, pp. 50–51). Thus the new technology may be proving a boon to crime syndicates across the world. Drug dealers can communicate anonymously with each other over telecommunication channels, and they have often been found to keep computerized records of their drug deals. A federal raid in Florida uncovered the names of two IBM employees who had been hired by a drug ring to help computerize its smuggling operations (Conly, 1989, p. 11).

A fake computer message allowed an alleged cocaine dealer, held on $3 million bail, to escape from the Los Angeles County Jail in August 1987. The authorities thought that the computer message had to be an "inside job" (though with computer ubiquity, it is not at all clear why they would have thought so). The most disturbing part of the report was that apparently no one discovered that the prisoner was missing for six days![46]

Counterfeiting   Counterfeiting has just recently gone from an art requiring highly skilled practitioners to an easy job for anyone with a high-quality copier or a computer, a scanner, and a laser printer. "Desktop forgery" is one of the up-and-coming new crimes of the era. The U.S. National Research Council reports that high-tech counterfeiting has doubled every year since 1989, and American currency is thought to be the most copied in the world, because it "uses only two colours and is exchangeable for almost any other"

(Hecht, 1994, p. 19). The technology of today's copiers and printers makes it possible to produce very accurate copies of paper currency,[47] tickets, cashier's checks, money orders, and credit-card receipts.[48]

The *Wall Street Journal* reported that the Russian authorities seized $539,000 worth of counterfeit banknotes and vouchers in the first five months of 1993, most of which were photocopied, and which exceeds the total seized over the previous five years.[49] There are other indicators that sophisticated computer crimes have risen very rapidly in Russia since the breakup of the former Soviet Union.

The Postal Service has been selling new money order forms since April 1991 that incorporate special paper with fibers that glow in ultraviolet light, metallic security threads, microline printing that can't be copied by photocopiers, and a watermark drawing of Benjamin Franklin to thwart counterfeiters.[50]

Officials at the University of Southern California investigated claims that counterfeit USC degrees were being sold, along with corresponding transcripts, for about $25,000 each (Bequai, 1978, p. 23). They probably would sell well, since in addition to not having to take a lot of exams and attend class, it would represent a substantial savings over the cost of the normal four years at USC to earn a degree! Apparently such documents were actually placed illegally into the university's computer system, so they would have been released, when requested, with the university's official seal, making them appear respectable.

It seems that people have also figured out how to copy "plastic"—including credit cards, ATM cards, and age IDs.[51] In 1992, Visa International said it expected to report worldwide counterfeit losses of $100 million for the year ending March 31, 1992, as compared to $55 million in losses for the previous year.[52] There were 13.2 billion ATM transactions in the United States in 2000, averaging approximately $60 each.[53] It was reported that U.S. commercial banks lost at least $568 million in fraudulent checks in 1991, most of which was blamed on copiers and desktop printers. New techniques to make check copying more difficult are using complex patterns and microscopic words that won't show up in a copy, and background designs that show up as the word "Void" when copied.[54]

In Philadelphia, ATM customers made fraudulent deposits—that is, they claimed a certain amount deposited but put in an empty envelope—and then withdrew money from the account against the fictitious deposit. When the banks started photographing people at the ATMs, the offenders would have an intermediary make the deposit for them (Conly, 1989, pp. 8–9). In Syracuse, New York, in 1992, a man used a stolen credit card in an ATM machine and, to his delight, it started ejecting $20 bills and did not stop until he had accumulated $5,600. He had stolen a woman's purse from her car, and the purse contained both her ATM card and her PIN (Personal Identification Number). Happy with this success, he hit several other ATMs at local grocery stores, collecting a total of $63,900. He was, however, apprehended, and later pleaded guilty to third-degree grand larceny and was sentenced to five years' probation. He returned all but $1,800 of the money.[55]

Efforts are being made on several fronts to stem the rising tide of high-tech counterfeiting. Xerox's Special Information Systems Division in Pasadena, California, received a $4 million contract in 1985 from the Treasury Department to develop holographic images that can be imbedded in currency to circumvent copying. "A holograph is a laser-generated 3-dimensional image that changes shape and color when held up to the light."[53] Developments in holographic technology for such purposes have been forthcoming since then.[54] Canon announced on September 29, 1992, that it had developed a new chip for its laser color copiers that will detect currency patterns from major nations and print black copies if it detects any such patterns.[55]

The Treasury Department has imbedded a polyester thread in all new bills of $10 or more. This thread can be seen when the bill is held up to the light, but does not show up in photocopying. It is imbedded in the pulp for the paper used to print U.S. currency. The National Research Council Report urges, in addition, the use of color-shifting inks (but these cost a hundred times as much as regular inks), moire patterns that vary the distance between lines and interfere with digital scanners, watermarks, and the like (Hecht, 1994, p. 19).

There is rampant copyright violation or counterfeiting in other areas besides the financial. Photographs, artworks, and books are being copied and sold on the black market using the same technologies. As useful as these advances are to the legitimate user, they are creating serious illegal activity, and creating a secondary market for new technology to detect or prevent the fraudulent use of the original devices. The biggest threat is not so much the high-quality copiers as it is the computer/scanner/laser printer technology, which allows the image or information from an original to be laser-scanned and recorded, and then to be stored or transmitted *anywhere* in the world at the touch of a button (Garn, 1992, pp. 75–76).

The Secret Service identified $80 million in counterfeit U.S. currency in 1990, but surely this was only the tip of the iceberg. Improving technology will only increase this amount. If someone is willing to use the counterfeit bills in small amounts, the odds are that they will go undetected at most places of business (your local grocery store, liquor store, gas station, pub, restaurant, or betting establishment) and the counterfeiter can go unrecognized. When the bills end up in a bank with fancy detection equipment and/or alert tellers, they may be spotted, but the person in possession of the bills at that time will most likely *not* be the counterfeiter.

Senator Jake Garn (R-Utah) urged tougher legislation regarding counterfeiters to keep up with this technology. He proposed raising the current criminal penalty from a $5,000 fine and/or 15 years in prison to a fine of $50,000 for each violation and/or 20 years imprisonment (Garn, 1992, p. 76). It is clear that something must be done, since undermining the currency undermines the stability of the state. Dante recognized this in 1314, and placed counterfeiters deep in Hell, deeper than thieves and sowers of discord. Any counterfeit bill that is passed devalues each legitimate dollar, and so harms the individual citizen as well as the state. Successful counterfeiting could lead to runaway inflation, which would hurt everyone (except, perhaps, the counterfeiters who could laser-print as much as they need).

It is our duty, as responsible citizens, to be aware of the implications of the increase in crimes such as counterfeiting brought about by the new technology, so that we can vote intelligently and support efforts to stem the tide.

Computer Crime Victims   Computer crime, a kind of "white-collar crime," is often said to be "victimless crime." But this is not the case. If there is embezzlement, it is always from someone or some institution. Fraud is perpetrated *against* individuals and/or companies. If software or hardware or information is stolen, it is stolen from some individual (or some institution) that has the right to it. And so on. The media tends to exaggerate the scope of computer crimes (Mandell, 1990, p. 345), and to glorify computer bandits as modern-day Robin Hoods, who rob the rich (the corporations and the government) and (sometimes) help the poor (at least the bandits help themselves!). The average reader is not very sympathetic to big business or big government, and so often gets a silent pleasure from seeing them taken down a peg.

However, such crime affects others as well—the stockholders who earn lower dividends, the insurance policyholders who must pay higher rates due to computer crime losses, the computer users who have to pay higher prices for software because of the extent of illegal copying, and more. And we all pay more in taxes to support the authorities who must track down and prosecute these criminals. We have seen that society, in order to work, must rest on certain implicit or explicit agreements (not to rob each other, not to kill each other, to drive on the right side of the road, and the like); the more these agreements are broken, the more the fabric of society is weakened, and we all suffer. Thus, though big business and the government may seem to be the victims of computer crime, in fact we are really all its victims.

Computer Criminals   Steven Mandell describes the typical computer criminal as someone that organizations are anxious to hire—"young and ambitious with impressive educational credentials" (Mandell, 1990, p. 343). Computer criminals view themselves (and often others view them) "as heroes challenging an impersonal computer as an opponent in a game" (Mandell, 1990, p. 344). Most often, they are employed by the institutions they attack. Computer crime is antiseptic and has none of the physical risks of normal crime. It also appears easier to rob someone you cannot see, through an inanimate device; it often doesn't seem like crime at all to the perpetrator, but more like a game, a test of skill and intelligence. Occasionally it is a way of "getting back" at an employer (who has fired, or not given a raise to, the employee) or at a bureaucratic government.

One of the problems with computer criminals is that often they are not severely punished. Embezzlers of millions of dollars may get light sentences; those who have committed damaging break-ins to computer systems often only pay a fine and serve a short time on probation or do community service. There is also a tendency for companies to hire the successful computer criminal to help them protect against similar break-ins. In the *Republic*, Book I, Socrates argues that the just individual is one who protects money when it is not in use, and the one best prepared to protect money is the one who knows well how to steal it—so the just individual turns out to be a kind of thief! Plato used this example to discredit an inadequate definition of justice, but in our times we see the thief being employed by the very types of organizations that he (much more often than she) stole from, and thus given a suit of respectability.

Computer Crime Stoppers   Not only are computers serving as the tools for criminals, they are also becoming the tools of the authorities for maintaining security and apprehending criminals. Computerized security checks can be instant checks of fingerprints, handprints, voice prints ("Computer, this is Captain Kirk"), lip prints,[59] or even eye prints (as in the James Bond movie *Thunderball* or its remake, *Never Say Never Again*). However, there are devious and/or violent means around all of these checks, as demonstrated by Wesley Snipes' character, Simon Phoenix, in the movie *Demolition Man*.

Computers can be used to track criminals' patterns, to figure out where they may strike next (as seen in many movies, including *Silence of the Lambs, Hannibal,* and *January Man*). Computers are used to check on the financial dealings of mobsters; often, if the government cannot find convincing evidence of criminal activity, they may be able to find proof of tax evasion (as with Al Capone), and at least put the gangster behind bars. They are also in effective use tracking terrorists and their networks and financial dealings.

Computers can also be used to track a person's movements and financial transactions (as we will examine in more detail in the Chapter 7, where privacy is discussed). This can also be used by law enforcement to establish whether someone's alibi stands up or not. Use of an ATM card or credit card can place the user at a particular location at a certain time. Also, patterns of excessive spending or gambling can alert the authorities to a potential welfare cheat, or drug trafficker, or embezzler or other criminal.

Computerized fingerprint-identification systems have greatly improved the apprehension of criminals. In Los Angeles, using a newly installed Cal-ID system, authorities were able to identify and arrest a prime suspect for the Night Stalker killings of fourteen people. They commented that comparing the suspected Stalker's prints to records on file the old-fashioned way could have taken up to 67 years; the Cal-ID system came up with ten close matches, with one rated as four times as likely as any of the others, in three minutes (Hussain, 1986, p. 233). Computers are also able to simulate, from the photograph of a child, how that child will look in eight to ten years. This is very useful in tracking down children who have been missing for an extended time (Hussain, 1986, p. 232). *Computerworld* reports that computer forensics is a fast-growing new career field.[60] The March 19, 2001 issue reported that cybercrimes cost top U.S. companies a total of $3,778,000,000 in 2000.[61]

The dedicated computer crime law enforcement units mentioned earlier and profiled in reports from the National Institute of Justice are well trained in computer technology, both to be aware of the crimes that can be perpetrated using computers and to use the computer themselves in tracking down offenders. In a May 22, 2001, speech to the First Annual Computer Privacy, Policy & Security Institute, Attorney General John Ashcroft said that the FBI has Computer Crime Squads in sixteen metropolitan areas around the country to investigate cybercrimes, and that the Department of Justice has "dramatically increased" the training of prosecutors and agents in this area. The government is initially creating ten special CHIP (Computer Hacking and Intellectual Property) units. A relevant website is:

www.cybercrime.gov

Failure to Report Computer Crimes   Many computer crimes are not ever detected, because of their subtlety, or because those who have been violated sadly have very little knowledge of how their computer systems work. Even when crimes are discovered, they are not always reported to the authorities. There are a number of reasons for this. Banks, insurance companies, and other organizations who base much of their success on public trust, do not want the public to know that their security has been compromised. Often, institutions are afraid of being made to look foolish, and would rather absorb the loss than suffer loss of face.

Other reasons include a lack of confidence in the ability of the authorities to apprehend the criminal(s). There are still very few dedicated computer crime units that have knowledgeable personnel to deal with these matters. "Many victims state that they do not report computer-related offenses because of unsatisfactory responses by law enforcement agencies to previous complaints" (Conly, 1989, p. 42). Companies often do not know who they should contact. Investigations can be very time-consuming, and prosecutions even more so. Prosecutions can also be expensive and, as we have seen, sentences are often light. There is also a fear that publicizing the crime will give others ideas, including perhaps even ideas about methods of attack (Conly, 1989, pp. 42–43).

The existing laws do not seem to fit computer crimes neatly, and those sitting in judgment on these cases are generally not familiar with the underlying technology involved. Thefts of information may not seem so important to a judge or jury who have no personal use for such information. To courts that are overburdened with violent crimes, a little pilfering of funds where no one is hurt or even threatened may not seem very serious. So, for a variety or reasons, many computer crimes are not discovered or, even if they are, are not fully prosecuted. This only gives rise to an increase in computer crimes which, as we have already discussed, are damaging to the stability of society.

The European Cybercrime Treaty   An international law enforcement treaty, led by the Council of Europe, and also involving the United States, Canada, Japan, and South Africa, was drafted in June 2001 and signed on November 23, 2001, by the countries involved. The articles of the treaty will regulate illegal access, data or system interference, "misuse of devices," computer-related forgery and fraud, child pornography, and copyright, among other items.[62]

 OBSERVATIONS

The activities discussed in this chapter are clearly *crimes*. They are not only immoral, they are illegal. Thus they pose no serious ethical dilemmas; we can clearly see that they are wrong. As Aristotle said in the *Nicomachean Ethics*, we recognize that murder is bad on its face, and we give it a negative name. The same is true of theft, fraud, and cheating; they are bad actions, and no less bad because they are committed with a computer instead of a knife or a gun. So what is ethically important about the material in this chapter is to make people aware of the extent and nature of computer crimes, and to point out that they *are* crimes, and not just intellectual games with no victims. It is also important to see that the present system is not set up to handle these crimes, and needs rethinking so that it can do so effectively. A move in the right direction may be the proposed Cyber Security Enhancement Act of 2001 (H. R. 3482) which would allow judges to consider factors such as the potential and actual loss from an online crime, the level of sophistication of the crime, whether the crime was committed for personal benefit, how it affects Internet privacy, and whether government computers were compromised.[63]

■ ENDNOTES

1. *Software Engineering Notes* 12, no. 2 (April 1987), 4.

2. Peter G. Neumann, "Fraud by Computer," *Communications of the ACM* 35, no. 8 (August 1992), 154.

3. "The Spreading Danger of Computer Crime," *Business Week*, 20 April 1981, pp. 86–88.

4. *Software Engineering Notes* 12, no. 4 (October 1987), 18.

5. Winn Schwartau, *Information Warfare: Chaos on the Electronic Superhighway* (New York: Thunder's Mouth Press, 1994), pp. 308–309.

6. *Software Engineering Notes* 17, no. 4 (October 1992), 9.

7. John Greenwald, "Your Chips or Your Life!", *Technology Review* 143, no. 18 (May 2, 1994), 69.

8. Found in notes I took a long time ago from *Computers and Society: A Reader*, ed. Robert Teague and Clint Erikson (St. Paul, MN: West, 1974).

9. "The Spreading Danger of Computer Crime," *Business Week*, 20 April 1981, p. 88; Martin Wasik, *Crime and the Computer* (Oxford, England: Clarendon Press, 1991), pp. 193–94; and Donn B. Parker, *Computer Crime* (Washington, DC: National Institute of Justice, 1989), pp. 166–67. See also Bruce Henderson and Jeffrey Young, "The Heist," *Esquire*, May 1981, pp. 36–47.

10. *Business Week*, 20 April 1981, p. 88; Thomas Whiteside, I, "Annals of Crime," *New Yorker*, 22 August 1977, pp. 42–49.

11. *Business Week*, 20 April 1981, p. 88.

12. *Software Engineering Notes* 17, no. 3 (July 1992), 10. In 1990, the General Accounting Office (GAO) warned that a serious breach of the U.S. banking system for EFT could be possible, because of inadequate security to prevent sabotage, fraud, or backup in case of breakdown (Steven Mufson, "GAO Calls Security Inadequate in Electronic Fund Transfers," *Washington Post*, 21 February 1990, sec. C, p. 3).

13. Ann W. O'Neill, "Man Pleads Guilty to Role in Illegal Wire Transfer," *Los Angeles Times*, 28 March 1995, p. B2.

14. Bernd Debusmann (Prague, 2 November 1993), "Czech Transition Spurs Boom in Economic Crime." Retold in *Software Engineering Notes* 19, no. 1 (January 1994), 7.

15. *Software Engineering Notes* 19, no. 1 (January 1994), 6.

16. *Software Engineering Notes* 23, 1 (January 1998), 14.

17. Jerry Knight, "SEC Finally Takes Up Halifax Embezzlement," *Washington Post*, 11 January 2001, p. E9ff.

18. "Bank Swindle Undone by Guilt: Vault Manager Turned Himself In," *Times-Picayune* (New Orleans, LA), 17 April 2001, p. A01.

19. *Software Engineering Notes* 16, no. 4 (October 1991), 8. See also Andy Zipser, "Terrible Toll," *Barron's*, 25 November 1991, p. 24.

20. *Software Engineering Notes* 12, no. 2 (April 1987), 8–9.

21. *Software Engineering Notes* 17, no. 4 (October 1992), 10.

22. "Criminal-History Data Leakage and Tampering," *Software Engineering Notes* 18, no. 4 (October 1993), 3.

23. *Software Engineering Notes* 12, no. 1 (January 1987), 13–14.

24. *Software Engineering Notes* 19, no. 2 (April 1994), 9.

25. *Software Engineering Notes* 19, no. 2 (April 1994), 7.

26. Michael Allen, "To Repair Bad Credit, Advisers Give Clients Someone Else's Data," *Wall Street Journal,* 14 August 1990, sec. A, p. 1. See also Michael D. Hinds, "The New-Fashioned Way to Steal Money: Fake Credit," *New York Times,* 31 December 1988, sec. A, p. 28; Simson L. Garfinkle, "Putting More Teeth in Consumer Rights," *Christian Science Monitor,* 8 August 8 1990, p. 13; and *Software Engineering Notes* 13, 4 (October 1988), 6–7.

27. *Software Engineering Notes* 16, no. 2 (April 1991), 16.

28. John T. McQuiston, "Four Charged with Theft Via Computer," *New York Times,* 18 March 1995, p. A25.

29. Ashley Dunn, "On Line, and Inside Credit Card Security," *New York Times,* 19 March 1995, sec. 1, p. 37.

30. *Software Engineering Notes* 18, no. 1 (January 1993), 14.

31. Arthur Goldsmith, "Photos Always Lied," *Popular Photography* 98, no. 11 (November 1991), 68–75. See also Malcolm W. Browne, "Computers as Accessory to Photo Fakery," *New York Times International,* 24 July 1991, sec. A, p. 6.

32. Paul McCarthy, "Antimatter: UFO Update," *Omni* 13, no. 6 (March 1991), 73.

33. Peter G. Neumann, "RISKS in Computerized Elections," *Communications of the ACM* 33, no. 11 (November 1990), 170. Cf. *Software Engineering Notes* 15, no. 1 (January 1990), 10–13.

34. "U.S. Study Faults Vote-Count Systems That Use Computers," *Wall Street Journal,* 7 November 1988, sec. B, p. 5. See also Ivars Peterson, "Making Votes Count," *Science News* 144, no. 18 (October 30, 1993), 282–83, which mentions a St. Petersburg, Florida, municipal election in which there was concern about possible computer tampering. For example, in the mayoral race, a precinct with no registered voters "suddenly acquired 7,331 voters, of whom 1,429 had cast ballots. The controversial incumbent mayor had won the race by just 1,425 votes" (p. 283).

35. I owe this analysis of auditing techniques to Jerry Erion, a double major in both accounting and philosophy, who graduated in May 1994, attended graduate school in philosophy at the University of Buffalo (SUNY), and is now teaching at Medaille College. He also helped me track down a number of the case references for this book.

36. Karen A. Frenkel, "Computers and Elections," *Communications of the ACM* 31, no. 10 (October 1988), 1182–83.

37. Christopher B. Daly, "IRS Charges Tax Preparer with $1.1 Million Fraud." Reported in the *Washington Post* newswire, and retold in *Software Engineering Notes* 19, no. 2 (April 1994), 5–6. The next *SEN* report on p. 6 tells of a man who had collected half a million dollars by filing W-2 forms and tax returns for *real* people who were too poor to file returns and collecting their rebates. All of this was done electronically on computerized returns. He was sentenced to 2 1/2 years in jail; he estimates that no more than 25 percent of fraudulent returns are detected. One consultant estimates that the true cost of such returns could be billions of dollars.

An IRS investigation reported that 350 of its workers had been investigated for snooping through IRS files of acquaintances and celebrities, and that at least six employees had used the IRS computers to prepare bogus returns yielding refunds (Rick Wartzman, "IRS Probe of Snooping by Employees Will Be Focus of Senate Panel Hearing," *Wall Street Journal*, 4 August 1993, sec. C, p. 24).

The first detected case of computerized tax return fraud was a Boston bookkeeper charged with filing $325,000 in fraudulent tax-refund claims electronically, reported in 1989 (*Wall Street Journal*, 17 August 1989, sec. A, p. 7).

38. *Software Engineering Notes* 22, no. 2 (March 1997), 24.

39. *Software Engineering Notes* 23, no. 1 (January 1998), 14.

40. *Software Engineering Notes* 22, no. 5 (September 1997), 14.

41. Daniel Kadlec, "Crimes and Misdeminors," *Time*, 2 October 2000, pp. 52–4.

42. Dan Verton, "The Enemy Within," *Computerworld,* 9 July 2001, pp. 34–5. See also Matthew L. Lease, "Identity Theft: A Fast-growing Crime," *FBI Law Enforcement Bulletin* 69, 8 (August 2000), 8–13. Celent Communications analyst Sang Lee predicts that reported incidents of identity theft will more than triple, from 500,000 in 2000 to 1.7 million by 2005, and that the biggest threat is from online information brokers (W. A. Lee, "Tripling of Identity-Theft Cases Projected by '05'," *American Banker* 167, 200 (October 18, 2001), 18.

43. "Couple Convicted of Pornography Sold Over Computer Network," *New York Times*, 31 July 1994, p. 15.

44. Philip Elmer-Dewitt, "On a Screen Near You: Cyberporn," *Time Magazine*, 3 July 1995, pp. 38–45.

45. For example, see the writings of Catharine MacKinnon, including *Only Words* (Cambridge, MA: Harvard University Press, 1993).

46. *Software Engineering Notes* 12, no. 4 (October 1987), 6.

47. "Cunning Copiers," *Wall Street Journal*, 31 December 1992, sec. A, p. 1; Andrew Pollack, "Computers Used in a New Crime: Desktop Forgery," *New York Times*, 8 October 1990, sec. A, p. 1; "Technology Is Called Aid to Counterfeiting," *New York Times*, 15 July 1990, Sec. 1, p. 16; "Information Age: Color Copiers Make It Easy to Counterfeit," *Wall Street Journal*, 21 April 1992, sec. B, p. 7. In Rick Wartzman's article, "Counterfeit Bills Confound Detectors at the Fed, Sleuths at the Secret Service," *Wall Street Journal*, 3 July 1992, it was reported that even the Federal Reserve Board was having difficulty recognizing a batch of counterfeit $100 bills, and that the quality of the counterfeit bills was so good that the FRB was not holding the institutions where they were deposited responsible but was absorbing the loss itself.

48. "Technology: Forgery in the Home Office," *Time* 135, no. 13 (March 26, 1990), pp. 69–71. But see also Lamont Wood, "Don't Try This at Home," *Compute*, August 1993, pp. 61–64.

49. "World Wire: Forgeries Soar in Russia," *Wall Street Journal*, 7 July 1993, sec. A, p. 6.

50. Bill McAllister, "Postal Form Aimed at Counterfeiters," *Washington Post*, 27 March 1991, sec. A, p. 21.

51. Kelley Holland, "Stalking the Credit-Card Scamsters," *Business Week [International Edition]*, 17 January 1994, pp. 68–69; Jerry Knight, "On PINs and Needles Over ATMs: Counterfeiting Scams Raise Security Worries," *Washington Post*, 21 May 1993, sec. G, p. 1.

52. "Visa International," *Wall Street Journal*, 28 February 1992, sec. C, p. 11.

53. www.aba.com/Press+Room/ATMfacts2001.htm

54. Mark Trumbull, "Rise in Check Fraud Puts Banks on Guard," *Christian Science Monitor*, 12 January 1993, p. 7.

55. *Software Engineering Notes* 17, no. 2 (April 1992), 12–13.

56. *Wall Street Journal*, 4 April 1985, p. 10.

57. "Business Bulletin: Holograms Help," *Wall Street Journal*, 9 September 1993, sec. A, p. 1.

58. Kenneth N. Gilpin, "Canon's Copiers Leave Money-Making to the Mint," *New York Times*, 1 October 1992, sec. D, p. 4.

59. According to Tom Forester and Perry Morrison, *Computer Ethics* (Cambridge, MA: MIT Press, 1994), p. 49.

60. Zachary Tobias, "Deadly Pursuit," *Computerworld*, 9 July 2001, p. 44. See also James R. Borck, "Leave the Cybersleuthing to the Experts," *Infoworld*, 9 April 2001, p. 54.

61. Dan Verton, "Cybercrime Costs on the Rise in U.S.," *Computerworld*, 19 March 2001, p. 10.

62. Pimm Fox, "Riding the Cybercrime Wave," *Computerworld*, 9 July 2001, p. 56. See also Brian Krebs, "Thirty Nations Sign Global Cybercrime Treaty," *Post-Newsweek Business Information Newsbytes*, 26 November 2001.

63. "Bill Strengthens Internet Criminal Sentencing," *Newsbytes*, 20 December 2001.

■ SHORT ESSAY QUESTIONS

1. A federal statute requires banks to give their customers "quick access" to funds from deposited checks. Given the problems we have seen with counterfeit checks, do you think this is a good law? Carefully assess all sides of the issue. If you could influence the federal government, how would you advise it to change or improve the law?

2. Reports on computer crime (not including software piracy and hacking among computer crimes) in newspapers and journals seem to be decreasing. Do as thorough a search as you can for, say, the past six months and document the most recently reported occurrences. Does a pattern seem to emerge about the kinds of reported computer crime that are popular this year?

3. If you were the manager of a bank, how would you try to protect your bank against computerized embezzlement and fraud?

4. You run a big insurance company and you are concerned about security. You have the opportunity to hire someone who pulled off a $4 million computer "heist" from another insurance company, has "paid his debt to society," and is just coming off his six-month stint in jail. Would you hire him as the security expert to protect your company? Discuss.

5. Chapter 4 deals with software piracy, this chapter deals with computer crime, and Chapter 6 deals with hacking and computer break-ins. Carefully examine the similarities and differences among these three classes of "computer abuse."

■ LONG ESSAY QUESTIONS

1. Comment thoroughly and critically on a proposal to keep many convicted criminals on an "out-patient" ("out-convict"?) basis by fitting them with nonremovable remote computer monitoring devices (perhaps even implants) that will report to a central computer on their whereabouts, activities, and so on.

2. A committee of Congress has been presented with a proposal for a "crime-prediction" program (something like the Inslaw "tracking" software discussed in Chapter 4) that would "pattern-match" data on suspicious characters and attempt to predict whether, when, and where they might commit crimes. Discuss both sides of this proposal critically.

3. Discuss critically the proposal that a crime should be tried and punished in exactly the same way, whether it involved the use of a computer or not (that is, penalties shouldn't be lighter for computer-aided crimes). Imagine a range of computer-aided crimes that might be committed, from the obvious robbery to arson and murder.

4. There are various theories of punishment (including vengeance, restitution, and deterrence). Read the article on "Punishment" in the *Encyclopedia of Philosophy*, track down at least two of the references on the topic that appear in the bibliography, and write a carefully considered essay on what the proper function for punishment should be. Try to connect your thinking and examples to possible applications of your theory (the one you choose after comparing the alternatives) to the area of computer crime and punishment.

■ REFERENCES AND RECOMMENDED READINGS

Allen, Michael. "To Repair Bad Credit, Advisers Give Clients Someone Else's Data." *Wall Street Journal*, 14 August 1990, sec. A, p. 1.

Bakewell, Eric J., et al. "Computer Crimes." *The American Criminal Law Review* 38, 3 (Summer 2001), 481–524.

Bequai, August. *Computer Crime.* Lexington, MA: Lexington Books, 1978.

Bequai, August. *Technocrimes*. Lexington, MA: Lexington Books/D.C. Heath, 1987.

Bliss, Edwin C., and Isamu S. Aoki. *Are Your Employees Stealing You Blind?* Amsterdam, Netherlands: Pfeiffer & Co., 1993.

Bloombecker, Buck. *Spectacular Computer Crimes: What They Are and How They Cost American Business Half a Billion Dollars a Year!* Homewood, IL: Dow Jones-Irwin, 1990.

BloomBecker, Jay, ed. "Computer Crime, Computer Security, Computer Ethics." Los Angeles, CA: National Center for Computer Crime Data, 1986.

Borck, James R. "Leave the Cybersleuthing to the Experts." *Infoworld*, 9 April 2001, p. 54.

Chantico Publishing Co., Inc. *Combating Computer Crime: Prevention, Detection, Investigation*. New York: McGraw-Hill, 1992.

Churbuck, David. "Desktop Forgery." *Forbes*, 27 November 1989, 246–54.

Computer Crime and Computer Security: Hearing Before the Subcommittee on Crime, U.S. House of Representatives, May 23, 1985. Washington, DC: U.S. Government Printing Office, 1986.

Computer Professionals for Social Responsibility (CPSR). "Vulnerable on All Counts: How Computerized Vote Tabulation Threatens the Integrity of Our Elections—An Election Watch Report." In *Ethical Issues in Information Systems*, eds. Roy DeJoie, George Fowler, and David Paradice (Boston: Boyd & Fraser, 1991), pp. 155–66.

Conly, Catherine H. *Organizing for Computer Crime Investigation and Prosecution*. Washington, DC: National Institute of Justice, July 1989.

Drucker, Susan Jo. "Cybercrime and Punishment." *Critical Studies in Media Communications* 17, 2 (June 2000), 133–158.

Elmer-Dewitt, Philip. "On a Screen Near You: Cyberporn." *Time*, 3 July 1995, pp. 38–45.

Forester, Tom, and Perry Morrison. *Computer Ethics: Cautionary Tales and Ethical Dilemmas in Computing*. 2nd ed. Cambridge, MA: MIT Press, 1994, ch. 2.

Frenkel, Karen A. "Computers and Elections." *Communications of the ACM* 31, no. 10 (October 1988), 1176–83.

Garn, Jake. "The U.S. Must Tighten Laws to Punish Counterfeiters." *USA Today*, May 1992, pp. 75–76.

Goldsmith, Arthur. "Photos Always Lied." *Popular Photography* 98, no. 11 (November 1991), 68–75.

Greenwald, John. "Your Chips or Your Life!" *Technology Review* 143, no. 18 (May 2, 1994), 69.

Hatcher, Michael. "Computer Crimes." *The American Criminal Law Review* 36, 3 (Summer 1999), 397–444.

Hecht, Jeff. "U.S. Counts Cost of Computer Counterfeiting." *New Scientist* 141, no. 1907 (January 8, 1994), 19.

Hussain, Donna S., and Khateeb M. Hussain. *The Computer Challenge: Technology, Applications, and Social Implications.* Santa Rosa, CA: Burgess Communications, 1986.

Johnson, Deborah G. *Computer Ethics.* 2nd ed. Englewood Cliffs, NJ: Prentice-Hall, 1994, ch. 6. Or see ch. 4 in 3rd ed. (2001).

Kadlec, Daniel. "Crimes and Misdeminors." *Time*, 2 October 2000, pp. 52–54.

Kizza, Joseph M. *Ethics in the Computer Age: ACM Conference Proceedings* (November 11–13, 1994). New York: ACM, 1994.

Kling, Rob. "When Organizations Are Perpetrators: Assumptions About Computer Abuse and Computer Crime." In *Computerization and Controversy: Value Conflicts and Social Choices*, eds. Charles Dunlop and Rob Kling. Boston, MA: Academic Press, 1991, pp. 676–92.

Lease, Matthew, "Identity Theft: A Fast-growing Crime." *FBI Law Enforcement Bulletin* 69, 8 (August 2000), 8–13.

The Ladykillers (British movie, 1955).

Mandell, Steven M. "Computer Crime." In *Computers, Ethics and Society*, eds. M. David Ermann, Mary B. Williams, and Claudio Gutierrez. New York: Oxford University Press, 1990, pp. 342–53.

McEwen, J. Thomas. Report Contributors: Dennis Fester and Hugh Nugent. *Dedicated Computer Crime Units.* Washington, DC: National Institute of Justice, June 1989.

Nicholson, Lauren J. "Computer Crimes." *The American Criminal Law Review* 37, 2 (Spring 2000), 207–59.

Parker, Donn B. *Computer Crime: Criminal Justice Resource Manual.* Washington, DC: National Institute of Justice, 1989.

Parker, Donn B., and Susan H. Nycum. "Computer Crime." *Communications of the ACM* 27, no. 4 (April 1984), 313–15.

Parker, Donn B. "Fighting Cybercrime: Good and Bad Objectives." *Computer Security Journal* 15, 1 (Winter 1999), 11–24.

Peterzell, Jay. "Spying and Sabotage by Computer." *Time* 133, no. 12 (March 20, 1989), 25–26.

Philippsohn, Steven. "Trends in Cybercrime." *Computers & Security* 20, 1 (February 2001), 53.

Power, Richard. "2001 CSI/FBI Computer Crime and Security Survey." *Computer Security Journal* 17, 2 (Spring 2001), 29–51.

Rosen, Jeffrey. "Cheap Speech: Will the Old First Amendment Battles Survive the New Technologies?" *New Yorker*, 7 August 1995, pp. 75–80.

Saltman, Roy E. "Accuracy, Integrity, and Security in Computerized Vote-Tallying." *Communications of the ACM* 31, no. 10 (October 1988), 1184–91, 1218. Available online at: **www.itl.nist.gov/lab/specpubs/500-158.htm**

Schwartau, Winn. *Information Warfare: Chaos on the Electronic Superhighway*. New York: Thunder's Mouth Press, 1994.

Steier, Rosalie, ed. "Congress Tackles Computer Abuse." *Communications of the ACM* 27, no. 1 (January 1984), 10–11.

Tinnin, David B. "How IBM Stung Hitachi." In Ermann et al., 1990, pp. 331–42.

Wasik, Martin. *Crime and the Computer*. Oxford, England: Clarendon Press, 1991.

Whiteside, Thomas. "Annals of Crime: Dead Souls in the Computer. I & II." *New Yorker*, I: 22 August 1977, pp. 35–65 passim; II: 29 August 1977, 34–64 passim.

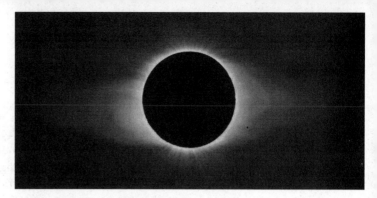

Chapter 6

Computer Intruders, Viruses, and All That

*T*here are many ways in which the significant potential of the computer for good can be misused. We saw a number of abuses in the chapters on piracy and computer crime. This chapter is devoted to other computer misuses, generally carried out by people who are very good with computers. Many of these abuses are done in the spirit of a game, or a challenge, or just as an intellectual exercise. Most of the perpetrators do not feel that they are doing any real harm. Nevertheless, the various kinds of misuses of the computer discussed in this chapter all have the potential to cause harm. Though some are amusing, and most are clever, the reader should keep in mind throughout the moral implications of these activities.

MORE WAYS TO STEAL USING COMPUTERS

Chapter 5 included many examples of embezzlement, theft of information or services, and fraud by computer. A few cases have been saved for this chapter, because they are generally carried out by knowledgeable programmers whose main motivation may well be the thrill of "beating the system" rather than monetary gain.

Thefts of Money

Generally, thefts of money involve banks (because "that's where the money is," as Willie Sutton once sagely observed) or electronic funds transfer (EFT) to and from banks. This "invisible" money wafting through the airwaves provides an often irresistible temptation to an enterprising programmer to intercept a transmission and reroute the funds, usually to his or her own account. Just having computers handle the payrolls and deposit accounts for large companies provides a significant potential for program modification that may manipulate these funds in ways not intended by the companies.

Roundoff Errors   There is a story, though we have no particular names or places to cite, about programmers taking advantage of computer "roundoff errors" to their own advantage. The fact that we have no names to put to the story may mean that it is apocryphal, or it may just mean that they got away with it.

A computer stores values in binary notation (0s and 1s), as we have seen. Any integer (whole-number) value can be stored precisely in binary, as long as it does not exceed the size of a "word" (or location) in computer memory.[1]

Matters are not so accurate when it comes to fractions. The only decimal fractions that can be stored precisely on a finite binary machine are those that are combinations of negative powers of 2, such as 1/2 (0.5), 1/4 (0.25), 3/8 (0.375), etc. Obviously, then, only 50 cents, 25 cents, and 75 cents in decimal money amounts can be represented exactly in binary. The algorithm to convert a decimal fraction to binary is to multiply by 2, collect the whole number part of the result, retain the fractional part of the result, and repeat (from "multiply by 2") until *either* you reach a fractional part of 0 (zero), in which case you have an exact binary equivalent, *or* carry out the result to a predetermined number of places.

For example, 0.40 (or 40 cents) converts to the infinitely repeating binary fraction 0.011001100110... (the pattern 0110 repeats forever). Thus, on a binary computer with only a few bits (binary digits, stored in binary devices) to represent the fraction, the rest of it will be "lopped off" and treated as if it were zero. So the binary value actually stored is *less than* the decimal value 0.4. If this is then used in a calculation, say, of the pay of a worker who receives $6.40 an hour and works 40 hours, on a computer that allows only eight bits for the fractional part of a value, instead of receiving a paycheck for a gross amount of $256.00, the check may be only for $255.94; if 12 bits are used for the fractional part, it will be for $255.97, and so on.[2]

An employee is not likely to make a fuss about the lack of 6 cents, 3 cents, or less in a paycheck, and may not even bother to calculate it out to note the discrepancy. Even if the slight error is noted, the employee is most likely to chalk it up to "computer error" and grumble a bit, but not make waves. There *are* ways to handle this calculation so that the amounts come out correct, such as calculating the amount of cents per hour times the hours worked, and placing the decimal point before the check is written (since the integer 640 can be represented precisely in binary, as 1010000000).

The story goes, however, that the programmers writing the payroll program did not try to rectify the paycheck errors, but rather wrote a program patch that would divert the extra 6 cents or less that was not put into each employee's paycheck into their own accounts! On the surface, everything looked all right, since the accountants expected to pay out the full amounts (in our example's case, the full $256.00), and so it was there to be paid.

The Salami Technique The "*salami*" technique gained considerable notoriety when it was first discussed in Donn Parker's 1976 book, *Crime by Computer*. It is a method of "slicing" small amounts that will not be noticed off many accounts and accumulating the totals in your own account. Thus, the "roundoff error" approach discussed in the previous section is a kind of salami technique. Generally, the slices taken are not due to a computer roundoff error, but rather are very small amounts in an actual account that will go unnoticed. If one were to "slice" 10 cents off of each of 150,000 accounts, the net gain would be $15,000 (with no effort other than writing the original program patch). If this were done every other month, it would represent a quite comfortable income!

We are reminded here of the argument Alec Guinness used on Mrs. Wilburforce in *The Ladykillers*, a film discussed in the previous chapter. If no one notices the little bit that he steals from each of them, does that make it all right? What if everyone (or even just 10,000 people) did the same thing? Then certainly the discrepancies would be noticeable, even missing from the original criminal's own accounts! What sort of character is one developing by doing this? It undermines trust and the financial structure of our society, on which the lives and health of many depend.

Parker notes, "Salami techniques are usually not fully discoverable within obtainable expenditures for investigation. Victims have usually lost so little individually that they are unwilling to expend much effort to solve the case" (Parker, 1976, p. 19). The criminals are more often caught because of inexplicable changes in their lifestyles (fast cars, expensive houses, large losses at gambling, and so on).

Rounded-Down Bank Interest Mungo and Clough (1992, pp. 161–62) tell of a bank employee who discovered that the bank he worked for, in calculating interest on its millions of accounts, only rounded up if the fraction of a penny was 3/4 (0.75) or more (the usual approach is to round up anything 1/2 or more), and anything less than that went back to the bank. The employee wrote a program modification that transferred these interest amounts of less than 3/4 of one cent into his own account. Again, this story is based on hearsay, but it does point out how simple it is to commit fraud in computerized bank accounts.

Breaking In and Entering

Phreaking Then and Now The word 'phreak' seems to be an amalgamation of 'phone', 'free', and 'freak'. It is used to describe people who access the telephone services illegally and run up considerable calling bills for which they are never charged. In the 1950s, Bell Telephone Company decided to base its direct-dial system on a set of twelve electronically-generated tones. The tones were supposed to be a company trade secret, but Bell published information about the tones used to route long-distance calls in an article in the *Bell System Technical Journal* in 1954, and more information on actually dialing using the tones in another article in 1960. "The journal was intended only for Bell's technical staff, but the company had apparently forgotten that most engineering colleges subscribed to it as well" (Mungo and Clough, 1992, p. 7) The result was that many bright young engineers began constructing "blue boxes" to create Bell's tones, and thus access the phone lines for free. They called these blue boxes MF-ers—for "multifrequency transmitters"—and perhaps to convey a double meaning as well (Mungo and Clough, 1992, p. 7).

In the October 1971 issue of *Esquire* magazine, Ron Rosenbaum wrote an article on "The Secrets of the Little Blue Box," and the secret came out in the open. The article made famous a young blind college student, Joe Engressia, who had perfect pitch, and discovered that he could whistle the Bell tones for long-distance calling. An even more infamous early phreaker was John T. Draper, a friend of Joe Engressia's, nicknamed "Captain Crunch" because he discovered that a toy whistle in the box of Cap'n Crunch cereal could be used to create the Bell long-distance tone. Working with another man, he began building and selling blue boxes, many to blind people, in California. Draper liked to play games with long-distance calls, sending them around the world.

Draper was eventually caught and sent to jail, where he was coerced into telling many criminal elements how to "phreak" out Ma Bell. Draper was closely monitored after his jail term, was sent to jail a second time in 1979, and seemed to give up phreaking after that. Before his first arrest, "Captain Crunch" had hung around the Personal Computer Company (PCC) and the Homebrew Computer Club; two members of Homebrew were Steve Jobs and Steve Wozniak, who began manufacturing blue boxes at an assembly-line rate. They next built the line of Apple computers, which were a greater success than anyone had imagined. Draper even wrote software for the Apple II—one of the first word-processing programs, called EasyWriter.[3]

Although Draper and his cronies no longer seem to be in business, there have been many to take their place recently. The computerized handling of telecommunication has opened the door for new kinds of phreaking, or gaining free access to telecommunication lines. Voice mail and e-mail are especially tempting targets, especially for nuisance value, but the PBX lines for big businesses are even more lucrative. A PBX often has a Remote Access Unit for employees to call from outside the office and access a long-distance line that is charged to the company. Someone who is not an employee who figures out how to do this can run up huge phone bills against the company. Some hackers run "call-sell" operations, where they sell access to a company's long-distance PBX, often on the street (Mungo and Clough, 1992, p. 155).

A plethora of different-colored "boxes" like the original "blue box" seems to have developed. They include a "green box" that lets the user emulate the coin return and coin collect signals, a "red box" and an "aero box" that let the user make free phone calls from a pay phone, a "mauve box" that lets the user tap a phone, a "gold box" that lets the user trace a call or tell if a call is being traced, a "rainbow box" that kills a trace, a "black box" that lets the user place a call without being billed for it, a "tron box" that supposedly makes your electric meter run slower, and a number of different boxes that allow the user to do various mischief (including listening in) to a neighbor's phone line.

Leslie Lynne Doucette, a 36-year-old Canadian living in Chicago sometimes described as the "female Fagin" of the computer underworld, ran a large-scale business in illegal credit cards, telephone credit cards, PBX access codes, and so on, in 1988 and 1989. She involved as many as 150 young people (all minors) in her racket. When her apartment was raided, the authorities found numbers for 171 phone credit cards, authorization codes for 39 PBXs, and numbers for 118 Visa cards, 150 Master Charge cards, and 2 American Express cards. It was estimated that she had accounted for $1.6

million in charges to credit card companies and telephone charges. Her lawyer plea-bargained her case, and she received 27 months in prison, "one of the most severe sentences ever given to a computer hacker in the United States" (Mungo and Clough, 1992, pp. 153–161).

Ten students from the University of Kent (England) admitted making long distance calls valued at roughly $1 million in 1991.[4] In 1988, *Software Engineering Notes* reported Nevada teenagers using a "blue-box" to make $650,000 in illegal phone calls, and the arrest of teenagers in Corte Madera, California, for making $150,000 in illegal calls. The *Houston Chronicle* reported on December 6, 1990, that computer intruders had stolen roughly $12 million in free telephone service through the Johnson Space Center, using a long-distance credit-card number and NASA's phone lines. NASA denied that there was a theft.[5] Two young Norwegian males, living in a wealthy area outside of Oslo, were accused of stealing telephone services, and using phone lines to perpetrate a fraud that involved ordering items from a transport company.[6] As in other similar areas, the public probably sees only a few of the many occurrences like these, the few that get reported and the few offenders who get caught.

Software Engineering Notes reported a demonstration of a Telecom Information Service that read Prince Philip's mail and altered a financial database.[7] Investigative reporter Jeffrey Rothfeder's book, *Privacy for Sale* (1992), is full of examples of how he or people he worked with got unauthorized access to records about people, including Dan Quayle and Dan Rather, using the phone and computer. Many of these concerns about invasions of privacy will be discussed in Chapter 7, but it is appropriate to mention them here as misuses of the phone system.

Tampering with Communication Signals At the 1984 Rose Bowl, there was a scoreboard takeover to display "Cal Tech vs. MIT" as the game was in progress.[8] "Captain Midnight" preempted an HBO program for a four-minute protest against HBO scrambling its signal so that satellite owners had to pay "$12.95 a month" to receive it.[9] The Playboy Channel was illegally preempted and replaced by a religious message that warned viewers to "repent your sins"; a CBN (Christian Broadcast Network) employee was convicted, and faced up to 11 years in prison and up to a $350,000 fine (Playboy plays hard ball!).[10] In November 1987, two Chicago television channels (WGN-TV and WTTW) were taken over for short unauthorized broadcasts, in one of which the masked bandit "mooned" the audience.[11] These incidents are generally amusing, though they do have the potential to be quite disruptive and even dangerous.

The disruption of financial transmissions through satellite or other telecommunication tampering has obvious negative impact, in a world where split-second timing often makes or breaks a deal. If transmissions of information or energy to hospitals are disrupted, the health and even lives of many can be put in danger.

Roughly $2 billion of software was stolen over the Internet in 1993, and the Software Publishers Association estimates that $7.4 billion was lost to piracy that year. In 2000, the estimate of computer software losses due to theft was $12.2 billion.[12] Proprietary software has occasionally been uploaded from break-ins to computers on college campuses.

A "HACKER" BY ANY OTHER NAME

The Original, "Good" Hackers

The *Oxford English Dictionary* defines a *hacker* as a person who hacks (cuts, mutilates), or hoes with a hack (a tool for breaking earth), or picks a quarrel, or mangles words (does not make sense). A new meaning for the word grew up in the 1950s and in the MIT Artificial Intelligence Laboratory culture in the 1960s. According to Steven Levy, in *Hackers: Heroes of the Computer Revolution*, hackers were "adventurers, visionaries, risk-takers, artists . . . and the ones who most clearly saw why the computer was truly a revolutionary tool" (Levy, 1985, p. ix). Levy characterizes the **Hacker Ethic** of the 1950s as follows:

> Access to computers—and anything which might teach you about the way the world works—should be unlimited and total. Always yield to the Hands-On Imperative. (p. 40)

It was the hackers' version of Kant's Categorical Imperative—always act so as to promote knowledge, especially of computers, for everyone. Hackers truly wanted this maxim of behavior to be universalized, so that everyone would behave as they (who had already seen the light) did. This would create the best world for all, in which the computer could be truly used to benefit humanity, and everyone would share in the benefits.

The proponents of this view believed that art and beauty could be created on a computer, and that a hacker should be judged strictly on performance (hacking on the computer), not by "bogus criteria" such as race, sex, age, position, or degrees, according to Levy. The hacker dream was realized—for a while—at the MIT Artificial Intelligence Lab, which had government grants for project MAC (Multiple-Access Computing, and Machine-Aided Cognition).

Here hackers could work freely with sophisticated machines, "shielded from the bureaucratic lunacy of the outside world" (Levy, 1985, p. 56).

These old-style hackers certainly were not immoral; they harmed no one. They were interested in furthering knowledge (their own and that of others), and stood for a principle—that information and computer access should be freely available to all.

Levy describes Richard M. Stallman (RMS) as "the last of the true hackers." Stallman stayed at MIT from 1971 through 1983, and saw it undergo a transformation from a hacker heaven (and haven) to a more bureaucratic, profit-minded entity that he came to hate. Stallman grieved at the "fall" of the AI Lab, and during that period would tell strangers that his wife had died. He wrote that he used to wander through the halls of the AI Lab at night and think, "Oh my poor AI lab! You are dying and I can't save you!" (Levy, 1985, p. 431). While at the AI Lab, Stallman had created the free software EMACS, to be freely shared with and modified by anyone, as long as they contributed their improvements to the "EMACS commune." He left MIT so that they could claim no proprietary control over his effort to promote free software (Levy, 1985, Epilogue, pp. 421–440).

We see, from Levy's account and others, that the early hackers were just very talented computer programmers and designers (of both hardware and software), who felt that this "brave new world" was full of wonderful opportunities, and that no restrictions should be placed on anyone trying to take advantage of them. Hackers were "a breed apart," huddled over their computers from morning well into the night, enjoying the challenges that this new medium gave them. Sometimes they were considered computer "nerds." They certainly were not destructive; much the opposite, they were interested in what they could do constructively with this marvelous new tool.

The part about "free access" to computer technology for all is what gets carried over from this older breed of hackers (of which Stallman may well have been the last, as Levy claims) to the new class of people that are currently called hackers.

The New Breed of Destructive Hackers

Today, anyone who breaks into, or in any way gains unauthorized access to, a computer system is called a "hacker." The term *hacker*—which was originally rather complimentary, referring to someone who was really good at doing amazing things with a computer—in current usage has negative connotations. It refers to anyone who breaks into a computer and/or damages data, programs, or the system.

Why do these less creative and more destructive hackers do what they do? The reasons seem to be much like those we discussed for the computer criminals—"because it's there!", it's a game, it's a challenge, you can "beat the system," you can get back at monolithic institutions like the bank or the phone company or the government, you can use it to make a political statement, and so on. Regardless of their success, we should look at the intentions of these hackers to assess their moral worth. Do any of the reasons suggested pass moral muster, especially when weighed against the value of a stable community?

There are a number of different forms that bad hacking can take, and we will examine those next.

Scanning A computer program that automatically generates a sequence of phone numbers, credit card numbers, passwords, or the like to try against some system entry test is performing a procedure called "scanning." An example of this occurred in the movie *War Games*, where the young hacker used a scanning program to search for phone numbers that responded with a computer data carrier tone. These programs are sometimes referred to as "Demon Programs." The best way to protect against one of these programs that just keeps trying card numbers or passwords until one works is to limit the number of attempts, cutting off the option to access the system after a certain number of failures (say, three) (Parker, 1989, p. 10).

Cracking Passwords To enter a computer system, one usually needs a usercode and a password. Usercodes are often the person's name or a variant on it, and so are relatively easy to get. The user has picked a password, so one must guess or use some other method to "crack" the password code. This is a little bit like safe-cracking—you can make a good guess, try out a number of combinations, look for the combination (password) written someplace nearby, or use some other means to get around the lock. In safecracking, a thief might blow the lock; in the computer case, a hacker might try to find an alternate way into the system, a "back door." [13]

Of course, the most direct way to get into someone's account is to find out the password. Movies have shown us many instances where the intruder just rummages around the person's desk and finds a slip of paper with the password written on it. This is harder to do if you are trying to break into the account from a distance, such as operating over phone lines. Other techniques involve trying the person's first name or a nickname, names of spouse, children, or pets. There are some very popular passwords that get used quite often. Some people use 'password' or 'passport' or just 'pass'; we are told that the favorite passwords in Great Britain are 'fred', 'god', 'genius', and 'hacker', and that the top two in the United States are 'love' and 'sex'.[14]

Robert T. Morris, Jr., who perpetrated the infamous Internet "worm" (a self-replicating, destructive program), had a list of common passwords for gaining access to a system; some of these you might not think are so common, such as 'anthropogenic', 'baritone', 'beowulf', 'campanile' (probably popular on campuses like Morris' Cornell University, which have bell towers), 'gryphon', 'rachmaninoff', 'vertigo', and 'wombat'. Another trick is if the usercode has the form 'abc' to try 'abc', 'cba', or 'abcabc' as the password.[15] Cracking passwords has been dramatized in a number of movies, such as *War Games* (1983) and, more recently, *Sneakers* (1992), *A Clear and Present Danger* (1994), *Hackers* (1995), and *Antitrust* (2000).

Cracking a password by guessing or by scanning a pre-stored list automatically can work, but there are other means as well. Some crackers get the user to reveal the password. They may telephone the user, pretending to be a system operator, and say that there has been some trouble with the accounts and they want to check out this user's account, but they need the usercode/password to do so. Another tricky method involves creating a program that pretends to be the system log-in, and then the program just collects usercodes and passwords as people try to log on. Another method would be to inform people that the telephone number to access the computer has been changed to the number of your computer, which has a pseudo log-in program (see Parker, 1989, pp. 10–11, on "masquerading").

Once the usercode and password are determined, the system or individual user's account can be accessed. The cracker may just browse through to see what is there, or may copy files, or modify information stored there. In bank or credit accounts, or in other records on individuals, this can be done to their detriment (such as transferring money from the account) or to someone else's benefit (such as doctoring some data in school grade records or credit records). For example, in a case in Fairbanks, Alaska, a computer specialist was charged with changing the grades of a female student at the University of Alaska (two "F"s and a "D" to two "A"s and a "C").[16]

Espionage   Computer hackers belonging to the West German Chaos Computer Club broke into NASA's data network (looking for files with such key words as 'shuttle', 'challenger', and 'secret') from May through August 1987. The news report indicated that they accessed files on space shuttles and "booster rocket incidents" and that they had the ability to "manipulate at will" the data in NASA's memory banks and to paralyze the network.[17]

Cliff Stoll, an astronomer who was a computer systems manager at Lawrence Berkeley Laboratory in 1986, was led on a merry chase through computer networks worldwide to track down an intruder to the Berkeley Lab computers and over thirty others (the same person also tried to access about 400 computers on MILNET). When Stoll found a 75-cent error in the accounting for the computer at the Lab, he traced it to an unauthorized user. Instead of blocking this user out, he decided to see what he was up to, and this led him through a maze of networks following the intruder's activity.

This hacker was snooping for whatever he could get, but was primarily interested in military computers with information on SDI, the Strategic Defense Initiative ("Star Wars"). After ten months of tracking the hacker and discussing the matter with the FBI, NSA, and the CIA, Stoll learned that he had been caught. But it was not until somewhat later that Stoll learned the identity of the hacker—a West German named Markus Hess, who (along with a few cohorts) had apparently been selling printouts of the files he had broken into, as well as details on breaking into Vax computers, which networks to use, and how MILNET operates, to the KGB (Russian secret service).

When Stoll was asked by friends *why* he had pursued this hacker so relentlessly, since he had been an advocate of "creative anarchy" himself, he did some soul-searching and realized why it had been important. He writes in *The Cuckoo's Egg*: "I learned what our networks are. I had thought of them as a complicated technical device, a tangle of wires and circuits. But they're much more than that—a fragile community of people, bonded together by trust and cooperation. If that trust is broken, the community will vanish forever."[18] Stoll's ideas of *community, friendship,* and *trust* are ones we should all keep in mind when examining the ethical issues related to today's computer networks, and those who hack about in them.

A report of extensive break-ins appeared in the *New York Times* in February 1994. Security experts "citing computer-security violations of unprecedented scope" warned that intruders have been breaking into "scores of government, corporate and university computers" connected to the Internet.[19] Such break-ins continue. The "attack of the wily hackers" may be just beginning.

Other Methods of Illegal Access　Piggybacking is getting into a secured area by slipping in right behind someone who *is* cleared for access. Piggybacking access to a computer can happen if the person who was previously using a terminal did not log off properly, and the account is thus still active; one could go in and read files and the mail, and, if one were vicious, change or destroy files. Another kind of piggybacking can be done by having a second computer secretly tied into the same line as a legal user (through switching equipment), and making use of the connection when the authorized user is not active (Parker, 1989, p. 11).

Tailgating "involves connecting a computer user to a computer in the same session as and under the same identifier as another computer user whose session has been interrupted" (Parker, 1989, p. 11). This can happen when a dial-up or direct connect session is abruptly terminated, and the second user is allowed to patch into the legitimate user's account.

Superzapping comes from the name of an IBM utility program that could bypass all system controls in case of an emergency. It also could bypass the copy-protection on IBM-type software. A number of commercial Superzap programs are available, and they create a serious problem for system security if they wind up in the wrong hands. Parker discusses a classic example of superzapping, where a manager of computer operations in a New Jersey bank used a superzap-type program to make corrections in erroneous customer accounts. Impressed by how easy it was to do this, he used the program to transfer money ($128,000) into the accounts of three friends. When a bank customer noticed a shortage, the fraud was detected and the perpetrators were convicted. "The use of the Superzap program, which left no evidence of data file changes, made discovery of the fraud through normal technical means highly unlikely" (Parker, 1989, p. 13).

Once in, an unauthorized user can delete or change files, or just read or copy them. Parker says that false data entry (or "data diddling") is "usually the simplest, safest, and most common method used in computer abuse" (Parker, 1989, p. 12). He gives an example of a timekeeping clerk who filled out forms claiming overtime hours for workers who often did work overtime, but put his own employee number on the forms; the people who looked at the books looked only at the names, which seemed to represent reasonable time charges; the computer, which dealt only with the employee numbers, paid the money to the timekeeper.

 POTENTIALLY DESTRUCTIVE ACTIVITIES

Vengeance Is the Computer's

One man sent his ex-wife a diskette that destroyed her entire hard disk.[20] A number of instances of damaging computerized records occur because of disgruntled employees who have been fired or passed over for advancement (unfairly, they think). Such an employee may plant a **logic bomb** to go off after he or she leaves the company. A logic bomb is code set to "go off" on a particular cue (such as on a certain date, which will be reflected in the computer's clock) and destroy files, erase tapes, or even sabotage the operating system itself. A logic bomb is a kind of Trojan horse, discussed next.

Trojan Horse

A **Trojan horse** is the disguised inclusion of program instructions or data in a program that otherwise functions normally. Named after the wooden horse that the Greeks left as a gift for Troy but was full of Greek soldiers and caused the fall of Troy, the Trojan horse lies dormant in the code until the proper time comes for it to be activated. It may leap into action on a specified date, or when a certain account number comes up, or when funds credited reach a certain amount, and so on (the possibilities are endless). Often the purpose of the Trojan horse code is destructive, as in the logic bomb vendettas we just discussed.

The Christmas Tree Trojan Horse   The Trojan horse may be embedded as part of a program from the start, or added by a clever programmer, or it may come as part of an electronic message sent to the terminal. Such an "electronic letter bomb attack" has control characters at the end of the message that will cause its embedded program to be executed. A "Christmas tree" Trojan horse appeared in German computers in 1987 connected to an e-mail message. It encouraged the recipient to type in 'Christmas', after which a large Christmas tree was drawn on the screen. The recipient then deleted the e-mail message, only to receive more copies of the Christmas tree message.

The program that drew the tree had also read the recipients' files containing e-mail addresses of their correspondents, and sent all of them the letter bomb as well. The message reached the United States academic community, and the IBM VNet, which sent it to thousands of computers around the world. The traffic generated by this "chain letter" brought the IBM systems to a halt right before Christmas, and kept many troubleshooters at IBM busy killing all copies of the file over the Christmas season (Mungo and Clough, 1992, pp. 102–3).

The Cookie Monster   Another Trojan Horse program is the "cookie monster," which announces "I want a cookie." If the nonplussed user does not respond, a few minutes later it displays "I'm hungry; I really want a cookie!" If the user still does not comply, more insistent demands escalate to a threat to wipe out some of the user's files if the monster doesn't get a cookie. The monster can, of course, be placated by the user simply typing in 'cookie'.[21]

The "Twelve Tricks Trojan" Horse An alert was sent out on a "Twelve Tricks Trojan [Horse]" in 1990, describing it as "very interesting, very nasty, and quite complex." It apparently was appended to a program to test hard disk performance (something called CORETEST). The Trojan Horse used a random number generator to select one of its twelve "tricks" to perform on the unsuspecting victim:

1. Inserts a random delay loop that executes 18.2 times a second, and causes the machine to slow down considerably and perform "rather jerkily."
2. Inserts an End-of-Interrupt in the timer that interferes with servicing hardware interrupts, and the floppy drive motor is on all the time.
3. Every time a key is pressed or released, increases the timer tick count by a random number, which sometimes causes programs not to run, file copying not to work, and a call for TIME to create a divide overflow.
4. Every time an interrupt 0dh is executed (for the fixed disk or the parallel port), does the routine only three times out of four.
5. Every time an interrupt 0eh (for floppy disks) is executed, does the routine only three times out of four.
6. Every time interrupt 10H (for video) is called, inserts a random delay loop that causes the video to be slow and/or jerky.
7. Every time the video routine to scroll up is called, the whole scrolling window goes blank.
8. Every time a request is made to the diskette handler, it is turned into a write request, which can overwrite the boot sector or directory or file allocation table of the diskette, and will create various errors and damage if you try to read a diskette.
9. Every time interrupt 16h is called (to read the keyboard), the Caps Lock, Num Lock, and other flags are set randomly, making the keyboard unusable, and perhaps restarting the system.
10. Everything that is sent to the printer is garbled.
11. Every letter that is sent to the printer has its case reversed (upper to lower or vice versa), line feed characters won't feed lines, and a space becomes a 0.
12. Every time the Time-of-Day interrupt is called, it does an End-of-Interrupt instead, "which means you can't set the system clock, and the time is set permanently to one value." [22]

The "Twelve Tricks Trojan" was apparently spotted in Surrey, England. It is just one example of the kind of malicious mischief (or worse, deliberate destruction) that can be caused by this kind of unseen program sabotage.

The AIDS Virus (Trojan Horse)   In December 1989, an American anthropologist (Harvard PhD, 1979) named Joseph L. Popp sent out an infected diskette that purported to contain information on AIDS to tens of thousands of people and organizations on a PC mailing list. It was shrink-wrapped, and contained Popp's own version of a shrink-wrap license, which said that if the reader did not agree with the terms, s/he should not use the disk. The terms were that the user could run the program for a year's worth of times (365) for $189, or could have lifetime rights to use it for $389. The money was to be sent to "PC Cyborg Corporation" at a post office box in Panama City, Florida. If one were to use the disk without this authorization, the threat was that "your computer will stop functioning normally."

The first companies to receive copies of the AIDS disk were Chase Manhattan Bank, the London Stock Exchange, British Telecommunications, Lloyds of London, the Midland Bank, and other major financial institutions, as well as the Imperial Cancer Research Fund organization in England. Computer security expert Jim Bates "found that the program had been written to behave almost like the real AIDS virus. It was opportunistic, just like its biological counterpart; it spread its infection slowly; and [it] was ultimately fatal to its hosts" (Mungo and Clough, 1992, p. 144). The New Scotland Yard Computer Crime Unit discovered Popp acting strangely at an Amsterdam airport; when his bags were checked, they found evidence linking him to PC Cyborg Corporation. The FBI arrested him at his home in Cleveland, Ohio, on February 3, 1990. Popp was extradited to Britain for prosecution, "the first person ever to be extradited for a computer crime and the first ever to be tried in Britain for writing a malicious program" (Mungo and Clough, 1992, p. 150). His defense presented evidence that he was mentally unfit to stand trial, and in November 1991 the prosecution concurred.[23]

The Burleson Blackmail   Donald Burleson, the director of computer security for the insurance firm USPA & IRA, set a Trojan Horse program that destroyed 75 percent of the "detail files" for accounts that netted the company commissions of $2 million a month. He was convicted in September 1988 of the criminal act of destroying crucial data (the first such computer criminal conviction), fined $11,800, and given seven years of supervised probation. He was also convicted in civil court of illegal trespass, breaking of "fiduciary duty," and gross negligence (and fined $12,000) (McEwen, 1989, p. 38, and Lore et al., 1988, p. 10).

Other "Bombs"   Perhaps the most damage done so far by a "logic bomb" was set by a former network administrator for Omega Engineering of Bridgeport, New Jersey (a firm supplying NASA and the navy), that caused $10 million in damage. This was listed on the website **cybercrime.gov** and also reported in *Computerworld* (February 23, 1998).

In October 1990, the London publication *The Independent* reported that a mysterious group of hackers had broken into the computers of five London banks over the previous six months. They had the potential to steal or alter bank data and disrupt systems, but their action to that point had been to demand large amounts of money from the banks to reveal how the bank computer systems had been penetrated. (None of the banks had paid the extortion to that point.) The banks called in private investigators in an attempt to avoid public disclosure and weakening of confidence.[24]

There is a wide range of types of break-in, and they vary widely in impact. As in the cases of software piracy discussed in Chapter 4, it is difficult to know where the line should be drawn. The extreme cases are clear. Messages that simply spread a rumor (such as the one that Bill Gates and Microsoft intend to acquire the Roman Catholic Church) are harmless and sometimes amusing. A "cookie monster" is an annoyance, but no serious harm is done. On the other extreme, Burleson's activity was blackmail, clearly wrong both ethically and legally, as would be murder by the computer (depicted occasionally in movies, such as *The Ghost in the Machine*).

It is, as always, the cases in the middle part of the range that will be difficult to decide on moral grounds. We should keep in mind whether they do harm, and whether they undermine any of the fundamental goods, as we examine different cases.

Worms

In a sense, a Trojan Horse has to be invited in to your system (as the wooden horse was pulled within the gates of Troy). The recipients of the Christmas Tree message had to take the bait and type in 'Christmas'; someone had to get and use the program containing the "Twelve Tricks Trojan"; and so on. A worm, however, can come into your system completely unbidden (just as a live worm can sneak into your apple). A **worm** is a program "that can run independently and travel from machine to machine across network connections; worms may have portions of themselves running on many different machines." [25] A worm is self-replicating; it makes copies of itself and spreads them throughout available memory.

John F. Shoch and Jon A. Hupp of Xerox's Palo Alto Research Center (PARC) worked on early versions of worm programs in the early 1980s as a positive experiment in the development of distributed computing, to make use of available memory space on a number of machines, wherever it could be found. They describe a worm as "simply a computation that lives on one or more machines; . . . the programs on individual computers are described as the *segments* of a worm" (Shoch and Hupp, 1982, p. 173). John von Neumann proved some time ago that there could be self-reproducing automata (computers); all you needed was a room full of spare computer parts and a computer that carried a copy of its own blueprint in memory. An interesting programming exercise is to write a program that will print itself out. Those of us who had to work with large programs on machines with limited memory capacity in times before memory was so plentiful used to have to learn to write our programs in segments so that a later segment could be "overlaid" on an earlier segment in memory that had already finished executing. This worked effectively, and Shoch and Hupp were merely applying the same principle, but using multiple computers.

Shoch and Hupp begin their *CACM* article with a reference to *Shockwave Rider*, a 1975 science-fiction book by John Brunner that described a "tapeworm"—the "father and mother of all tapeworms"—that the protagonist had just loosed on the net:

> My newest—my masterpiece—breeds by itself . . . By now I don't know exactly what there is in the worm. More bits are being added automatically as it works its way to places I never dared guess existed . . . And—no, it can't be killed. It's indefinitely self-perpetuating so long as the net exists. Even if one segment of it is inactivated, a counterpart of the missing portion will remain in store at some other station and the worm will automatically subdivide and send a duplicate head to collect the spare groups and restore them to their proper place.[26]

Just another example of yesterday's science fiction becoming today's science!

Shoch and Hupp also compared their worm program research to a science-fiction movie, *The Blob* (1958). My recollection of that movie is of a reddish goop that kept getting bigger and getting into everything—perhaps not a bad model for a worm program after all. Their model was of a program that begins by running on one machine, but then spreads (as its "appetite" grows) to other machines, making use of available resources, and doing its work. In the morning, it "retreats" leaving the machines free to do their normal jobs, having saved its results of the night's work. Their article describes how their research effectively used multimachine worms to accomplish big jobs.

They admit that a big problem in "worm management" was "controlling its growth while maintaining stable behavior," and they told of one night when they left a small worm running and came back in the morning to find "dozens of machines dead" (Shoch and Hupp, 1982, p. 175). They had provided an emergency plan for just such an occasion, and sent a program into the net that stopped all segments of the worm from operating.

The most famous (and infamous) example of a worm program is the **Internet Worm**. This worm program was released on the ARPANET by Robert T. Morris Jr., a first-year graduate student at Cornell University, on November 2, 1988. Morris, a Harvard graduate, is the son of a chief computer security officer at the National Computer Security Center of NSA (the National Security Agency). Thus, Morris' father's job is to protect government computers against just the sort of intrusion that his son created over ARPANET.

The worm reached from 2,500 to 3,000 computers, including those at Berkeley, MIT, Purdue, and the University of Utah (teams at these universities worked to analyze the worm and put in the required fixes), as well as NASA, Lawrence Livermore Laboratory, and Los Alamos National Laboratory. The worm's purpose was to propagate, making thousands of copies of itself as it moved. These copies clogged the systems it invaded, and rendered them essentially inoperable. Though initial estimates were much higher, it probably caused a loss on the order of $1 million due to lost computer time. No files or operating systems were destroyed.

Morris apparently wanted to run an experiment in which the worm penetrated the computers on the net, to expose several "holes" in the system, but he did not intend for any computers to crash. The worm propagated faster than he had anticipated, and it got out of hand. At one point, he tried to post a message on a bulletin board to the computers on the net telling them how to disable the worm, but they could not access it because their systems were down. The federal government apparently tried initially to suppress or restrict information on the worm; the National Security Center of NSA asked Purdue University officials to remove information on the worm (incorrectly categorized in their report as a virus).[27]

The worm entered a system through one of three paths: finding a password that worked that was either a permutation of the usercode or among its dictionary of names to try; exploiting a bug (error) in the finger protocol; and exploiting a trap door in the debug process of Sendmail.[28]

Once in, the worm issued commands to the system to execute it and copied the parent worm (a 3,000-line C program) into memory. The parent then issued commands to create a new worm and execute it. Peter Denning reports:

> The worm also made attempts at population control, looking for other worms in the same host and negotiating with them which would terminate. However, a worm that agreed to terminate would first attack many hosts before completing its part of the bargain—leaving the overall birthrate higher than the deathrate. Moreover, one in seven worms declared itself immortal and entirely bypassed any participation in population control." [29]

The worm program was well camouflaged and enciphered; it left no traces in the system file directories of its existence.

The Internet Worm got considerable media coverage, and received very different responses from people. Some considered Morris a folk hero, a hacker in the old tradition, doing brilliant things to help point out weaknesses in large computer systems. But by far the majority deprecated his actions. The Computer Professionals for Social Responsibility issued a statement condemning the action. It said in part:

> This was an irresponsible act that cannot be condoned. The Internet should not be treated as a laboratory for uncontrolled experiments in computer security. Networked software is intrinsically risky, and no programmer can guarantee that a self-replicating program will not have unintended consequences.
>
> The value of open networks depends upon the good will and common sense of computer users. Computer professionals should take upon themselves the responsibility to ensure that systems are not misused. (CPSR, 1989, p. 699)

They went further to encourage the teaching of ethics in the computer community, and pointed out how the Worm exposes our "increasing dependence on computer networks." They also mention the government's attempts to conceal information about the worm as "short-sighted."

Morris was tried and convicted under the 1986 Computer Fraud and Abuse Act, given three years' probation and a fine of $10,000, and was sentenced to 400 hours of community service. It may be that the court stretched the literal coverage of this law to fit Morris, since his act was so well publicized and they wanted to make an example of him. The Act is aimed at those who gain unauthorized access to a system, but Morris was an authorized user of the system on which he unleashed the worm. This just emphasizes the fact that the laws need to be more finely tuned to deal with the new issues brought up by modern computing.

Pamela Samuelson, an insightful writer on computer hacking, computer crime, software piracy, and the legal system, provides some perspective on the Morris case in an article, "Computer Viruses and Worms: Wrong, Crime, or Both?", written for Peter J. Denning's collection, *Computers Under Attack*, which was an effort to make the information on the

Internet Worm and the response of the computing community to it more widely available. She points out that the Computer Fraud and Abuse Act was designed to punish those who break into federal computer systems and do damage to data or commit other malicious acts. But Morris had access rights to the system, which "gave him the right to create and distribute programs on the network," so the current law does not seem to have had someone like him in mind. There also is an open question whether Morris had malicious intent in committing the act; everything he said indicated that he did not.

Samuelson then analyzes two bills that were under consideration in Congress in 1990 that would broaden the legal coverage in computer misuse cases. The first bill "would create criminal liability for anyone who knowingly and maliciously altered computer hardware or software so as to disable a computer"; it is a "consequences-oriented approach." "The second bill focuses on the action of inserting material into a computer system with knowledge that some harm is likely to arise as a consequence (a conduct-oriented approach)."[30]

Samuelson points out that a law must not be too broad, so that it penalizes more people than it was intended to cover. It also should be enforceable. Illegal access is easier to prove than malicious intent, and it may not be possible to prove that an act has had disabling results to a system. She also raises the question whether someone who, through negligence or lack of knowledge that an action will cause harm (in this case, to a computer system), causes damage or disruption should receive the same punishment as one who has acted maliciously. These are serious questions, but one can also ask whether the person who is negligent *should not have been negligent* (a question of a violation of responsibility); there also exists a legal category of *criminal negligence* that is punishable. Aristotle points out that we are responsible for acts we initiate.

In the case of a person who *does not know* that the action will cause harm, the question arises whether the person *should have known*. In Morris' case, someone knowledgeable enough about computer systems to write an intricate, encrypted program like the worm certainly should have had knowledge of the disruption it could produce. A responsible computer professional (and Morris was in a graduate program at Cornell to become just that) should make it his or her business to know, or investigate, the possible consequences of any contemplated computer activity.

Samuelson points out that Morris did have access to the system that was compromised, but that he used a "hole" or a "back door" in the security system to bypass the security; thus the actual access gained for the worm was not that for which Morris was authorized. Samuelson comments:

> Given that his father is a computer security expert, Morris must have known that there were other ways to deal with a potential network security problem than to plant a worm in the system. It is hard to believe that Morris could have thought that the university or the government sponsors of the network would have thought it acceptable for him to introduce a worm into the system to test out its effectiveness without telling them beforehand."[31]

With regard to the hackers' defense of Morris, that he was doing the university and the network users a favor by exposing a hole in the security for the system, Samuelson remarks that "we would hardly let a bank robber off the hook for demonstrating that a bank needed a new safe."[32] It is useful in these cases to draw the analogies with other more familiar instances of negligence or lack of knowledge. Just because the computer technology is new and raises some new possibilities for improper action does not mean that we cannot use established moral principles to deal with these violations. Good laws arise out of sound moral principles, or out of practical exigencies (such as deciding on which side of the road everyone should drive). We should ask in these new cases whether the actions undermine any fundamental goods, such as health, friendship, or knowledge. We should look at the consequences of the actions under consideration, and ask "what if everyone were to do this?"

The law may need to be made more clear to deal with these new wrinkles, but the basis on which the law should be drawn is still the same—it is wrong to violate the rights and damage the property of others, it is bad to undermine the basic goods. Questions regarding the proper definition of *property* need to be dealt with, so that laws dealing with just *tangible* property are expanded to include programs and data in a computer system.

The newsweekly *Computerworld* interviewed a number of people in influential positions in the computing community right after the Internet Worm had hit, and asked them whether they would hire Robert T. Morris, Jr. or not. Several said "yes," that they were looking for creative people, but the majority said strongly that they would not, for security reasons or because they thought he had a "bad attitude." Typical of these responses was that of Gene Spafford, a computer science professor at Purdue:

> We would not hire him. We wouldn't do business with any firm that did. Just because you have the means to invade somebody else's domain and damage

their work doesn't mean you become a vandal. There are many computer scientists who would no sooner dream of unleashing a virus than you would burn
down a neighbor's house just because you know how to strike a match.[33]

What is interesting is that there *are* companies who would hire him, because
they think he has demonstrated that he is clever. The problem is that he
demonstrated this at the expense of others. But here again we have the problem we saw with regard to computer criminals—they get light sentences and
then are often hired to work for the very sort of company they victimized.
This is not sending a desirable message (from society's point of view) to
potential computer criminals or destructive "hackers."

More and More Worms   A later worm struck the Space Physics Astron-
omy Network (SPAN) of NASA in October 1989 with a protest:

> WORMS AGAINST NUCLEAR KILLERS
> Your System Has Been Officially WANKed.
> You talk of times of peace for all, and then prepare for war.

The WANK Worm affected several hundred computers at NASA and the
Department of Energy (Mungo and Clough, 1992, pp. 104–5).

A nasty worm called SirCam surfaced in mid-July 2001. It arrived as an
e-mail beginning "Hi! How are you?" followed in most cases by "I send you
this file in order to have your advice" and ending with, "See you later.
Thanks." If the recipient opened the attached file, the worm would append a
random document (which could be secure) to itself and send this new
infected file to everyone in the victim's address book. Thus the e-mail would
seem to be coming from someone the recipient knew and had previous communication with. According to a Symantec report, the worm also had a 1 in
20 chance of deleting all the files and directories on the C drive (only on
systems using the D/M/Y date format) and a 1 in 33 chance of filling all the
remaining space on the hard disk by adding text to the file c:\recycled\sir-
cam.sys at each restart (this happened to several people I know at my college). It was also said that if SirCam was not completely removed, it might
wipe out one's hard drive on a certain date of the next month. It was difficult to remove.

Close on the heels of SirCam came "Code Red." The ZDNet report on it
by Rob Lemos begins "For one moment last week, the Internet stood still."
Unleashed on July 18, 2001, the worm, after it had infected a server (due to
a Microsoft flaw) would scan the Internet using 100 "threads," or subprograms, looking for vulnerable computers to infect. Each copy of the worm,

writes Lemos, would send out 400 megabytes of garbage every 4.5 hours; at its peak, it infected more than 2,000 servers every minute. It defaced websites with the message "Hacked by Chinese!" Hotmail and FedEx were infected, and a flood of data attack aimed at the White House site was only averted by its administrators changing its Internet Protocol address.

A new version, called "Code Red II," hit in early August, moving faster than its namesake and establishing "back doors" that would allow hackers to gain access to infected systems. Whereas the original Code Red looked for 100 systems at a time to infect, Code Red II searched for 300 at a time (or 600 in some cases). A Reuters report (August 8, 2001) on the Internet estimated the economic damage caused so far by the Code Red worms was close to $2 billion, and that it might well in time exceed the $8.7 billion in estimated damages caused by the "Love Bug" virus.

On September 18, 2001, a new worm called "Nimda" (for "admin" spelled backward) was reported spreading to both servers and PCs running Microsoft software. It attaches to e-mails, but can also spread through Internet relay chat, and return Web pages requested that are infected. Connections to the September 11 terrorist attacks in New York and Washington were denied by officials.

Another worm was reported in the February 13, 2001 *Wall Street Journal* (p. B5) that was spread when a recipient of an e-mail opened an attachment that claimed it contained a sexy photo of tennis star Anna Kournikova.

Virus

A virus is a segment of code that copies itself into a larger program and, when that program is executed, the virus is activated, does its work, and copies itself into other programs. Unlike a worm, which can run independently, a virus requires a "host" program to infect; the virus will not be executed or make more copies of itself until the host is run.

The first use of the term 'virus' for undesired computer code appeared in David Gerrold's 1972 science fiction novel, *When Harlie Was One* (HARLIE stood for Human Analogue Robot Life Input Equivalents). But the more recent use of the term is traceable to Fred Cohen, who formally defined the term 'computer virus' in 1983, when he was doing work that would lead to a dissertation on computer viruses. Cohen (1991, p. 24) pointed out that viruses could be innocuous, or malicious (like wiping out disk storage), or even helpful (he demonstrated a virus program that reduces the disk space needed to store programs). The name was chosen because of their similarity to biological viruses. They need a larger "host" to infect, they spread rapidly to other hosts by replicating themselves, and their spread is enhanced by increased contact between hosts, as when programs are shared.

The Latin word *virus* means slime, or poison (venom), or a harsh, bitter smell. All have very unpleasant connotations, which are appropriate to the use of viruses in computers. Some symptoms that indicate your system may have "picked up" a virus are reductions in available memory, change in length of any program, strange screen graphics, reduction in system performance (such as operations taking longer), errors cropping up in software that has been reliable in the past, new files appearing on your disk, or a system that will not restart.[35] There has been considerable activity in the development of anti-viral software programs, creating an "immune system by observing viruses at work and collecting their "signatures" on a "wanted list" (Beard, 1994, pp. 18–19). Some anti-viral programs are in the public domain or available as shareware. The problem is that the software must be continually updated as new, more lethal and more subtle forms of viruses are developed. Some people speak of "exorcising" a virus from a system.[36]

Historically, viruses can be traced back to a couple of games. The first, mathematician John H. Conway's "Game of Life," was presented in the October 1970 issue of *Scientific American* (p. 120). The "game" models the growth and changes in a complex collection of living organisms; the model can be interpreted as applying to a collection of microorganisms, an ecologically closed system of plants or animals, or an urban development (and, perhaps, to the spread of a computer virus). Its implications were the inspiration for a book by William Poundstone, *The Recursive Universe*. It makes a nice example for a programming problem:

> You have a 50 × 50 board (of course, you can make it larger) on which entities are to be placed. Allow the user to pick how large the population will be (but don't make it too small for the space, or the population will die out rapidly from loneliness, or too large, in which case it will die of overcrowding). Each location (except those on the borders) has exactly 8 neighbors. Entities are born, die, or survive during each generation according to the following rules:
>
> > *Birth.* Each empty location with exactly three neighbors in its immediate (8-location) neighborhood is a birth location. A new entity is placed in this space for the next generation.
> >
> > *Death.* Entities with four or more immediate neighbors die from overcrowding and are removed for the next generation. Entities with one or zero neighbors die of loneliness.
> >
> > *Survival.* Entities with two or three neighbors survive to the next generation.

Assume the edges of your board are infertile regions; nothing is born or dies in this region. After you have set up this game to run on your computer, it is interesting to watch the different patterns that develop, as well as the cases of population growth and those of annihilation of the entire population.

The other game, called "Core Wars," was also published in *Scientific American*, in 1984. In this game, computer programs compete for memory (territory).[37] Ideas that started out as just interesting games and intellectual challenges have been transformed into potentially deadly attackers of computers.

Brain Virus The *Brain* virus—the first virus documented to have attacked outside a laboratory—hit the University of Delaware on October 22, 1987, and spread to several other universities after that. It originated in Pakistan; its authors (Basit Alvi, 19, and his brother Amjad, 26) apparently created it "for fun," and it was intended to be innocuous—just giving its own label, "Brain," to the floppy disks it infected. But it had unwanted side effects, accidentally overwriting parts of some disks it entered. Basit had given a copy of the virus on a disk to a friend, who traveled to the United States. At the University of Delaware, it was said to have made 1 percent of the disks unusable, and to have destroyed one graduate student's thesis; at the University of Pittsburgh it was reported to have affected work of several hundred graduate students in business.[38]

The Brain virus caught the attention of *Time* magazine, which published an article titled "Invasion of the Data Snatchers!" that hyped a swarm of contagious viruses striking the country.[39]

Lehigh Virus Lehigh University, in Bethlehem, Pennsylvania, where Fred Cohen was a professor of computer science and electrical engineering, was hit with a more destructive virus in November 1987. This virus replicated itself, and used a counter so that after a disk had been accessed four times, it zeroed out the first 50 sectors on the disk, making it unusable. It "infected thousands of disks and caused hundreds of systems to lose all of the data on their disks before it was detected."[40] A modified version of the virus hit the campus again in 1991, but this time it waited until a program had been accessed ten or more times before actually doing any damage to the disk, which meant it had much more opportunity to spread before being detected. Peter Denning wrote that Lehigh students "lost homework"[41] to the virus. This gives a variant on the old excuse: "I'm sorry, professor, but the virus ate my homework!"

The Israeli Virus The Jerusalem virus, or Israeli virus, was discovered in December 1987 at the Hebrew University in Jerusalem. It would wipe out entirely any program files used on a Friday the thirteenth (the first target date was May 13, 1988); at other times it would just slow programs down considerably. It often added itself to the same program files a number of times, resulting in a glut in computer memory. It spread rapidly from Israel to Europe and North America, and "a year after its discovery it had become the most common virus in the world" (Mungo and Clough, 1992, pp. 108–9).

The Malta Disk Destroyer A nasty virus struck the main bank on the island of Malta on January 15, 1991. It temporarily destroyed the File Allocation Table (FAT) on a disk, and then asked the user to gamble (as at a casino) to restore the information. Without the FAT, the files could not be found on the disk. If the user won, the FAT was replaced on the disk; if not, too bad! The Maltese bank ended up having to restore damaged files on two-thirds of their infected computers (Mungo and Clough, 1992, 112–13).

The Ping-Pong Virus Also called the Italian virus, the Ping-Pong virus was reported in March 1988. It caused a circular ball to bounce around the text that was on screen.[42]

The Datacrime Virus This virus, which says it was released on March 1, 1989, formats part of the hard disk and destroys important information including that in the File Allocation Table.[43]

The Bulgarian Dark Avenger This virus, which called itself "Eddie" ("Eddie Lives . . . Somewhere in Time!") and indicated it was written in the city of Sofia (the capital of Bulgaria), attached itself to executable files and randomly deleted files and portions of the hard disk. It took 700 hours for the financial organization that it hit in 1989 to eliminate "Eddie" (they thought!), but it popped back up in less than a week. They estimated they lost half a million dollars in direct business during the period, and at least another half a million in customers that would not come back (Mungo and Clough, 1992, pp. 118–21).

Many other viruses seemed to originate in Bulgaria, including one that hit the English House of Commons library and destroyed valuable statistical information. During a period when viruses were relatively rare worldwide, it was said that two new viruses were being discovered every week in Bulgaria. By the middle of 1990 "there were so many Bulgarian viruses that one researcher was moved to refer to the existence of a 'Bulgarian virus factory'" (Mungo and Clough, 1992, p. 124).

There may be an analogy here to the rapid increase in computer crimes that we noted in countries like the Czech Republic and Slovakia which had during that period emerged from under the yoke of Soviet communism. Bulgaria was coming out from under communist rule between 1989 and 1990. Perhaps Bulgarian youths, with no KGB breathing down their necks, were just exercising their newfound freedom.

The Michelangelo Virus A computer "alarm" was sounded in early March 1992, warning of the Michelangelo virus that would wipe out the hard disks on any infected IBM PC-compatible computer on March 6, which was the artist Michelangelo's 517th birthday. The reality turned out not to be as dire as the threat, but the widespread publicity it got considerably raised consciousness about the potential dangers of computer viruses. In the 1995 movie *Hackers*, the major culprit is called the "da Vinci virus."

Macintosh Viruses Though the virus activity is much greater on IBM-type personal computers, viruses have attacked Macintosh computers as well. One (the *Peace virus*) displayed a message of world peace on March 2, 1988, and then removed itself from any system on which it appeared. A much more destructive virus, the *Scores virus*, spread to applications programs, caused system crashes, and destroyed data. It targeted a particular company, perhaps as an ex-employee's revenge.[44] The Peace virus, true to its name, was benign, but most of the viruses we have considered did damage, wasted valuable time, and in some cases destroyed valuable information and programs.

It seems that Robert T. Morris Jr.'s inspiration "spread" to other students at Cornell. On February 14, 1992, a virus created by two Cornell undergraduates (David Blumenthal, '96, and Mark Pilgrim, '94) infected games for the Macintosh, disrupting computers in Japan and Stanford, California. These two students were arraigned on charges of "second-degree computer tampering" (a misdemeanor) and were sentenced to pay restitution to people whose systems were affected. Each of them also had to perform ten hours of community service a week for a year. In their community service, they worked on developing a program to make it easier for a quadriplegic to use a computer. When asked to comment on the damage caused by the virus, M. Stewart Lynn, vice president for information technologies at Cornell, said, "At Cornell we absolutely deplore this kind of behavior."[45]

The Health-Care Plan Virus The Clinton Health-Care Reform plan (1993) was the first government proposal to be made available to reporters on computer disks. It was said that the disks (two 3 1/2-inch floppies containing the

1,336-page report) might have carried a virus being called "Stoned III," which (according to the *New York Post*) could affect the functioning of the computer, as well as display: "Your PC is Stoned—Legalize Marijuana."[46]

Operation Moon Angel Hackers broke into a NASA computing facility that controlled the Hubble telescope and changed its orientation toward Earth to spy on a nudist colony near Camden, Maine. One of the hackers, called Brain Dead, said when arrested: "Getting arrested for hacking is the first significant step in my career goal of becoming a highly paid security consultant."[47]

Kevin Mitnick Kevin Mitnick, who had already been in jail once for his illegal hacking activities, broke in and erased the accounting records for the online service the WELL. Following Robert Morris Jr. as an example, he capitalized on weaknesses in the Sendmail program, and hacked into the home computer of computer crime expert Tsutomo Shimomura. Shimomura was instrumental in tracking down Mitnick, who was arrested two months after the break-in, and indicted on March 9, 1995 on 23 counts of fraud involving computers. At the time of his first arrest in 1992, Mitnick said: "I was just an electronic joyrider having fun in cyberspace." He seems to treat the whole thing as a game, a big challenge. He would stash stolen software in files belonging to Computers, Freedom, and Privacy, and broke into the computer of cryptography expert John Gilmore.[48] It seemed to be a matter of always raising the stakes, seeing who he could outsmart.

Melissa Virus On March 26, 1999, network users began receiving e-mails with a subject line that began "Important Message From," followed by the name of the last victim, whose address book had sent the message, and a message that said "Here is that document you asked for" and an attachment supposedly containing usernames and passwords for pornographic websites. The attachment, when opened, sent itself to the first 50 names in the victim's address book and also infected the Word document template, so that if documents were created by Word and sent as attachments, the virus would travel along with them. As it propagated, the Melissa virus began to overwhelm e-mail servers; it created "serious disruptions" at duPont, Honeywell, Lockheed, Lucent, Microsoft, and the Marine Corps. It took advantage of the capability of a macro language like Microsoft's Visual Basic for Applications that allows a user to program executable functions into a document (that was then made into an e-mail attachment). It is estimated that it cost between $249,000 and $269,000 to fix (Garber, 1999, 16–17) and that losses due to Melissa were on the order of $80 million (**cybercrime.gov**). It is believed that the perpetrator of this virus was caught, though he denied all charges. In a recent speech, Attorney General John Ashcroft claimed this capture as one of the FBI's major achievements in fighting computer crime.

Chernobyl Virus   A more deadly virus, created by a student in Taiwan, had infected close to 700,000 computers in Asia and the Middle East in April 1999. It deleted data and corrupted programs, and forced the closure of a number of businesses (Langford, 2000, 163).

The Love Bug   In May 2000, a rapidly spreading virus referred to as "super-Melissa" that carried the message "I Love You" downloaded its files onto the recipients' hard disks. The Love virus forced the State Department to disconnect its files from the Internet and cost 45 million users billions of dollars in damages.

Viruses Make It to the Big Screen   In the 1996 movie *Independence Day* the earth is under attack by deadly invading aliens. It is a computer *virus* that is used to disable the communication system of the "mother ship" and allow the earth forces to fight back and win. This correlates with Cohen's view that viruses can be helpful; unfortunately, most of what we have seen is the harm they can do.

MISUSE OF THE (ELECTRONIC) MAIL

Electronic mail (e-mail) has rapidly established itself as one of the preferred methods of communication on college campuses and in businesses. It presents a great convenience but also many drawbacks. It seems that people are willing to put in e-mail messages things they would never say to someone directly, or even put in writing. Just as with long-distance weapons, one tends not to think of the "victim" as a real person when you are just staring at the screen of a machine, and so some very damaging things may be written. Also, one does not *sign* the message with a handwritten signature, and so can always deny being the one who sent it. It is also easy to "masquerade" as someone else over the wires by stealing someone's password or just by taking on a different "persona."

One occasion of the latter is reported by Lindsy Van Gelder in "The Strange Case of the Electronic Lover," a true story that appeared in *Ms*. magazine in 1985.[49] We are told about a person communicating online with many others; she said "she" was Joan Sue Green, a woman who had been badly disfigured in an automobile accident that killed her boyfriend and affected her ability to speak and walk. She, however, wrote very well and affectingly through e-mails, and made many friends. It was finally revealed that "Joan" was a prominent New York male psychiatrist who had been doing this as a "bizarre, all-consuming experiment to see what it felt like to be female." All those who had corresponded with "Joan" felt "betrayed." "Joan" had even pressured her correspondents to have "compusex" (typing out their hot fantasies), and had arranged for one of them to meet this "great guy"–the New York psychiatrist himself![50] They got rather involved before the deception was revealed.

Although the psychiatrist may have rationalized to himself that he was doing it all for the good of science, a "science" that undermines the trust and self-esteem of other people to achieve its ends must be judged immoral. It violates friendship.

We can see from the "electronic lover" that it is very easy to dissemble on the Net. One can play gender-role games in MUDs,[51] or pretend to be rich and famous, or poor but talented, or to be a spy (a kind of air-waves *True Lies* or *Total Recall*), or . . . the possibilities are endless. The problem is that many people can get hurt by such deceptions, like those who corresponded with "Joan." The point is well-made in the *New Yorker* cartoon with a dog explaining to his canine friend that on the Net no one knows you're a dog.

In the fall of 1993, the University of Wisconsin provided students at its Madison campus with e-mail accounts, encouraging them to use the accounts to interact with their instructors. A small group of students forged messages including a letter of resignation from the Director of Housing to the new Chancellor, and a message "from the Chancellor" saying he was going to "come out of the closet" on September 25.[52] This gives you a small taste of the kinds of message-tampering that can go on.

"Flaming" is sending someone a nasty e-mail. Often such a message is bracketed by <FLAME ON> . . <FLAME OFF>. An article, "My First Flame," in the *New Yorker* in 1994 brought flaming to more general public attention. The author, John Seabrook, had recently been flamed by a colleague (a tech writer), or someone impersonating him on the Internet. In the article, Seabrook published the contents of the message–a painfully aggressive (and apparently undeserved) attack with no holds barred, full of offensive language. He said that "To flame, according to 'Que's Computer User's Dictionary,' is 'to lose one's self-control and write a message that uses derogatory, obscene, or inappropriate language'" (Seabrook, 1994, p. 70). The message he received certainly fit that description like a glove. Seabrook was shaken by the message, an upset that did not go away.

Seabrook wrote of his fascination on first going on Internet with the possibilities it offers. He thought that "I was going to be sheltered by the same customs and laws that shelter me when I'm talking on the telephone or listening to the radio or watching TV" (Seabrook, 1994, p. 71); but he quickly found out that is not the case. There are no FCC regulations governing what goes over the Net. He contacted CompuServe to ask whether subscribers were allowed to "talk" to each other like this, and received the answer that these mail messages "are private communications, [so] CompuServe is unable to regulate their content" (Seabrook, 1994, p. 72).

Seabrook said this was the only medium through which he would have received such a message, which elsewhere would be, "literally, unspeakable. The guy couldn't have said this to me on the phone, because I would have hung up and not answered if the phone rang again, and he couldn't have said it to my face, because I wouldn't have let him finish" (Seabrook, 1994, p. 71). Face-to-face, such things would be much more difficult, if not impossible, to say. Seabrook's size might have intimidated the speaker, as a possible audience or even the flamer's own conscience might have as well. Even in a letter he might not have used the same language, and there is the matter of actually *signing* one's own name in ink, and the time it takes actually to mail the letter, which allows reflection that might conclude that sending the letter was not prudent. None of those considerations deter the e-mail flamer. There is no audience but the intended target, he doesn't have to face the victim, he can always claim that someone else sent it if pressed legally, and there is no time lag in which to think. As soon as the last character is typed in, the message can be sent to its destination at the speed of light.

As Seabrook pointed out, the normal laws do not seem to apply here, in what is characterized as *cyberspace*. The bad language does not constitute an FCC violation, and it is not clear whether a recipient of an attack can charge defamation of character or libel. Another problem is that many "flames" are not sent directly to the target, but rather are posted on a public "bulletin board" for all to read. The ease with which one can publish a thought (good or bad, friendly or destructive) to hundreds, thousands, or more readers is frightening.

A community with no laws quickly becomes an anarchy, which might be all right if everyone in the group was morally responsible and rationally competent. But if we live in a community (in this case, that of the Net) in which not everyone acts ethically and rationally, and there are no laws to constrain hurtful behavior, the community will self-destruct.

Should there be laws in cyberspace? If so, to what extent? If we operate on a libertarian principle that you should be free as long as you don't harm others, then close attention must be paid to what counts as *harm*. The harm problem comes down to creating degrees of evil in the hierarchy of evils (the opposites of the fundamental goods). Thus, what causes death, pain, illness, frustration, ignorance, weakness, or enmity is evil, and should be avoided, and forbidden by law in cases where human choice brings these evils about. Such ethical deliberations lay the groundwork for whether we should have laws, and what those laws should be. We are in new territory where there are no existing laws to which we can appeal; we must appeal to ethical principles.

The issues connected with laws and the Internet will be examined further in Chapter 10.

IS HACKING MORAL, VALUE-NEUTRAL, OR BAD?

Harper's magazine ran a *Forum* article in March 1990 called "Is Computer Hacking a Crime?" which raised and discussed some very interesting aspects of hacking. The discussion group included hackers and former hackers (most notably, Richard Stallman and Cliff Stoll), three people connected with *Whole Earth Review*, the editor of *W.O.R.M.* (a cyberpunk magazine), a columnist for the *San Francisco Chronicle*, a lyricist for the Grateful Dead, and others. The Hacker Ethic was mentioned first, with emphasis on its principle of *avoiding waste*—that means using computer time that no one else is using, so the machine would otherwise be idle; of course, this just *might* involve getting on to the computer illegally. The second goal of the hacker ethic is free exchange of information, and the third is "the advancement of knowledge for its own sake." [53]

At the Harper's forum, Lee Felsenstein, designer of the Osborne–1 computer and a cofounder of the Homebrew Computer Club, talked about the *creativity* of computing design, creative art for its own sake. Richard M. Stallman said that "there's nothing wrong with breaking security if you're accomplishing something useful" [54]—like breaking the lock on your toolbox to get at a screwdriver you badly need. Cliff Stoll disagreed with Stallman, saying that if breaking security involves invading someone's privacy, then there *is* something wrong with it. Breaking into systems can reveal someone's personal letters, or their financial records, or their medical records—does anyone have a right to read those?

Richard Brand stressed the importance of *invariance*—if you enter someone's house (or files) and leave everything undisturbed when you leave, that is all right. However, he wants certain *information* kept private, because it could be misused to his detriment. He suggests that the solution to the problem of the theft of some of this data is that it not be collected in the first place. Emmanuel Goldstein, editor of *2600* ("the hacker's quarterly"), said that "electronic rummaging is not the same as breaking and entering."[55] It was suggested that locked doors and locked security systems on computers just provide a challenge, a temptation, primarily to young people, and that the answer is to leave everything open. Stallman said that British law has treated these matters sensibly, in not viewing an action as worse (or more innocent) if committed by a computer than without one. Thus trespassing and theft should have the same status in a court of law, whether accomplished with or without a computer.

The rest of the discussion centered primarily on claims that hacking was a defense—perhaps the only, or at least the most effective defense—against the government and private data-gathering organizations collecting, disseminating, manipulating, and comparing information on private citizens. Kevin Kelly, editor of *Whole Earth Review*, summed up this position:

> Hackers are not sloganeers. They are doers, take-things-in-handers. They are the opposite of philosophers. They don't wait for language to catch up to them. Their arguments are their actions. You want a manifesto? The Internet Worm was a manifesto. It had more meaning and symbolism than any revolutionary document you could write. To those in power running the world's nervous system, it said: Wake up!
>
> ("Is Computer Hacking a Crime?", p. 55)

It may be stylish to contrast thinkers with doers, to the detriment of the thinkers, but action without thought is rash and potentially dangerous. If there are serious problems regarding privacy and "Big Brother," we should confront them openly with argument in what we can only hope will remain an open society. One of the potential reactions against the "doers" who assault the barricades is to make the barricades much stronger—and those in power have the money to command the technology to do so—and to post guards with lethal weapons to protect them.

As history should have taught us, violence only breeds more violence. Even if the "violence" is not physical, but only assaults on entities in cyberspace, the reaction may be just as strong as if it had been buildings or machinery that had been destroyed and not data or programs. We are living in an age where information and the tools to manipulate it are among the more valuable commodities. The best way to protect what is valuable is to build a rational foundation for rights and duties, one that recognizes that human goods (such as life, health, freedom, satisfaction, knowledge, and friendship) and related states such as privacy deserve the greatest protection.

Thus, to the provocative opening question—"Is Computer Hacking a Crime?"—the answer would seem to be that it is a crime if it violates any of the basic rights of individuals or if it undermines the fabric of society. Stallman had a good point in noting that an action should be treated the same way, whether it is done with or without a computer. If it is harmless, then it is not a crime. And we should make the question broader.

Crimes are generally defined as violations of the law, and sometimes the law is unfair or needs to be modified to meet new situations that it was not originally designed to cover. The more basic question regarding any action (be it hacking or driving or throwing) is whether it is ethical, neutral, or bad. This can be determined by holding it up to ethical analysis. We may examine its consequences and, if we find them unacceptable, outlaw it. We may ask whether we could will that everyone should act thus; if so, it is either ethical or neutral (like putting on your pants right leg first), and the law does not need to get involved. We might ask if it contributes to or hinders the overall virtue of its performer; if it leads to bad character, it should be discouraged. Most basically, we can ask whether it destroys any fundamental goods.

The law should be based in what is moral, and occasionally it needs to be updated to do just that. We have seen that hacking refers to a wide spectrum of activities, some innocent, some quite destructive. It would be foolish to try to treat them all the same. A careful examination of the problem cases in the middle of the spectrum, and holding them up to ethical analysis, should help determine where the bad cases lie.

The Computer Abuse Amendments Act of 1994 changes the term 'intent' in computer abuse cases to 'reckless disregard', and broadens the machines covered from only "federal interest computers" (primarily those belonging to government agencies or financial services firms) to any computers "used in interstate commerce," which will cover any personal computer that is hooked up to the Internet.[56] This toughening up of the law and broadening its scope allows the courts to be more tough on destructive hackers.

Hacking as Civil Disobedience   Abby Goodrum and Mark Manion of Drexel University raise an interesting point regarding what they call "hactivism." They suggest that there is a recognized role in society for the peaceful disagreement, through protest, of objectionable practices of the government and society (Goodrum and Manion, 2000). Historically, this has been carried out through marches, or "sit-ins," or actual blocking of access to buildings; some of these actions have been technically illegal, but the law tends to look (in most cases) leniently on such actions if they are done with the intent of improving the society. Some hacking has not been just childish "games" or destructive pranks; some has been deliberately used as a form of civil disobedience.

Goodrum and Manion specifically mention the Electronic Disturbance Theater (to help the Zapatista rebellion in Mexico), Milw0rm (to protest nuclear testing at India's Bhabba Atomic Research Centre), the Hong Kong Blondes (hacking China's "Human Rights" website), and Kaotik Team (that attacks Indonesian government websites over the occupation of East Timor), and suggest that such civil disobedience can play a forceful and effective role. They outline five basic tenets of civil disobedience: (1) no intentional damage done to persons or property, (2) nonviolence, (3) no personal profit, (4) ethical motivation, and (5) willingness to accept personal responsibility for the outcome of actions (Goodrum and Manion, 2000, p. 53). It would seem that hackers, who generally try to remain anonymous, do not meet the fifth criterion (unlike their compatriots in the past, who have been willing to go to jail for their protests). But this may be the case because too lenient an eye is turned on such acts if they are in civil disobedience, as in other areas, and all are considered *cyberwarfare*. According to Goodrum and Manion (2000, p. 55), "organizations such as RAND and NSA have categorically ignored the existence of hactivism as an act of civil disobedience and repeatedly refer to all acts of hacking as info-war or info-terrorism in an attempt to push for stronger penalties for hacking regardless of ethical motivations." Perhaps, as in other areas we have examined, the emergence of new technologies demands a new look at old problems.

 ## THE SORCERER'S APPRENTICE

In Goethe's story "The Sorcerer's Apprentice," the young apprentice tries to use his master's magic without fully understanding it or its consequences, and the results are disastrous. The story might be more familiar to you in the Walt Disney version, with Mickey Mouse as the apprentice in the movie *Fantasia* (and repeated in *Fantasia 2000*), to the music of Paul Dukas. The problem is an old one (faced by Pandora and others) of unleashing a power that the agent then cannot control. As Norbert Weiner and others have noted, we humans may have done that with nuclear power. Is it possible that the computer may have provided another such magic chest full of demons?

The computer has given us amazing capabilities to store and manipulate information that are just beginning to be tapped. It can be used (in super-computer form) to design airplanes or to predict the weather; it can aid greatly in scientific research and in writing; it can make registration and record-keeping at schools much easier than ever before; it can perform sim-ulations that allow people to train (to fly airplanes or to do surgery) without damaging anything or anyone, or to estimate the effects of going to war ("war games") without firing a shot. It has these and many more marvelous capabilities. But the capability of the computer to store and analyze and alter such vast amounts of information also has the potential for evil, if used to spy into people's private lives or to control them, or to do damage to the property of others. We should not destroy the tool just because it has bad possibilities as well as good, but it is crucial to educate those who use it to avoid the applications that are negative, and to understand *why*.

 ## WHAT IS TO BE DONE?

In 1990, the British passed the Computer Misuse Act. It describes a "com-puter misuse offence" as follows:

(1) A person is guilty of an offence if—
   (a) he causes a computer to perform any function with intent to secure access to any program or data held in any computer;
   (b) the access he intends to secure is unauthorised; and
   (c) he knows at the time when he causes the computer to perform that that is the case.

(2) The intent a person has to have to commit an offence under this section need not be directed at—
   (a) any particular program or data;
   (b) a program or data of any particular kind; or
   (c) a program or data held in any particular computer.

(3) A person guilty of an offence under this section shall be liable on summary conviction to imprisonment for a term not exceeding six months or to a fine not exceeding level 5 on the standard scale or to both." (Wasik, 1991, p. 211)

The first person to be convicted in Britain of offenses under the new law was Nick Whiteley, a young man known as the "Mad Hacker," who worked as a computer operator at a chemical supply store. He hacked into the Queen Mary College computers, and those at the University of Glasgow and Hull University. He put a "rabbit" (a program that gives the computer useless tasks that keep multiplying) into Hull's system.

The Mad Hacker left messages at Queen Mary College for the system manager such as "WILL E.T. PLEASE PHONE HOME" and "WILL NORMAN BATES PLEASE REPORT TO THE SHOWER ROOM." Occasionally he copied reports, tied up the system, and even caused it to crash once. It was alleged he broke into the computers of the Ministry of Defense and MI5. Scotland Yard finally tracked him down in 1990, and he received a sentence of one year in prison, but actually served only two months (Mungo and Clough, 1992, pp. 38–52). Whiteley's reported view—that what he had been doing was some kind of game, like playing chess—is illuminating:

> The excitement comes from knowing that a computer in the bedroom at home can be used to break into multimillion-dollar installations. There's the thrill of exploration, of going around the world electronically. The objective is to try to gain the highest status within the system, that of system manager, and once there, to begin making the rules instead of following them. If the system manager blocks one way in, then you find another. It becomes a game with the systems manager; the hacker's goal is simply to try to persuade the computer that he should have increased privileges. (Mungo and Clough, 1992, 44)

Hackers often think of what they do as a game, an intellectual challenge where they can succeed. Perhaps they also feel a surge of creativity when they write a devious worm or virus program. They will gain some notoriety, and perhaps they feel they will gain a shred of immortality by leaving something behind. It is vital that these people (and others) come to see the importance of creating something positive, something of value, rather than doing something destructive.

Thus one of the most important factors in what to do about the problems that arise with computers lies in good education. People should be taught about the wonderful capabilities of the computer, which can open up new worlds of creative, scientific, and social possibilities. This is the technological aspect of the education, and the only issue here is to see that everyone has a fair access to this. The other crucial aspect of education is the part that teaches about the nature of social communities, the problems they face and possible solutions to these problems, and the foundations for moral choice.

If we are sensitive to the ethical obligations we have to others—to individual humans and to the community—we will not engage in activities that hurt others or undermine the society. When issues arise—such as the proper status of information and software as property, or what rights individuals should have to privacy, or who should control the information superhighway—the well-educated, thoughtful person will have a sound basis on which to deliberate the issues and come to well-grounded conclusions.

Fred Cohen has suggested emphasizing positive uses of computer viruses, such as distribution of work to many computers (like the original worm programs) or an automated bill collector. His publisher (ASP Press) was offering a $1000 prize annually for the most useful computer virus submitted to the contest. Cohen offers this solution:

> If the inventors of malicious viruses were given a legitimate outlet for their talents, they might willingly forgo damaging other people's computer systems—not to mention the risk of arrest, prosecution and punishment. Positive recognition and financial rewards for the development of beneficial viruses could lead to a dramatic decline in the global appearance of malicious viruses and simultaneously harness the creative efforts of virus writers for useful applications.
> (Cohen, 1991, p. 28)

To this, Gene Spafford of Purdue says, "It's like publicizing in the paper that anyone who comes up with the best use for a handgun should be given an award for firing it within the city limits" (Markoff, 1991, p. 18). Even if the gun analogy is a good one, isn't it more like a target-shooting contest with guns, where no one gets hurt, and skill can be demonstrated and rewarded? The problem is the same in both cases: What is to keep the expert from exercising this skill *outside* of sanctioned competitions, to the detriment of others?

"Tiger Teams" are groups of "reformed" (?) hackers who test the vulnerability of corporations and banks to computer break-ins for a handsome fee. Since recent estimates on losses in the United States due to various computer intrusions range from $150 billion to $300 billion a year,[57] hiring such consultants is an investment in protection. In 1992, a group of hackers called the Legion of Doom "went legit," and began offering their services to check out computer security systems for customers (something like the team in the 1992 movie *Sneakers*).

Many companies are hesitant to trust former hackers in their system. Large management-consulting firms, like Price Waterhouse and Coopers & Lybrand, are now offering this sort of system-penetration security check for their clients, again for a fee. The article on "Hacking Goes Legit" (by Steffora and Cheek) says that these companies do not hire hackers, but rather "technically skilled people." One has to wonder how they tell the difference, since surely there are many "closet hackers" who do not publicly declare their avocational activity, and work normal jobs.

Some suggested applications for the "beneficial" use of viruses are anything but benign. One idea is that they be used to discourage unauthorized copying of software by infecting the copier's disk. Reportedly, Amjad Alvi said that the purpose of his Brain virus was to punish people who illegally copy software.[58] Others suggest using viruses as *weapons* by sending a "commando virus" by radio waves or phone lines to infiltrate enemy computers. This was being investigated by a specialist in electronic warfare at Booz, Allen & Hamilton, by Sparta (a consulting firm for the Army in McLean, Virginia), and by Application Configured Computers in Baldwin, New York. The response by CPSR (Computer Professionals for Social Responsibility) is, "Do we really want to escalate a war where we are more vulnerable than anyone else?"[59] Some people are skeptical about the possibilities of such virus-at-a-distance capabilities, but who knows what the future may develop.

Michael Gemignani pointed out that there are legal problems pinning down just *where* and *when* a computer break-in has taken place, when the perpetrator was not at the scene but at a computer miles away, and the program that carried out the theft was activated at a later date than it was written and incorporated into the system. It is also difficult to present evidence connecting the perpetrator to the break-in (no paper trail, no fingerprints) and to assess the amount of the damages. Perhaps the current law only considers break-ins to *federal* computers a criminal act, and this was a private corporation computer. One can only be convicted of breaking a law *as the law is stated*, and most current laws are not clear on computer trespass (Gemignani, 1990, pp. 489–94). The requisite laws must not be too broad (and catch too many actions in their net, as well as interfere with normal activity) or too narrow (and let too many criminal actions slip through). Gemignani raises some serious questions that must be faced in framing these laws:

> Would an expert be able to circumvent the statute by designing a harmful program that would not be covered by the statute? Does the proposed statute clearly define the act that will be punished so as to give clear notice to a reasonable person? Does the statute distinguish between intentional acts and innocent programming errors? Does the statute unreasonably interfere with the free flow of information? Does it raise a First Amendment free speech problem? (Gemignani, 1990, p. 493)

It is clear that the laws must be designed thoughtfully and carefully, and be based on an appreciation of the technology. They must take into account the rights of both programmers and users, and distinctions as to what is unlawful must be clearly drawn. Once this is done, the importance of violations of the laws must be recognized by the courts, which currently view computer crime as only slightly more serious than shoplifting and illegal immigration (Gemignani, 1990, p. 491).

Theft and invasion by computer are relatively easy and safe at this time. One can break into a computer across the country or halfway around the world from the comfort of home, at no physical risk. The crime can be carried to completion with no one seeing the agent do it. It provides the kind of cloak of invisibility given by Gyges' ring.[60]

Socrates maintained that the truly good individual would behave the same way with or without the ring of Gyges. There are many in the computer community who behave ethically even though no one is watching them, because they know it is the right thing to do. The ideal would be if the entire community were composed of such individuals, and then no laws or regulations would be required. However, not everyone *does* act ethically when given the cover of invisibility, and so we need good laws to deal with those who violate the rights and the trust of others.

If violations of the law occur, the punishment should fit the seriousness of the crime. To this point, it seems that sentences for computer crimes have been unusually light. We should not, however, go too far in the other direction, either. It was reported that an accountant at the Agricultural Bank of China had forged bank-deposit slips and embezzled more than 122,000 British pounds over a three-month period in 1991. He was caught when he tried to transfer some of the money to the Shenzhen province; he was convicted, and executed (!) "as a warning to others that computer crime does not pay."[61] China sentenced to death a pair of brothers, who had hacked into a state-owned bank and transferred funds into secret accounts, in 1998.[62] We should not go that far, but punishments should be commensurate with the damages inflicted in analogous non–computer-aided crimes. If *intent* is also to be taken into account, then we are fitting the punishment to the criminal, and not just the crime, as we have already discussed. This view seems evident in both the Robert Morris Jr. and the David LaMacchia cases.

In 1985, an ACM panel on hacking made a number of recommendations "to promote effective legal and ethical use of the technology." These included passing laws that are "consistent and enforceable"—consistent between federal and state laws, and across state lines, since computer communications traverse state borders. Legal definitions of terms such as "computer abuse" should be made clear. Curricula in computing should include discussions of ethical issues. Access to computing power should be made available to anyone interested. A system of apprenticeship of young people to professionals in the field should be established. An organization should be established for a program of education and development of skills in computing. There should be a central information resource on technological aspects of stories for the press.

In general, a system of good education (including a basis for moral decisions) and good law is needed. Plato and Kant would point out that laws do not make people moral, though they may prevent them from *acting* unethically (if it is against the law, and they fear punishment). But true morality must come from within. You *choose* to do the right thing *because it is good* and you recognize its goodness. Aristotle adds that you must act from a *fixed, unchanging principle* or a *fixed, virtuous character* for the action to be virtuous. Plato's Form of the Good and Kant's Categorical Imperative are attempts to provide such principles. However, Aristotle recognizes that not all are naturally good, or are brought up to respect argument, so we need laws, "for most people obey necessity rather than argument, and punishments rather than the sense of what is noble." The individual who wants to make people "better by his care must try to become capable of legislating, if it is through laws that we can become good" (*Nicomachean Ethics*, X, 9).

■ ENDNOTES

1. If one tried to store as an integer value the U.S. national debt, in trillions of dollars, it would exceed the storage capacity on a 16-bit microcomputer (which is $2^{15} - 1$, or 32,767) and could press the capacity on a 32-bit micro or mini (which is $2^{31} - 1$, or 2,147,483,647).

2. If the machine stores more than eight bits in the fractional part of the number, it may be slightly higher, but still not the exact $256.00.

3. Paul Mungo and Bryan Clough, *Approaching Zero* (New York: Random House, 1992), pp. 14–27; consult this book for many more fascinating details.

4. Forester and Morrison, *Computer Ethics,* 2nd ed. (Cambridge, MA: MIT Press, 1994), p. 77.

5. *Software Engineering Notes* 16, no. 1 (January 1991), 14.

6. *Software Engineering Notes* 19, no. 1 (January 1994), 8.

7. *Software Engineering Notes* 10, no. 1 (January 1985); from a report in the *London Daily Mail,* 2 November 1984.

8. *Software Engineering Notes* 9, no. 2 (April 1984). The scheme is not original with these perpetrators, however; the idea was used in the 1980 movie *Used Cars*, in which the "heroes" jam transmission of a pro football game and later interrupt a speech by then-President Jimmy Carter to air outrageous commercials for their used car lot.

9. *Software Engineering Notes* 11, no. 3 (July 1986), 20–21; *Software Engineering Notes* 11, no. 5 (October 1986), 24–25.

10. *Software Engineering Notes* 12, no. 4 (October 1987), 13; *Software Engineering Notes* 16, no. 1 (January 1991), 13.

11. *Software Engineering Notes* 13, no. 1 (January 1988), 7.

12. *Computerworld* 35, no. 22 (May 28, 2001), p. 42. See also Michael Myers, "Crimes of the 'Net'," *Newsweek*, November 14, 1994, p. 47.

13. A "back door" or "trap door" is often left in as a way for the system designer to get back into the system if the need arises. Generally, designers put in such a device to allow them to get around the protection against changing the code in an operating system, just in case they have to go in and make a modification or correct a "bug" (Parker, 1989, p. 20).

14. "UK Security Audit," *Software Engineering Notes* 12, no. 1 (January 1987), 17.

15. Donn Seeley, "Password Cracking: A Game of Wits," *Communications of the ACM* 32, no. 6 (June 1989), 700. Perhaps also try 'cab', 'bac', 'bca', or 'acb'? This gets more complex with a 4-letter code, of the form 'abcd', which has 24 permutations instead of 6. A string of length n has $n!$ (n factorial, or $n(n - 1)(n - 2)\ldots(2)(1)$) permutations.

16. *Software Engineering Notes* 16, no. 3 (July 1991), 13.

17. "West German Crackers Enter NASA Computers," *Software Engineering Notes* 12, no. 4 (October 1987), 14.

18. Cliff Stoll, *The Cuckoo's Egg* (New York: Pocket Books, 1990), p. 313. For a full and exciting account of Stoll's hunt for the hacker, reading this book is highly recommended; it is like a good detective story (but true). For a more technical account of the way in which he tracked the hacker, see "Stalking the Wily Hacker," *Communications of the ACM* 31, no. 5 (May 1988), 484–97.

19. "A Rise in Internet Break-ins Sets Off a Security Alarm," *Software Engineering Notes* 19, no. 2 (April 1994), 5. Excerpted from an article by Peter H. Lewis, *New York Times*, 8 February 1994.

20. *Software Engineering Notes* 18, no. 2 (April 1993), 4.

21. Ian H. Witten, "Computer (In)Security: Infiltrating Open Systems," *Abacus* 4, no. 4 (Summer 1987), 13.

22. Electronic file received through a friend at Cornell; the file originated with SQUID::"VALERT-L@IBM1.CC.LEHIGH.EDU". A report on this also appeared in *Software Engineering Notes* 15, no. 2 (April 1990), 16–18.

23. For a more detailed version of the incident, see Mungo and Clough, 1992, pp. 141–152; cf. *Software Engineering Notes* 17, no. 2 (April 1992), 18–19.

24. *Software Engineering Notes* 16, 1 (January 1991), 22.

25. Eugene H. Spafford, Kathleen A. Heaphy, and David J. Ferbrache, "A Computer Virus Primer," in *Computers Under Attack: Intruders, Worms, and Viruses*, ed. Peter J. Denning (Reading, MA: Addison-Wesley, 1990), p. 317.

26. John Brunner, *Shockwave Rider* (New York: Ballantine Books, 1975).

27. John Markoff, "U.S. Is Moving to Restrict Access to Facts About Computer Virus," *New York Times*, 11 November 1988, sec. A, p. 28.

28. Eugene H. Spafford, "Crisis and Aftermath," *Communications of the ACM* 32, no. 6 (June 1989), 678–79.

29. Peter J. Denning, "The Internet Worm," in *Computers Under Attack*, ed. Peter J. Denning, 1990, p. 195. The *finger* utility program allows a user to get information about other users—their full names, whether they are currently logged in, when they last accessed the system, and possibly even telephone numbers where they can be reached. The *fingerd* program, or *finger daemon*, is a background process to service remote users. The bug in *fingerd* allowed the worm to overrun the input buffer and insert a command of its own for the system. The *Sendmail* program routes mail to and from the system; the bug in Sendmail allowed the worm, by issuing the *DEBUG* command to it, to give it commands instead of a user address.

30. Pamela Samuelson, "Computer Viruses and Worms: Wrong, Crime, or Both?", in Denning, p. 481.

31. Samuelson, p. 484.

32. Samuelson, p. 484.

33. *Computerworld*, 14 November 1988, p. 8.

34. Spafford, Heaphy, and Ferbrache, p. 318.

35. Ibid., 333–34.

36. Witten, p. 19.

37. A. K. Dewdney, "Computer Recreations," *Scientific American*, May 1984, pp. 15–19, and March 1985, pp. 14–19.

38. Harold Joseph Highland, "Computer Viruses—A Post Mortem," in Denning, p. 304. Originally appeared in *Computers & Security* (August 1988), 367–70. See also Anne E. Webster, "University of Delaware and the Pakistani Virus," *Computers & Security* 8 (1989), 103–5.

39. Philip Elmer-DeWitt, Scott Brown, and Thomas McCarroll, "Invasion of the Data Snatchers!", *Time* (September 26, 1988), p. 63.

40. Fred Cohen, "Implications of Computer Viruses and Current Methods of Defense," in Denning, p. 388. See also Kenneth R. van Wyk, "The Lehigh Virus," *Computers & Security* 8 (1989), 107–10.

41. Denning, p. 286.

42. Spafford, Heaphy, and Ferbrache, p. 344. It is also referred to as the "bouncing ball" or the "Vera Cruz" virus.

43. Spafford, Heaphy, and Ferbrache, p. 346.

44. Spafford, Heaphy, and Ferbrache, pp. 351–52; Cohen, pp. 388–89; both articles are in Denning.

45. *Software Engineering Notes* 17, no. 2 (April 1992), 19; *Software Engineering Notes* 18, no. 2 (April 1993), 15.

46. "Health-Care Plan on Computer Disks Spreading 'Virus'?", *Editor & Publisher* 126, no. 45 (November 6, 1993), 13.

47. Michael Alexander, "Feds Crack Hacker Gang," *Datamation* 41, no. 6 (April 1, 1995), 15.

48. Jeff Goodell, "The Samurai and the Cyberthief," *Rolling Stone* 707 (May 4, 1995), p. 43; Paul Wallich, "A Rogue's Routing," *Scientific American* 272, no. 5 (May 1995), p. 31; John Markoff, "Hacker Case Underscores Internet's Vulnerability," *New York Times*, 17 February 1995, p. D1; "A Hacker Is Indicted in Computer Fraud Case," *New York Times*, 11 March 1995, p. A25.

49. Lindsy Van Gelder, "The Strange Case of the Electronic Lover," *Ms.*, October 1985, p. 99.

50. Van Gelder, pp. 103–4.

51. A MUD is a "Multi-User Dungeon" (an outgrowth of the "Dungeons and Dragons" game); it is also used to stand for "Multi-User Domain" or, for those into virtual reality, "Multi-User Dimension."

52. *Software Engineering Notes* 19, no. 1 (January 1994), 7–8.

53. Richard Brand, in "Is Computer Hacking a Crime?", *Harper's*, March 1990, p. 47.

54. Richard M. Stallman, in "Is Computer Hacking a Crime?", p. 48.

55. "Is Computer Hacking a Crime?", p. 49.

56. *Information Week* (September 12, 1994), 10.

57. Ann Steffora and Martin Cheek, "Hacking Goes Legit," *Industry Week* 243, no. 3 (February 7, 1994), 43.

58. Chris Johnston, Mark Fleishman, and Bruce Eder, "Wired: Just Say No to Computer Paranoia," *Village Voice* 33, no. 43 (October 25, 1988), S4.

59. G. Pascal Zachary, "Computer Viruses May Win Military Role," *Wall Street Journal*, 11 November 1991, sec. B, p. 1; Mark Lewyn, "'Killer' Computer Viruses: An Idea Whose Time Shouldn't Come," *Business Week* (July 23, 1990), 30.

60. In Book II of Plato's *Republic*, the story of Gyges' ring is related by Glaucon. Gyges, a shepherd, was tending his flocks one day when he came upon a crevice created by an earthquake in which he found a corpse wearing a beautiful ring. Gyges took the ring and wore it when he went back to town. When sitting with some acquaintances, he began twisting the ring on his finger, only to discover that this made him invisible! Taking advantage of this invisibility, Gyges seduced the queen, killed the king, and took the throne of Lydia.

Glaucon's point in the tale is that, he claims, if two men (one of whom is considered just and the other is thought unjust) each had a "ring of Gyges," they would behave exactly the same way, both acting unjustly and taking advantage of the cloak of invisibility. The implication here is that those who *are* just—that is, act in a just manner—only do so because they are afraid of being caught. Take away the threat of being caught, and they will cease to be just. This also connects with the teachings of the sophists, since they teach men how to cover their actions (through persuasive speech and devious action) with a similar "cloak of invisibility" that allows them to *appear just* while they are being unjust.

Socrates strongly disagrees, and says that the truly just individual will always behave the same way (justly), whether he has the ring of Gyges or not, because he is acting in the way that his reason tells him is best. The laws of justice are "written in his heart" (as is the new covenant God makes in Jeremiah 31: 31–33), and they, not external laws and forces, determine his actions. He is Kant's *autonomous* agent.

61. "China Executes Hacker," *Software Engineering Notes* 18, no. 3 (July 1993), A–12.

62. John Gittings, "China Sentences Bank Computer Hackers to Death," *The Manchester Guardian,* 30 December 1998, p. 16.

■ SHORT ESSAY QUESTIONS

1. Assess critically Richard Brand's claim in the "Is Computer Hacking a Crime?" forum that the solution to the threat of invasions of privacy and theft of private data (such as credit records and medical records) is that it not be collected in the first place. Would/could this work? What kind of a society would function effectively without the collection of such data?

2. Write a personal letter (as if to a friend) to a hacker (in the new, "bad" sense, not in the old Stallman sense) which tries to convince your friend to discontinue hacking activities. Use the best arguments and persuasion you can.

3. Check out the current concerns of the Computer Professionals for Social Responsibility (CPSR) on their website: (www.cpsr.org). Pick a topic and research it. What is at stake? How serious is the concern?

Join the CPSR. Their address is P.O. Box 717, Palo Alto, CA. 94302–0717. (Student memberships are only $20 a year.) Examine their most recent newsletters and the information they put out on Listserv on the Net.

4. The use of e-mail is becoming more and more prevalent in our society. An estimated 15 million people employed in Fortune–2000 companies were using it in 1992, and many more now. Do you see any potential disadvantages other than those discussed in this chapter? If so, what are they? Do you think the benefits outweigh the potential dangers? Assess both sides critically.

■ LONG ESSAY QUESTIONS

1. Do a literature search to see what you can find out about the newest instances of hacking, viruses, worms, and the like. Document interesting cases that have occurred since those written about in this book.

What sort of a trend do you see based on your research? Is destructive hacking on the rise, or is it becoming less prevalent? Try to assess why it is taking the direction that you find it has moved in.

2. Get copies of the Clinton administration's two volumes on the National Information Infrastructure (NII); see the text for information on how to do this. Read carefully for crucial points, and then draft a serious, critical letter to the Secretary of Commerce indicating what you support in the proposal and what you think its weaknesses (if any) are. You may want to make reference to commentaries on NII such as those by CPSR.

3. In Pamela Samuelson's discussion in Denning of the Internet Worm, she argues that there should be new legislation to deal specifically with computer intrusions like the worm, without trying to make them fit under current laws whose designers did not conceive of this technology. Discuss (based on what you learned in Part One) the various advantages of a "consequences-oriented" approach (like Utilitarianism), a "conduct-oriented approach" (like Kantian ethics), a "virtue ethics" position (following Aristotle), or the goods view. Samuelson mentions the first two approaches, but not the latter two. Are there any other viable moral approaches to this problem? If so, what are they? Just what sort of legislation might each approach give rise to? (If you come up with a good answer here, please share it with the Congress of the United States.)

4. The issue of punishment is a very knotty one. It is alternately justified as retribution (proportional), restitution, revenge, utilitarian (promoting the greatest good for the greatest number), or as a deterrent. What (if anything) justifies punishment, and what determines which punishment is appropriate for a given crime? Which view of punishment seems most apt for destructive hacking, and how do you think the severity of the punishment should be determined? Should the *intentions* of the hacker be taken into consideration? In your discussion, include perspective from at least *one* of the following:

Plato, *Gorgias* (472a–477a, 507a–e, 525a–527d)—punishment *benefits* the criminal.

Plato, *Laws* (V, 735; IX, 853–863b, 872a–873a, 880e–881a)—laws on crime and punishment in the *real* (not the *ideal*) state.

H.L.A. Hart, "Prolegomenon to the Principles of Punishment," in *Proceedings of the Aristotelian Soc.* 60 (1959–60)

John Rawls, "Two Concepts of Rules," in F. A. Olafson, ed., *Society, Law, and Morality* (Englewood Cliffs, NJ: Prentice-Hall, 1961)—

basically deals with the problem of a utilitarian view allowing the punishment of a totally innocent person for the overall good.

Walter Berns, "The Morality of Anger," in Robert M. Baird and Stuart E. Rosenbaum, eds., *The Philosophy of Punishment* (New York: Prometheus, 1988)

W. D. Ross, *The Right and the Good* (Oxford: Clarendon Press, 1930), Appendix II

A. R. Manser, "It Serves You Right," *Philosophy* 37, 142 (1962), 293–306.

5. University of Michigan student Jake Baker posted at least three "grisly" rape-and-murder stories on the Internet BBS alt.sex.stories; one of the stories used the name of a female classmate of Baker's. A Michigan alum read the story and alerted the campus administration. Baker was arrested by the FBI and charged with making interstate threats to injure someone (see *People Weekly* (March 6, 1995), pp. 59–60). When university police searched his room, they found e-mail he had sent describing his fantasies about abducting another female Michigan student, also named. Baker's case was dismissed on June 21, 1995, because "his words were a fantasy rather than a true threat" (Jeffrey Rosen, "Cheap Speech," *New Yorker*, 7 August 1995, p. 78). Assess Baker's actions from a moral perspective.

■ REFERENCES AND RECOMMENDED READINGS

Anthes, Gary H. "Newspapers Go Digital." *Computerworld* 28, 8 (February 21, 1994), 58.

Anthes, Gary H. "Virus Fighters Face Expanding Threat." *Computerworld* 28, 25 (June 20, 1994), 39, 41.

Beard, Jonathan. "Virus Busters Get a Shot in the Arm." *New Scientist* 141, 1908 (January 15, 1994), 18–19.

Betts, Mitch. "Critics Anticipate Privacy Abuses on Superhighway." *Computerworld* 28, 5 (January 31, 1994), 27.

Bruno, Maria. "Hackers Steal 1 Million Card Numbers." *Book Technology News* 14, 4 (April 2001), 6.

CPSR Newsletter. Winter 1994 and Summer 1994.

CPSR (by Gary Chapman). "CPSR Statement on the Computer Virus." *Communications of the ACM* 32, 6 (June 1989), 699.

Cavazos, Edward A., and Gavino Morin. *Cyberspace and the Law: Your Rights and Duties in the On-Line World.* Cambridge, MA: MIT Press, 1994.

Cerf, Vint. "Ethics and the Internet." *Communications of the ACM* 32, 6 (June 1989), 710.

Cohen, Fred. "Friendly Contagion." *Sciences* 31, 5 (September 1991), 22–28.

Coldwell, R. A. "Some Social Parameters of Computer Crime." *Australian Computer Journal* 22, 2 (May 1990), 43–46.

Cosentino, Victor J. "Virtual Legality." *Byte* 19, 3 (March 1994), 278.

Coughlin, Ellen K. "Proposed Rules on Government Data Worry Librarians and Scholars." *Chronicle of Higher Education* (June 12, 1985), 11.

Dehaven, John. "Stealth Virus Attacks." *Byte* 18, 6 (May 1993), 137–142.

Denning, Peter J., ed. *Computers Under Attack: Intruders, Worms, and Viruses.* Reading, MA: Addison-Wesley, 1990.

Dery, Mark, ed. *Flame Wars: The Discourse of Cyberculture.* Durham, NC: Duke University Press, 1994.

Eisenberg, Ted, David Gries, Juris Hartmanis, Don Holcomb, M. Stuart Lynn, and Thomas Santoro. "The Cornell Commission: On Morris and the Worm." *Communications of the ACM* 32, 6 (June 1989), 706–9.

Elmer-DeWitt, Philip, Scott Brown, and Thomas McCarroll. "Invasion of the Data Snatchers!" *Time* (September 26, 1988), 62–67.

Emmeche, Claus. *The Garden in the Machine.* Princeton, NJ: Princeton University Press, 1994; discusses the Game of Life.

Farber, David J. "NSF Poses Code of Networking Ethics." *Communications of the ACM* 32, 6 (June 1989), 688.

Forester, Tom, and Perry Morrison. *Computer Ethics: Cautionary Tales and Ethical Dilemmas in Computing.* 2nd ed. Cambridge, MA: MIT Press, 1994, ch. 4.

Garber, Lee. "Melissa Virus Creates a New Type of Threat." *IEEE Computer* 32, 6 (June 1999), 16–19.

Gemignani, Michael. "Viruses and Criminal Law." In Peter J. Denning, ed., *Computers Under Attack* (Reading, MA: Addison-Wesley, 1990), 489–94.

Goodrum, Abby, and Mark Manion. "The Ethics of Hactivism." *Journal of Information Ethics* 9, 2 (Fall 2000), 51–59.

Gould, Carol C., ed. *The Information Web.* Boulder, CO: Westview Press, 1989, essays 1, 5, 7, 8, 13.

"Health-Care Plan on Computer Disks Spreading 'Virus'?" *Editor and Publisher* 126, 45 (November 6, 1993), 13.

"Is Computer Hacking a Crime?" (Harper's Forum) *Harper's Magazine* (March 1990), 45–57.

Johnson, Deborah G. *Computer Ethics.* 2nd ed. Englewood Cliffs, NJ: Prentice-Hall, 1994, ch. 6.

Kane, Pamela. *V. I. R. U. S. Protection: Vital Information Resources Under Siege.* New York: Bantam, 1989.

Langford, Duncan, ed. *Internet Ethics.* New York: St. Martin's, 2000.

Lee, John A. N., Gerald Segal, and Rosalie Steier. "Positive Alternatives: A Report on an ACM Panel on Hacking." *Communications of the ACM* 29, 4 (April 1986), 297–300.

Levy, Steven. *Hackers: Heroes of the Computer Revolution.* New York: Doubleday, 1985.

Lewyn, Mark. "'Killer' Computer Viruses: An Idea Whose Time Shouldn't Come." *Business Week* (July 23, 1990), p. 30.

Lore, Lew, Douglas Stanglin, Joseph L. Galloway, Robert Rosenberg, Michael Satchell, et al. "Vengeance by 'Virus'." *U.S. News & World Report* 105, 13 (October 3, 1988), p. 10.

Markoff, John. "Can Computer Viruses Be Domesticated to Serve Mankind?" *New York Times,* 6 October 1991, sec. 4, p. 18.

McEwen, J. Thomas (report contributors: Dennis Fester and Hugh Nugent). *Dedicated Computer Crime Units.* Washington, DC: National Institute of Justice, June 1989.

Moore, Thomas H. "Colleges Seem Vulnerable to Legal Actions Arising from Computer Viruses." *Chronicle of Higher Education* 35, 42 (June 28, 1989), A1, A20.

Mungo, Paul, and Bryan Clough. *Approaching Zero: The Extraordinary Underworld of Hackers, Phreakers, Virus Writers, and Keyboard Criminals.* New York: Random House, 1992.

Negroponte, Nicholas. *Being Digital.* New York: Knopf, 1995.

Parker, Donn B. *Computer Crime: Criminal Justice Resource Manual.* 2nd ed. Washington, DC: National Institute of Justice, August 1989, sec. 2.

Poundstone, William. *The Recursive Universe.* New York: Morrow, 1985.

Raymond, Eric, ed. *The New Hacker's Dictionary.* Cambridge, MA: MIT Press, 1991.

Rochlis, Jon A., and Mark W. Eichin. "With Microscope and Tweezers: The Worm from MIT's Perspective." *Communications of the ACM* 32, 6 (June 1989), 689–98.

Rosenberger, Rob, and Ross M. Greenberg. "Computer Virus Myths." March 1992.

Samuelson, Pamela. "Can Hackers Be Sued for Damages Caused By Computer Viruses?" *Communications of the ACM* 32, 6 (June 1989), 666–69.

Samuelson, Pamela. "Copyright and Digital Libraries." *Communications of the ACM* 38, 3 (April 1995), 15–21, 110.

Schemo, Diana Jean. "Software Maker Accused of Using Virus to Compel Client to Pay Bill." *New York Times,* 23 November 1993, sec. A., p. 1.

Seabrook, John. "My First Flame." *New Yorker* (June 6, 1994), 70–79.

Shoch, John, and Jon A. Hupp. "The 'Worm' Programs—Early Experience with a Distributed Computation." *Communications of the ACM* 25, 3 (March 1982), 172–80.

Seeley, Donn. "Password Cracking: A Game of Wits." *Communications of the ACM* 32, 6 (June 1989), 700–703.

Slatella, Michelle, and Joshua Quittner. *Masters of Deception: The Gang that Raided Cyberspace.* New York: HarperCollins, 1995.

Spafford, Eugene H. "The Internet Worm: Crisis and Aftermath." *Communications of the ACM* 32, 6 (June 1989), 678–87.

SQUID: "VALERT-L@IBM1.CC.LEHIGH.EDU." "Twelve Tricks Trojan." (1990)

Steffora, Ann, and Martin Cheek. "Hacking Goes Legit." *Industry Week* 243, 3 (February 7, 1994), 43–46.

Stoll, Cliff. *The Cuckoo's Egg: Tracking a Spy Through the Maze of Computer Espionage.* New York: Pocket Books, 1990.

Stoll, Clifford. *Silicon Snake Oil: Second Thoughts on the Information Highway.* New York: Doubleday, 1995.

Stoll, Clifford. "Stalking the Wily Hacker." *Communications of the ACM* 31, 5 (May 1988), 484–97.

Sudetic, Chuck. "Bulgarians Linked to Computer Virus." *New York Times,* 21 December 1990, sec. A, p. 9.

Sussman, Vic. "Policing Cyberspace." *U. S. News & World Report* (January 23, 1995), 55–60.

Thompson, Ken. "Reflections on Trusting Trust." (Turing Award Lecture) *Communications of the ACM* 27, 8 (August 1984), 761–763.

Trumbull, Mark. "Computer 'Viruses' Infiltrate Government." *Christian Science Monitor*, July 14, 1988, p. 3.

Van Gelder, Lindsy. "The Strange Case of the Electronic Lover." *Ms. Magazine* 14, 4 (October 1985), 94, 99, 101–4, 117, 123–24.

Wasik, Martin. *Crime and the Computer.* Oxford, England: Clarendon Press, 1991, ch. 3.

"The Worm Story" (Special issue on the Internet Worm). *Communications of the ACM* 32, 6 (June 1989), 677 ff.

Chapter 7

Privacy

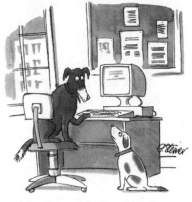

"On the Internet, nobody knows you're a dog."

> *I give the fight up: let there be an end, A privacy, an obscure nook for me.*
> *I want to be forgotten even by God.*
>
> —Robert Browning, Paracelsus
>
> *The grave's a fine and private place,*
> *But none, I think, do there embrace.*
>
> —Andrew Marvell,
> "To His Coy Mistress"

*H*uman beings may invade the privacy of other human beings, but in our modern technological society it is a variety of fancy monitoring devices and computerized record-keeping and record-processing procedures—initiated, run, and analyzed by humans—that pose the greatest threats to personal privacy by greatly enhancing the possibilities of invasion. One cannot help but think of the two-way telescreens in George Orwell's *1984* or the "Boss" monitoring Charlie Chaplin's bathroom break in *Modern Times*, if the potential of much of today's technology is examined closely.[1]

An analogy can be drawn with the right to own guns. Defenders of this right say, "It's not guns that kill people—people kill people." Similarly, one can say, "it's not computers that invade privacy—people invade privacy." However, the storage, processing, and monitoring capabilities of today's computers make these invasions of privacy much easier and perhaps more likely.

WHY IS PRIVACY OF VALUE?

In the *Second Treatise of Government*, John Locke argued that anyone who threatens your (private) property potentially threatens your life, and so you are justified in using the same measures against such a person (including killing him) that are permissible in protecting your life. To Locke, the most fundamental human rights were to life, liberty, and property. The defense of private property put forward by Locke connected it with one's right to own one's own body, and any natural extensions of that body through one's labor.

The right to one's own, if valid, can be interpreted to include one's thoughts and actions. Thus one would seem to have a right to protect those thoughts and actions against unwanted intrusions; for, just as no one should violate someone else's body (by rape or murder, for example), no one should violate someone else's thoughts or actions. The logical exceptions to this are if one's actions infringe on another's rights; then they are subject to control by others. We have a notion of having a personal "space" into which we can invite others, but into which no one should trespass unbidden. Yet modern surveillance techniques and methods of record analysis and "matching" pose a threat to invade our personal spaces, often without our knowledge and certainly without our permission.

The Stoics found that in bad times, even though their bodies might be in chains, their minds could still be free, and it was on this presupposition that they turned inward to engage in the freedom of their thoughts. If one's mental activity is also threatened, there is nothing left to make life worthwhile.

In order to be fully developed human beings, we must be free to choose. Kant says that the moral individual must be *rational* and *autonomous*. I cannot be autonomous if there are outside forces directing my decisions. My choices must be private to be truly *mine*, to be truly *choices*. One of the highest-level goods is the exercise of the will, displaying courage or fortitude. These are not group activities. One's courage, one's knowledge, even one's pleasure are all personal, private. They could not exist without privacy. Your courage may help others, and you can share your knowledge, but they originate and develop in your own private world. Thus if privacy is not intrinsically valuable in itself, it makes possible achievements that *are* intrinsically good.

Kant also stressed the value of a *person*, as an end in itself, and that persons should never be used as means. Constant surveillance diminishes your personhood. The world is no longer as you think it is, but rather a miniworld under the microscope of some larger world. You become a *means* to some other end—that of governmental power, or corporate profit. Even if you do not ever know you are being observed, the value of what you hold in high regard is diminished, made into a cold statistic. If you *do* realize that you are being observed, then this affects your actions, and you are no longer autonomous.

Charles Fried argues that privacy is essential to the fundamental good of friendship. Friendship entails love, trust, and mutual respect, and these can occur only in a *rational context* of privacy.[2] Trust presumes some things are secret or confidential and will not be revealed; if there is no privacy, there can be no such confidences. A love relationship involves a certain intimacy that is just between two people; if all of their actions, conversations, and special gifts are made public, something valuable has been lost.

Privacy may simply be necessary to mental survival, just as the body needs sleep. Much of the time we are on a public stage, performing in class, or in front of a classroom, or at work for an employer, or acting in a play. This requires concentration and effort; we work hard to put forward a certain appearance and a high level of performance to others. It would be very difficult, if not impossible, to do this all of the time. Thus we need some privacy in which to rest, to kick off our shoes, put our feet up, and do and think what we please, *in private*. We are talking about *preservation of mental health* here.

A utilitarian argument can be made that invasions of privacy cause more harm than good overall. There is the potential for inaccurate information being spread around about a person, or even information that is accurate, but is no one else's concern, being *misused*. Think carefully about the sorts of instances in which you value your privacy. Your bank account? Your grades? (Of course, you may have to disclose them to a potential employer or graduate school, and the administration knows them; but colleges, under federal law, must protect your records from casual prying.) Your bathroom activities? (Presumably, you would prefer not to have these broadcast over the airwaves.) Your sex life, or lack thereof? (There are legal protections in most states for what consenting adults do in the privacy of their own homes; these legal protections are grounded in fundamental ethical principles, which recognize privacy as a good, or as contributing to other goods.) Your medical records? Your private fantasies? What else would you add to the list?

What is it about each of the preceding cases that you value and that would be compromised if your privacy in these respects was invaded? A totalitarian government, like that of Nazi Germany or Orwell's *1984*, might want to know *everything* about its citizens. Those citizens would then cease to be autonomous, freely choosing beings; they would be more like animals in a laboratory, or cogs in a machine.

Alexis de Tocqueville, writing in *Democracy in America* about his observations of the United States in 1832, described the sort of despotism that he feared could overcome democratic nations:

> Above this race of men stands an immense and tutelary power, which takes upon itself alone to secure their gratifications, and to watch over their fate. That power is absolute, minute, regular, provident, and mild. It would be like the authority of a parent, if, like that authority, its object was to prepare men for manhood; but it seeks, on the contrary, to keep them in perpetual childhood: it is well content that the people should rejoice, provided they think of nothing but rejoicing. For their happiness such a government willingly labors, but it chooses to be the sole agent and the only arbiter of that happiness; it provides for their security, foresees and supplies their necessities, facilitates their pleasures, manages their principal concerns, directs their industry, regulates the descent of property, and subdivides their inheritances: what remains, but to spare them all the care of thinking and all the trouble of living? . . .
>
> It covers the surface of society with a network of small complicated rules, minute and uniform, through which the most original minds and the most energetic characters cannot penetrate, to rise above the crowd. The will of man is not shattered, but softened, bent, and guided; men are seldom forced by it to act, but they are constantly restrained from acting: such a power does not destroy, but it prevents existence; it does not tyrannize, but it compresses, enervates, extinguishes, and stupefies a people, till each nation is reduced to be nothing better than a flock of timid and industrious animals, of which the government is the shepherd.
>
> (Tocqueville, 1956, pp. 303–4)

You probably remember what it was like to be a young child. You don't get any privacy. Adults are constantly hovering over you, afraid you will hurt yourself or some object, and telling you "no" a lot. As you grow up, you are given more and more autonomy, control of your own life, and *privacy*. Who would want to give this up by going back to total surveillance?

"I'LL BE WATCHING YOU"

Gary T. Marx uses the lyrics from the rock song "Every Breath You Take" by the Police to point out the scope of current surveillance in our society:

every breath you take	[breath analyzer]
every move you make	[motion detection]
every bond you break	[polygraph]
every step you take	[electronic anklet]

every single day	[continuous monitoring]
every word you say	[bugs, wiretaps, mikes]
every night you stay . . .	[light amplifier]
every vow you break . . .	[voice stress analyzer]
every smile you fake	[brain wave analysis]
every claim you stake . . .	[computer matching]
I'll be watching you.	[video surveillance][3]

This is a very dramatic way to illustrate what Marx calls "the new surveillance." This might also be called "dataveillance"; we are living in a world where data, or information, has become the most active commodity. One buys and sells information—on which products the affluent neighborhoods are buying, on the "best buys" in goods (*Consumer Reports*), on who are the most likely prospects to buy into a land deal, and on and on.

Information about you is sold. The magazine you subscribe to sells your mailing address to other magazines, or to those who sell products that connect with the theme of the magazine. There is an increasing demand for information that can be found in government records, and a *New York Times* article comments that, "for government, selling data can provide extra revenue in times of tight budgets."[4] Vance Packard had noted as early as 1964, in *The Naked Society*, that privacy was becoming harder to maintain, and surveillance was becoming more pervasive.

SOME NOTEWORTHY VIOLATIONS OF PRIVACY INVOLVING COMPUTERS

Ed Pankau, the president of Inter-Tect, a Houston investigative agency, wrote a book called *How to Investigate by Computer*. In it, he describes how easy it is to sit at a computer terminal and gather information about someone, and how lucrative it can be for an agency like his. He says that much of his business comes from single women who want potential romantic partners investigated. "For $500, Inter-Tect investigative agency in Houston promises to verify within a week a person's age, ownership of businesses, history of bankruptcies, if there are any tax liens, appearance in newspaper articles, as well as divorces and children."[5]

Proctor & Gamble, disturbed when they discovered that someone had leaked confidential company information to the *Wall Street Journal*, got a court order for the phone company in Cincinnati, Ohio, to turn over the phone numbers of anyone who had called the home or office of the *Journal* reporter on the article. This involved scanning millions of calls made by 650,000 phone units.[6] However, this sort of search is the kind of thing that is made incredibly easy by computerization. What is scary is the impact on private lives of the ease of getting such information.

In California in 1989, Rebecca Schaeffer, a television actress, was murdered by a man who got her home address through the Department of Motor Vehicles records. Since then, California has restricted access to DMV files, but they can still be accessed readily by car dealers, banks, insurance companies, and process servers. Since anyone can register as a process server for a small fee, this does not afford much protection of such files.[7]

Although the following is not an invasion of *personal* privacy, it makes an interesting example of the power of computer correlation. The scholars working with the Dead Sea Scrolls had very slowly been releasing the documents as they finished working with them and had denied other groups any access to them. However, they did publish concordances of some of the scrolls that had not yet been published. The concordances list all the significant words and their place of occurrence in the text. A group at Union Hebrew College in Cincinnati "reverse-engineered" the concordance, by computer, to recreate one of the unreleased texts.[8] Again, this would not have been possible without the use of a computer. What the Dead Sea Scrolls scholars had hoped to keep private until they were ready to publish was made public through the use of a program that was able to manipulate and correlate the partial information they *had* released.

Software Engineering Notes reported on a middle school computer in Burbank, California, that calls the homes of absent students until it gets a live voice or an answering machine, to check on the validity of the absences.[9] This kind of surveillance could easily be extended to other areas—the workplace in particular.

Records disclosed in 1992 indicate that many employees of the Los Angeles Police Department ("dozens") had been using the police computer files to investigate babysitters, house sitters, and others (potential dates?) for personal reasons.[10] When we think of people in police departments and in tax return offices *snooping* into our files for their own personal reasons—people who are not authorized to process personal records—it should send chills up and down our spines.[11] Who is snooping into our bank records, our charge-card records, our phone records, and for what reasons?

In *The Naked Consumer*, Erik Larson describes an interview he had with Jonathan Robbin, president of Claritas, a Virginia "target-marketing company." The company uses computerized *cluster analysis* of census data into different neighborhood types and then examines (and predicts) their consumer habits. They call this analysis "geodemographics"; some of the categories identified are Blue Blood Estates (the richest), Gray Power (the oldest), Public Assistance (the poorest), Pools & Patios, Shotguns & Pickups, Tobacco Roads, and Bohemian Mix (Larson, 1992, pp. 46–47). Claritas has many customers, including the U.S. Army, ABC, American Express, Publishers Clearing House, and big manufacturers of consumer goods such as Coca-Cola, Colgate-Palmolive, and R. J. Reynolds Tobacco. Robbin calls his computer system "a 'prosthetic' device for the mind" (Larson, 1992, p. 47)—one that allows corporate minds to "perceive" new targets. For example, the new Saturn division of GM used the Claritas program PRIZM (Potential Rating Index for Zip Markets) "as part of its vast market research campaign to figure out what kind of car to build and how to sell it" (Larson, 1992, p. 48). You can check it out on their website (www.connect.claritas.com).

Lotus Corporation was going to market a software package called Lotus Marketplace: Households, which was a database containing information on 120,000,000 Americans, including names, addresses, incomes, consumer preferences, and other personal data. In January 1991, however, Lotus withdrew the package due to an avalanche of complaints about its invasion of privacy.

Jeffrey Rothfeder, in *Privacy for Sale*, describes how easy it is to access credit rating information on anyone; he was able to get extensive information on Dan Quayle and Dan Rather. He describes how Oral Roberts was able to buy lists of debtors whose accounts were overdue 60 days or more. Roberts used these lists to send letters addressing the person by first name, saying that he is a friend, and that "it's time to get out from under a load of debt, a financial bondage." The letter continued, commiserating with the recipient's financial burden, and then got to the point—to plant a seed to get out of the financial bondage by sending a gift of $100 to Oral Roberts, so he could intercede with God and "begin the war on your debt" (Rothfeder, 1992, pp. 23–24).

Rothfeder discusses the fact that your credit reports might not be private, but your video-rental records are. This is because of a personal incident involving a government official. When Robert Bork was a candidate for the Supreme Court in 1987, "an enterprising reporter" at a Washington weekly paper went to Bork's local video store and got a list of the movies that Bork had rented recently (nothing salacious; mostly John Wayne). The *City Paper* published the list of titles anyway, and "lawmakers were outraged—and quickly passed the Video Privacy Protection Act of 1988" (Rothfeder, 1992, p. 27).

Rothfeder describes a service called PhoneFile where for a fee you could get the address, telephone number, and "household makeup" of almost anyone in the United States, from just the name and the state of residence (1992,

p. 29). A New York City woman named Karen Hochmann received a call in the fall of 1988 from a salesman for ITT who wanted her to subscribe to their long-distance service. When she said no, that she didn't make many out-of-town calls, the salesman said, "I'm surprised to hear you say that; I see from your phone records that you frequently call Newark, Delaware, and Stamford, Connecticut." Hochmann was "shocked" and "scared" by this blatant invasion of her personal records (Rothfeder, 1992, p. 89).

Rothfeder reports on the case of a young man whose American Express card was cancelled because the company determined that he did not have enough money in his bank balance to pay his March bill (1992, p. 17). Apparently, American Express made regular checks into people's financial accounts to determine the likelihood of their being able to pay their AmEx tabs.

There exist databases on employees in heavy industries like construction, oil, and gas that are accessed regularly by employers—for example, Employers Information Service (EIS) in Louisiana. They contain information such as which employees have demanded workers' compensation; the employer consulting such a database may then decide not to hire such a potential employee (Rothfeder, 1992, pp. 154–57). There apparently are also databases maintained by landlords, which can be used to determine that they do not want to rent to people who show up in the database as having complained to previous landlords (even if such complaints are about lack of heat or water or rodent control).

The coming together of the information superhighway and the proposals for national health care raise serious problems in terms of the confidentiality of medical records. There is a principle that goes back to Hippocrates in the 5th century B.C. that a doctor should hold a patient's medical information to be confidential. But storing of patient records in electronic form and transferring them from one computer to another, perhaps across considerable physical distances, raises all of the difficulties that we have already seen with the security of *any* electronic data. A report was produced in 1991 called *The Computerized Patient Record: An Essential Technology for Health Care*; this raises serious issues of the accuracy, access, and privacy of such a record.[12]

Many corporations have a privacy officer, and the Clinton administration created a position of "chief counselor for privacy." However, the George W. Bush administration decided not to fill that position; rather, it put any privacy issues under the Office of Management and Budget (one might wonder just how much attention privacy issues will get *there*). In 1997–8, Congress took an interest in issues of medical privacy with the Medical Information

Privacy and Security Act (MIPSA), which gives patients the right to control access to their medical records. One area of concern is that physicians often send out their notes made on tape to be transcribed. The people doing the transcribing have no medical confidentiality obligation as would a doctor, and this raises serious possibilities for invasions of privacy.

Some people are so disturbed by the dehumanization they believe is being brought about by computers that they mount physical attacks against the machines; many of these incidents were described in Chapter 5. Other such attacks were perpetrated by the Committee for the Liquidation of Computers, which bombed the government computer center in Toulouse, France, on January 28, 1983. Bombings also took place at the Dusseldorf, Germany, offices of IBM and Control Data Corporation in 1982, the Sperry Rand office in West Berlin, and a Harrison, New York, office of IBM (Eaton, 1986, p. 133).

In 1974, Senators Barry Goldwater and Charles Percy proposed an amendment to a bill in Congress to stop the use of a Social Security number as a universal identifier, to "stop this drift towards reducing each person to a number":

> Once the social security number is set as a universal identifier, each person would leave a trail of personal data behind him for all of his life which could be immediately reassembled to confront him. Once we can be identified to the administration in government or in business by an exclusive number, we can be pinpointed wherever we are, we can be more easily manipulated, we can be more easily conditioned and we can be more easily coerced.[13]

The Pythagoreans thought that everything was number, especially souls (or personal identities). Think about the old phrase "I've got your number!"—a statement that implies that you know everything there is to know about a person. If we allow government and big business to have all of our numbers, will they gain control of our personal destinies?

In Aleksandr Solzhenitsyn's *Cancer Ward*, we are given a chilling view from the Stalinist Soviet Union:

> As every man goes through life he fills in a number of forms, each containing a number of questions . . . There are thus hundreds of little threads radiating from every man, millions of threads in all. If these threads were suddenly to become visible, the whole sky would look like a spider's web, and if they materialized like rubber bands, buses and trams and even people would lose the ability to move and the wind would be unable to carry torn-up newspapers or autumn leaves along the streets of the city.

This is also reminiscent of the network of rules that Tocqueville described; is it today the network of computers containing information on all the members of our society?

In Chapter 8, which discusses errors, we will see examples of cases of mistaken identity that have caused serious invasions of the privacy of the people concerned; a number of such cases have occurred because of errors in the National Crime Information Center (NCIC) database.

If you are interested in privacy issues, look into the work of several civil rights organizations, such as the Electronic Frontier Foundation (www.eff.org), the Electronic Privacy Information Center (www.epic.org), the Center for Democracy and Technology (www.cdt.org), and People for Internet Responsibility (www.pfir.org). You might also want to check out www.privacyfoundation.org .

 ## A NATIONAL COMPUTERIZED CRIMINAL HISTORY SYSTEM?

In 1986, Kenneth C. Laudon wrote a book called *Dossier Society: Value Choices in the Design of National Information Systems*; his purpose was primarily to examine the FBI's plan for a national computerized criminal history (NCCH) system, and the impact it would have on our society and on personal privacy. He first examines the positive side of such a proposal—"the professional record keeper vision," as he calls it. This would foresee "a more rational world in which instantly available and accurate information would be used to spare the innocent and punish the guilty" (Laudon, 1986, p. 18). He says that this vision is held primarily by police, district attorneys, and criminal courts. The question of whether such information could be accurate and instantly available should be examined in the light of the performance of similar smaller systems (issues of errors and reliability are addressed in Chapter 8); the odds of increasing errors and decreasing reliability go up alarmingly as the size of a system increases.

As Laudon points out:

> The significance of a national CCH extends beyond the treatment of persons with a prior criminal record. Creating a single system is a multijurisdictional, multiorganizational effort which requires linking more than 60,000 criminal justice agencies with more than 500,000 workers, thousands of other government agencies, and private employers, from the local school district to the Bank of America, who will use the system for employment screening. (p. 16)

Two questions immediately come to mind about such a system: (1) What kind of reliability can it possibly have (and what will be the magnitude of the consequences of system failures or reporting errors)? and (2) is it appropriate, or even legal, for a system designed for one purpose (criminal record-keeping for the justice system) to be used for such a different purpose (employment screening)?

Laudon also notes that, in addition to the fingerprint records on millions of people with criminal records, the FBI has fingerprints of over twice as many citizens who do *not* have any criminal record. These would include people who have had their fingerprints taken for the armed forces, or to work in nuclear plants or on defense contracts, or to obtain security clearance for a job. With the amazing capabilities of computerized fingerprint identifications, it would be quite feasible to run *all* of these prints—not just those of people with criminal records—in any investigation. This would greatly increase the chances of "false positives" and the resulting invasion of innocent people's privacy and equanimity.

The second perspective regarding the national CCH, Laudon writes, is the "dossier society vision" held by members of the American Civil Liberties Union (ACLU), state and federal legislative research staffs, and defense lawyers. This vision thinks in terms of a system with "imperfect information and incomplete knowledge," a "runaway" system that would be out of anyone's control. Linking this information (see the upcoming section on "computer matching") with that from other agencies such as the Social Security Administration, the IRS, and the Department of Defense, could create "a caste of unemployable people, largely composed of minorities and poor people, who will no longer be able to rehabilitate themselves or find gainful employment in even the most remote communities" (Laudon, 1986, pp. 20–21). He also points out that even the present system already discriminates against those who live in poor and ghetto neighborhoods, where the police may regularly make a pass down the street in the summer and haul everyone in for questioning, thus creating "criminal records" for many who violated no laws (Laudon, 1986, pp. 226–27).

We must also be keenly aware of the possible breaches of security in such a system. In Chapter 6, we examined the various ways in which intruders break into large computer systems and their databases and steal or alter information. This could have disastrous consequences in a CCH.

Laudon pessimistically concludes, "In the absence of new legislation, it is clear that national information systems . . . will continue to develop in a manner which ensures the dominance of efficiency and security over freedom and liberty" (Laudon, 1986, p. 367). This is a frightening prospect. Those running these systems would claim that they are the guards of our domestic and national security; but the old question echoes, "Who will guard the guards?" Hobbes would respond that it must be the Leviathan. What other possibilities are there?

The *Christian Science Monitor* (September 7, 2001) included an article entitled "Watch the Watchers," that discussed the networks of surveillance cameras trained on all of us, from those in post offices to the IKONOS satellite 400 miles overhead that was able to discover the secret location of "Survivor III" in Kenya. There are also cameras that photograph those who run red lights (discussed in Simson Garfinkel's *Database Nation* (2000)). Surveillance cameras scanned the crowd at the 2001 Super Bowl in Tampa with a system called Face-Trace. Three women brought suit against an engineering firm for a camera installed in the restroom (reminiscent of Charlie Chaplin in *Modern Times*!).

THE FBI WIRETAP LAW

A hotly contested FBI proposal called the Wiretap Bill, or the Digital Telephony (DT) bill, finally passed the Congress *unanimously* on October 7, 1994. The bill *mandates* that all communications carriers must provide "wiretap-ready" equipment. The purpose of this is to facilitate the FBI's implementation of any wiretaps that are approved by the courts. The bill was strongly opposed by Computer Professionals for Social Responsibility (CPSR), the Voters Telecomm Watch (VTM), the ACLU, and the Electronic Privacy Information Center (EPIC), among others, and much support for this opposition was marshalled in terms of letters and e-mail messages to congressional representatives.

CPSR sent out a list of "100 Reasons to Oppose the FBI Wiretap Bill"; for example, Reason 29 was that the bill contains inadequate privacy protection for private e-mail records. The estimated cost of enacting the law is (according to a CPSR report) $500 million, a cost that will be borne by "government, industry, and consumers." (This information came from their website, **www.cpsr.org**.) This is just another instance of an action of government that will infringe a right of the public (in this case, privacy) and require the public to pay for it.

THE CLIPPER CHIP PROPOSAL

Another disturbing government proposal is the "Clipper chip," a device to establish a national data encryption standard. The device would sell for about $30 (or less in large quantities) and allow the encoding of messages sent electronically, to avoid tampering. The objectors (some of whom are referred to as "cypherpunks") fear that the standard, developed by NSA, will have a "trapdoor" that will allow the government to eavesdrop on any transmissions they choose.[14]

Some fear that the Clipper Chip will create an "Information Snooper-highway," but NSA assures us that Clipper is "your friend." CPSR is at the forefront of the opposition, and made available an electronic petition against Clipper; the petition goes straight to the president, because the proposal does not require congressional approval, and states reasons for the opposition.

The Clipper petition said that the proposal was developed in secret by federal agencies (NSA and the FBI) whose main interest is in surveillance, not in privacy. The plan will create obstacles to businesses wanting to compete in international markets, and discourage the development of better technologies to enhance privacy; "citizens who anticipate that the progress of technology will enhance personal privacy will find their expectations unfulfilled." The petition goes on to say that the signees fear that if the proposal and the standard are adopted, "even on a voluntary basis, privacy protection will be diminished, innovation will be slowed, government accountability will be lessened, and the openness necessary to ensure the successful development of the nation's communications infrastructure will be threatened" (CPSR Clipper petition, available on **www.cpsr.org**). In spite of the opposition, President Clinton approved the Clipper program.

There is a moral dilemma arising between the desire for an open society and the need to reduce crime and disorder. This tension is never easily resolved. The ideal would be to have a society in which all people minded their own business, supported the state, and were truly just (Plato's ideal state). Since the real world is not like that, there must be some laws and restrictions to control wrongdoing. However, the laws must not suppress all freedom and undermine what openness is possible. The Wiretap Bill and the Clipper Chip lean too far in the direction of suppressing fundamental goods such as freedom. There is an increased danger of the misuse of such methods in the wake of the September 11, 2001 terrorist attacks. If all communications can in principle be monitored, that creates a closed society, not an open one. All of the arguments against invasions of privacy in the beginning of this chapter apply.

 ## COMPUTERIZED CREDIT

The consumers of today use credit cards to buy countless products and services—from groceries to clothing to doctors' services. The information from any of these credit cards, plus data on any loans from banks or other financial institutions, goes into several huge centralized credit bureaus. An institution (or, as Rothfeder demonstrated, an individual) can request this information on someone, usually if they are considering giving the person a loan or a credit line.

The Federal Trade Commission puts out informational pamphlets on credit bureaus, so that individuals will know what they are, how they operate, and what the individual's rights are with respect to credit bureaus. A credit bureau is a kind of "clearinghouse" for information on a person's financial history. The Fair Credit Reporting Act of 1971 (amended in 1997) attempted to regulate the credit bureaus' operation and provide some privacy for the personal information they handle. However, there is in reality very little private about this data. The regulations *do* provide that an individual should have access to the information and the opportunity to request correction of any erroneous information.

One of the largest credit bureaus is Experian (once TRW). At the time of the first draft of this book, they would provide you, on request, with one free copy of your credit report per year; however, that option no longer seems to exist. Under the Fair Credit Reporting Act (as amended), the only people entitled to a free disclosure are the following: those who are unemployed and intend to apply for employment within 60 days; those receiving welfare assistance; those who believe their file contains inaccurate information due to fraud; and those who have been the subject of adverse action, such as denial of credit. In most states now, a report costs $8.50 (less in some states).

To request a copy of your credit report, send a letter (with your check) indicating your full name, current mailing address (and any other addresses within the past five years), your Social Security number, and your date of birth. Send this to one of the major credit bureaus:

Experian, P.O. Box 2104, Allen, TX 75013–2104

www.experian.com

Equifax Credit Information Services, P.O. Box 105496,

Atlanta, GA 30348–5496

www.equifax.com

Trans Union Fraud Victim Assistance Department, P.O. Box 390, Springfield, PA 19064–0390

www.transunion.com

The report comes with a copy of your credit rights, and how to go about resolving any disputes.

The report I received contained a listing of recent (it seemed to cover about the past six years) charge accounts and bank loans. It contained a description of each account (revolving credit, car loan, mortgage, etc.), the current balance, and whether all payments had been made on time. It also contained a list of inquiries made into the credit record. Most of them were inquiries from financial institutions determining whether to send me an offer of a new charge card ("to develop a list of names for a credit offer or service"). Thus a credit bureau does not have to notify you every time an inquiry is made, but when you receive a credit report you get a listing of recent inquirers into your record.

Rothfeder says that TRW (now Experian) "upgrades and expands its files with information it purchases from the Census Bureau, motor vehicle agencies, magazine subscription services, telephone white pages, insurance companies, and as many as sixty other sources. 'We buy all the data we can legally buy,' says Dennis Benner, a TRW vice president" (Rothfeder, 1992, p. 38). TRW (Experian) also has a Highly Affluent Consumer database, from which it sells names, phone numbers, and addresses of people categorized by income to anyone (catalog company, telemarketer, or political group) that will pay for it (Rothfeder, 1992, p. 97). It will also screen out names of those who are late in payments, or likely to go bankrupt.

The storage, transfer, and analysis of all of this information is made possible by computers. Computers have thus presented us with the ethical concern of whether the handling and disseminating of this information creates a breach of our moral rights—in this case, the right of privacy.

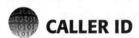 **CALLER ID**

A telephone service feature called "Caller ID" *sells* information on who you are (your phone number) when you make a phone call. Some states (such as California) have prohibited "Caller ID," but it is in place in most other states, including New York. The original idea behind Caller ID was to identify nuisance callers (who could simply avoid such devices by calling from pay phones) and to allow call recipients to screen their calls. However, in practice it represents an invasion of the caller's privacy, the right not to have one's number identified; many people pay to have unlisted phone numbers for just that reason. CPSR spoke out against it: "Caller ID, for example, reduced the privacy of telephone customers and was opposed by consumers and state regulators."[15]

There is also an option called "Call Return" (*66), which allows anyone you have called to call you back, whether they answered your call or not. In New York, they have a feature called "Per-Call Restrict," where you can *block* display of your number on the recipient's "Caller-ID" device, *if* you press *67 on a touch-tone phone, or dial 1167 on a rotary phone, before you place your call. That seems like an annoyance at the very least. In something that should by rights be private, you have to go to an extra effort every time you place a call to ensure privacy. And, given that feature, what nuisance caller (against whom the ID system was initially devised) would not use the call-restrict option to prevent identification?

To those who think that Caller ID is just a harmless convenience, consider some cases where it might be damaging.

1. A professor who values her privacy and quiet time returns the call of a student who has left a message of panic regarding the next day's exam. After the professor spends half an hour on the phone answering questions, the student lets classmates know that the professor helped, and gives out her (unlisted) phone number, obtained through Caller ID. The professor (who had more than adequate office hours all semester to help students) is harassed all evening with phone calls from other students in the class.

2. A consumer calls to make a telephone inquiry about the price of a product, but decides not to buy it. The organization that took the call begins phoning her every week, trying to talk her into their other products.

3. An informant who wishes to remain anonymous calls the Police Department to report a crime. The police record from Caller ID is used to track down the informant, and the phone number and address are also picked up by a nosy reporter who puts the person's name in an article.

 ## COMPUTER MATCHING

Computer matching involves the combining of information from several databases to look for patterns—of fraud, criminal activity, etc. It is most generally used to detect people who illegally take government money from more than one source—they are termed "welfare double-dippers."

The Reagan administration was quick to capitalize on the capabilities of computer matching. In March 1981, President Reagan issued an executive order establishing a President's Council on Integrity and Efficiency (PCIE) to "revitaliz[e] matching to fight waste, fraud, and abuse" (*Computer Matching*, 1986, p. 56). The major concern of this governmental committee was primarily to assess the cost-effectiveness of matching programs, rather than to look into how they may constitute serious invasions of personal privacy. The Long-Term Computer Matching Project published a quarterly newsletter, developed standardized formats for facilitating matching, created a "manager's guide" to computer matching, established Project Clean Data (a program that identifies incorrect or bogus social security numbers), and has looked into problems of security with the systems in which matching takes place, in order to promote "efficient and secure matches" (*Computer Matching*, 1986, pp. 59–60).

Some of the government agencies involved in computer matching include Defense, Veterans Administration, HEW, HUD, the Postal Service, Agriculture, Health and Human Services, Justice, Social Security, Selective Service, NASA, and Transportation. Examples of matches performed include matching Wanted and Missing Persons files with federal and state databases, detecting the underreporting of income by those receiving mortgage or rent subsidies (or food stamps or other aid), locating absent parents with child support obligations, matching wage reports against those receiving unemployment, and so on (*Computer Matching*, 1986, pp. 236–46). One can see that the possibilities here are practically limitless. Some of these matches may be perfectly justifiable, as in cases where Social Security fraud is being perpetrated against the government. But it will be easy to cross the line into blatant invasions of personal privacy, and the lines are not clearly drawn, or not drawn at all.

The American Bar Association (ABA) has identified seven distinct areas in which computer matching programs impinge on privacy.

1. *Fourth Amendment.* Privacy advocates have argued that the matching of databases containing personal information constitutes a violation of the Fourth Amendment right to security against unreasonable searches. Supporters of computer matching argue that the programs do not search in general, but rather "scan" for records of particular persons who are applying for benefits. That, of course, does not mean that such programs could not easily be modified to search in general.

2. *Privacy Act.* It is claimed by some that computer matching programs violate the Privacy Act of 1974, which provides that personal information collected for one purpose cannot be used for a different purpose without notice to the subject and the subject's consent. However, the Privacy Act has a "routine use" clause that has been used to bypass this consideration. "Congress has in fact authorized most of the ongoing matching programs, overriding whatever protection the Privacy Act afforded" (*Computer Matching*, 1986, p. 97).

3. *Fair Information Practice Principle.* Even if current computer matching practice does not violate the law, it does violate the fair information practice that information collected for one purpose should not be used for another purpose without due notice and consent. This is reflected in

the 1979 ABA resolution: "There must be a way for an individual to prevent information obtained for one purpose from being used or made available for other purposes without his or her consent" (*Computer Matching*, 1986, p. 97).

4. *Due Process.* Violations of "due process" have occurred in computer matching cases. For example, in 1982 the state of Massachusetts matched welfare records against bank accounts and terminated benefits without notice. In several cases, the "matches" were incorrect, and in others there were legitimate reasons for the money in the bank accounts that did not violate welfare restrictions.

5. *Data Security.* Unauthorized access to the databases in which this matching information is stored constitutes a real threat to the personal privacy of those whose records are stored there, and the government has not developed security measures adequate to protect them (*Computer Matching*, 1986, p. 98).

6. *Data Merging.* The government can query any number of files on a citizen; this leads to the possibility of a merged file in a new database containing information from various sources, which could violate (2) and (3). For example, there are rulings that allow the IRS to deduct debts owed the government from tax refunds, and the IRS proposed in 1986 to establish a "master debtor file" (*Computer Matching*, 1986, p. 98).

7. *Fundamental Privacy Rights.* What is to keep the government from linking personal data on medical records, financial records, reading and viewing preferences, and political and religious activities? This is all unsettlingly reminiscent of Orwell's *1984*. Ronald L. Plesser, who made the presentation to Congress as designee of the American Bar Association, said: "Substantive limits on data linkage have to be established. At some point, privacy and autonomy outweigh government efficiency" (*Computer Matching*, 1986, p. 99; general discussion, pp. 92–103).

When New York City and New Jersey compared their welfare databases, they discovered 425 people who were regularly collecting welfare in both areas using fake IDs, to the tune of about $1 million in unauthorized costs to the welfare system. The system is experimenting with using fingerprints as IDs for welfare recipients. Critics complain that it will discourage poor people from getting aid, since it carries with it the stigma of a criminal context. Soon after the fingerprint experiment was implemented, over 3,000 people dropped out of the system.[16]

Some might say "Good! Three thousand fewer leeches on society." The question comes down to the real purpose of our welfare system. Do we really want to help people in need, or not? A number of the ethical systems we examined would support this as the right thing to do, if one cannot have an ideal society in which there is enough for everyone to prosper. The utilitarian principle is clear—we should do what fosters the greatest good (pleasure and absence of pain) for the greatest number of people. Kant would emphasize that rational beings must be treated as ends in themselves, and this would include awarding them respect and humane treatment, since *they,* not dollars, represent what is intrinsically valuable. Certainly it develops virtuous character to be generous. And, on the goods view, we should do what maximizes the highest goods, such as friendship, knowledge, satisfaction, health, and life.

As it is, people who go for legitimate welfare support, or for temporary unemployment compensation when they unexpectedly lose their jobs in an unstable economy, may be made to feel demoralized as they are brought back repeatedly to fill out repetitive forms. If we add fingerprint identification, they will surely be made to feel like criminals, as the article suggests. If we *intend* to help those who need help, then we should do it with open hearts and efficient procedures, not grudgingly and in a demeaning way.

HOW THE INTERNET COMPLICATES PRIVACY CONSIDERATIONS

The amazing growth of the Internet in recent years has interconnected people in an unprecedented way. E-mail has become a major mode of communication (with some associated problems we have already discussed). Any business that hopes for continued success must now sport an elaborate website, and retailers must provide an easy way for customers to order from them online. Amazon.com is a prime example of the amazing success of an online business—in this case an online bookstore that expanded into music, video, tools, toys, electronics, and other areas as well.

The problem is that all this electronic communication leaves, as philosopher Jim Moor says, "electronic footprints" everywhere. We have a record on our computers of all e-mails we have sent and received until we delete them (and perhaps their "ghosts" remain behind). Our employers can monitor our e-mails and, in fact, all our computer activities (see Chapter 9). The websites we visit keep a record of our visit, some of which is even stored on our own computer on "cookies." And now the government can potentially monitor all e-mail through the use of "Carnivore."

Cookies

Our web browsing activity leaves a trail that tells a lot about us—our preferences, our varied interests. Many websites store information about our visits in an information packet called a "cookie." Did you ever wonder how a website knows what new suggestions to make to you about what you might like to buy? Your past purchases and also your browsing can be stored, as well as what website you transfer to when you leave. Any server that connects to or contributes to a website you visit can access your cookie information. If some sort of government oversight group took an interest in your web surfing activity, they might be able to piece together a very interesting picture of you (analogous to the "Daily Surveillance Sheet" discussed later in this chapter in "The Worst Scenario" section). Notice that these cookies are stored on *your* computer without your consent (and often without your knowledge).

Your web browser may have a security option that allows you to see a "cookie alert" when a website wants to set a cookie; you then have the option of accepting or rejecting the cookie. For more general information on cookies, see www.cookiecentral.com; some cookie managers include Cookie Cruncher (www.rbaworld.com) and Cookie Crusher (www.thelimitsoft. com). If you subscribe to www.anonymizer.com, it will prevent marketers and identity thieves from knowing where you surf.

Communications Decency Act (CDA) and CDA II (COPA)

In 1995, Congress passed the Communications Decency Act (CDA), a law that restricted written communication in an electronic medium (purportedly in the name of child protection). It was strongly opposed by supporters of free speech and was declared unconstitutional by the Supreme Court in 1997. Such a restriction on free speech would have been a serious abrogation of personal rights, and effectively an invasion of privacy (attempting to control what we could write in the privacy of our home or office by reading it).

The statement from the Supreme Court decision on the act is worth noting carefully:

> We are persuaded that the CDA lacks the precision that the First Amendment requires when a statute regulates the content of speech. In order to deny minors access to potentially harmful speech, the CDA effectively suppresses a large amount of speech that adults have a constitutional right to receive and to address to one another. That burden on adult speech is unacceptable if less restrictive alternatives would be at least as effective in achieving the legitimate purpose that the statute was enacted to serve.[17]

In 1998, another piece of legislation, the Child Online Protection Act (COPA, referred to by many as CDA II), was passed into law. This law makes it a crime for anyone to make any communication *for commercial purposes* that is "harmful to minors" by means of the Web (unless access by minors is restricted by demanding a credit card). It also raises many problems, including constitutional ones. It puts severe restrictions on constitutionally-protected speech, especially for medical information websites dealing with sexual awareness; it does not afford any protection against material originating from outside the United States. A number of civil liberties organizations are joining to challenge COPA in court. Information can be found at www.cdt.org/speech/copa. The legislation itself can be viewed at www.epic.org/free_speech/censorship/copa.html

Carnivore

In July 2000, the existence of an FBI monitoring system called "Carnivore" was revealed. It is installed at an Internet Service Provider (ISP), and then monitors e-mail traffic to intercept information relating to criminal suspects. The *Wall Street Journal* reported in July 2000 that Carnivore "can scan millions of e-mails a second" and "would give the government, at least theoretically, the ability to eavesdrop on all customers' digital communications, from e-mail to online banking and Web surfing." [18] After the revelation, the Electronic Privacy Information Center (EPIC) filed a Freedom of Information Act request for all FBI records concerning Carnivore. When the FBI finally responded, 254 pages of the responsive material were withheld entirely, and other pages were released only in part.

In July 2001, the House passed a bill to require federal officials to be more "forthright" in answering questions about electronic surveillance (it passed by a unanimous voice vote). It seems that the name "Carnivore" (admittedly an unfortunate choice) has been dropped, and its successor is called DCS1000. A statement made before Congress in July 2000 by the Assistant Director of the FBI can be found at

www.fbi.gov/congress/congress00/ kerr072400.htm

It emphasizes that applications for electronic surveillance must be made to the Department of Justice, and unauthorized surveillance is a criminal act. Carnivore is characterized as a "sniffer" that grabs only those packets fitting a "filter" that is in conformity with the court order. It is said to be a "small-scale device intended for use only when and where it is needed." Its use was claimed to be justified by the rapid growth of computer-related crimes.

The existence of such a "sniffing" device, small-scale or not, must give us pause. It apparently "sniffs" for certain *content* without attempting to distinguish communications from criminal suspects from those who are not. Its *potential* for widespread invasion of privacy is frightening.

 THE WORST SCENARIO

We have seen how records on us are kept, analyzed, sold, and transmitted. Most of this information is financial, but there are other records on us as well. *USA Today* estimated recently that the average adult American has computerized files in at least 25 different databases. The General Accounting Office, in 1990, reported that there were at least 2,006 federal computer databases, 1,656 of which were covered by the Privacy Act. These databases were under the various Cabinet departments (Defense, Health and Human Services, Justice, Agriculture, Labor, Treasury, Interior, Transportation, Commerce, Energy, Veterans Affairs, Education, and Housing and Urban Development—in order from most systems to least), and various independent agencies such as the Environmental Protection Agency, NASA, the FCC, the Nuclear Regulatory Commission, and the Federal Reserve System, to name a few. The odds are that your name (and data) shows up in a number of those databases. When the databases start "talking to" each other, they are doing "matching" on you for various purposes.

In the foreword to David Burnham's *The Rise of the Computer State*, Walter Cronkite wrote:

> Orwell, with his vivid imagination, was unable to foresee the actual shape of the threat that would exist in 1984. It turns out to be the ubiquitous computer and its ancillary communication networks. Without the malign intent of any government system or would-be dictator, our privacy is being invaded, and more and more of the experiences which should be solely our own are finding their way into electronic files that the curious can scrutinize at the punch of a button.
>
> The airline companies have a computer record of our travels—where we went and how long we stayed and, possibly, with whom we traveled. The car rental firms have a computer record of the days and distances we went afield. Hotel computers can fill in a myriad of detail about our stays away from home, and the credit card computers know a great deal about the meals we ate, and with how many guests.

The computer files at the Internal Revenue Service, the Census Bureau, the Social Security Administration, the various security agencies such as the Federal Bureau of Investigation and our own insurance companies know everything there is to know about our economic, social and marital status, even down to our past illnesses and the state of our health.

If—or is it when?—these computers are permitted to talk to one another, when they are interlinked, they can spew out a roomful of data on each of us that will leave us naked before whoever gains access to the information.

Cronkite, Burnham, and many others have seen the threat to our privacy and our autonomy that these systems present. Yet our complex world could not run as it does now without them. It has been suggested that the best way to cripple a country would be to take out its financial networks, and these are now totally dependent on computers. But this leaves us with the question (a very important and very difficult one) of how we can maintain some level of autonomy and some measure of privacy for ourselves and others in the face of this ever-growing "spider's web" (as Solzhenitsyn described it) of communication and *control*. How can we remain *persons* (with the rights and responsibilities that are entailed) when we are being reduced to mere *numbers* every day?

Dennie Van Tassel devised a very clever scenario for the collection he co-edited entitled *The Compleat Computer* (which is highly recommended reading).[20] In it he describes the "confidential" report on "Harry B. Slow," which tracks his every move through the use of his many credit cards. All purchases and bank transactions are listed, and from this record the computer analyzes that Harry drinks too much, is probably overweight, has a weakness for young blondes, and is probably having an affair with his secretary (a blonde).

The scenario is amusing, but it is also frightening. We are moving into an age where most of our purchases and activities can be tied to a record with our name (or number) on it, through credit cards, bank accounts, library cards, video rental cards, and other identifiers. We tend not to carry a lot of cash (fear of being robbed, perhaps) and so pay for most items by a traceable credit card. My grocery store has a record of what I buy because, even though I usually pay in cash, to receive their special discounts on items each week, I have to use a special coded card that identifies me as a member of their "club." Thus they have a record of my buying patterns to analyze and sell to various companies that manufacture the products I buy.

Van Tassel has shown us a picture that is not far from the truth today, and will most likely be very close to the truth in the future. Does this present a moral problem and, if so, is there anything we can do about it? Our political systems should have moral underpinnings, and it is through those political systems that we can try to make a difference. One of the problems is that many of the "technocrats" creating and using the computer systems that are invading privacy are not part of the government, and so are not accountable to the public as the government should be.

Some of you will become part of the technological force that creates and maintains elaborate computer systems, and so you, at least, will be aware of the dangers involved and your corresponding responsibilities. Others may not be so aware, and so the answer must lie in education and in making groups accountable. Some impact can come from the public "voting with its feet" and not buying certain products, or making public complaints, such as those against the Lotus Marketplace: Households project or the Clipper chip. But government must also be sensitized to the threats to the freedoms promised by the Constitution, and which it is the responsibility of the government to protect.

WHAT PROTECTIONS ARE THERE FOR PRIVACY?

The Bill of Rights of the U.S. Constitution has two Amendments which might be thought to relate to the privacy issue—the First Amendment and the Fourth. The First Amendment guarantees freedom of religion, speech, the press, and assembly. However, none of those freedoms mentions privacy or necessarily entails privacy. The Fourth Amendment says "the right of the people to be secure in their persons, houses, papers, and effects against unreasonable searches and seizures, shall not be violated." This relates to prohibiting anyone from looking for and/or taking anything from you or your home without a warrant issued upon demonstration of *probable cause*. However, it does not say anything regarding information about you that is not on your person or in your home, but which should be kept private, or at least not made public (such as your tax report, your medical records, your driving record, or the like). Notice also that your garbage is not considered private; it is no longer in your home, and someone can search it without violating any laws.

The point is that your tax report is private business between you and the IRS, your medical files are private business between you and your doctor, and your driving record is private business between you and the Department of Motor Vehicles. With few exceptions, no one outside of the offices mentioned has any *need-to-know*, or any *right-to-know*, such information about you. (Exceptions that arise because of "matching" programs between agencies raise problems discussed earlier.) Yet there are cases of people working at the IRS "snooping" into people's files (*not* the ones they are assigned to work on, but those of neighbors, or famous people), of medical information being sold to drug or insurance companies, and of drivers' records being available for a small fee to anyone in many states.[21] Medical records of political candidates have been compromised to leak stories about psychiatric counseling, or suicide attempts, or other damaging information. The press will claim the public's "right-to-know" in cases of public figures, but the fact remains that a fundamental guarantee of the privacy of information between patient and doctor has been violated.

In the *Roe v. Wade* (410 U.S. 113, 1973) abortion decision, Justice Harry A. Blackmun stated the opinion:

> The Constitution does not explicitly mention any right of privacy. In a line of decisions, however, . . . the Court has recognized that a right of personal privacy, or a guarantee of certain zones or areas of privacy, does exist under the Constitution. In varying contexts, the Court or individual Justices have, indeed, found the roots of that right in the First Amendment, . . . in the Fourth and Fifth Amendments, . . . in the Ninth Amendment, . . . or in the concept of liberty guaranteed by the first section of the Fourteenth Amendment . . . These decisions make it clear that only personal rights can be deemed "fundamental" or "implicit in the concept of ordered liberty" . . . are included in this guarantee of personal privacy. (Cited in Freedman, 1987, p. 73)

If the right to privacy is suggested in the Fifth Amendment, it would have to lie in the right of a person not to be compelled to be a witness against himself (or herself). The Ninth Amendment states: "The enumeration in the Constitution, of certain rights, shall not be construed to deny or disparage others retained by the people." This is too vague or too broad to be helpful. If it is interpreted to support privacy, it could also be construed to support an individual's right to a free car. The Fourteenth Amendment states that all citizens have the rights of citizens, but does not spell these out beyond the rights to life, liberty, and property. It does not seem that a right to privacy can be inferred as strongly from the Fifth, Ninth, and Fourteenth Amendments as from the First and Fourth Amendments.

WARREN AND BRANDEIS MAKE A CASE FOR PRIVACY

The beginning of the Court's recognition of the right to privacy lies in an article written by Samuel D. Warren and Louis D. Brandeis in 1890.[22] They suggest that the rights to life, liberty, and property as previously interpreted were seen to relate only to the *physical* side of human beings, and do not take into account their *spiritual* side. Gradually this spiritual side came to be recognized, and "Now the right to life has come to mean the right to enjoy life—the right to be let alone; the right to liberty secures the exercise of extensive civil privileges; and the term 'property' has grown to comprise every form of possession—intangible as well as tangible" (Warren and Brandeis, cited in Schoeman, 1984, p. 75).

Recognition of the "legal value of sensations" gave rise to laws against assault, nuisance, libel, and alienation of affections. The rights to property were legally extended to processes of the mind, works of literature and art, good will, trade secrets, and trademarks. They suggest that this development of the law was "inevitable"; the heightened intellect brought about by civilization "made it clear . . . that only a part of the pain, pleasure, and profit of life lay in physical things" (Shoeman, 1984, p. 76). Their concern is for the "right to be let alone"—to be free of the intrusions of unauthorized photographs and yellow journalism.

Warren and Brandeis point out that the law of libel covers only broadcasting of information that could injure the person in his relations with other people; but there are other personal items of information that no one else should be able to communicate, and libel does not cover these items. The very occasion of the article was untoward prying into the lives of Mr. and Mrs. Warren, and the wedding of their daughter, by the Boston newspapers. William L. Prosser, in commenting on privacy in the context of the Warren and Brandeis article, suggests that four torts (wrongful actions for which civil suit can be brought) arose out of their position and subsequent court decisions:

1. Intrusion upon the plaintiff's seclusion or solitude, or into his private affairs.
2. Public disclosure of embarrassing private facts about the plaintiff.
3. Publicity which places the plaintiff in a false light in the public eye.
4. Appropriation, for the defendant's advantage, of the plaintiff's name or likeness. (Prosser, cited in Schoeman, 1984, p. 107)

Warren and Brandeis close by saying that "the protection of society must come through a recognition of the rights of the individual." Each individual is *responsible* for his or her own actions only; the individual should resist what he or she considers wrong, with a weapon for defense.

> Has he then such a weapon? It is believed that the common law provides him with one, forged in the slow fire of the centuries, and to-day fitly tempered to

his hand. The common law has always recognized a man's house as his castle, impregnable, often, even to its own officers engaged in the execution of its commands. Shall the courts thus close the front entrance to constituted authority, and open wide the back door to idle or prurient curiosity?" (Warren and Brandeis, in Schoeman, 1984, p. 90)

The subtitle to "The Right to Privacy" is "The Implicit Made Explicit." It would seem that what Warren and Brandeis tried to do (and most courts subsequently followed their lead), was to point out the strong connection between holding an individual *responsible* for actions and allowing him or her the *privacy* of thought and control of action to exercise such responsibility.

The Warren and Brandeis analysis deals only with the harm that can be done if someone *uses* information about you, and suggests that merely possessing that information is not a harm. However, one can think of many instances when someone merely possessing private information about you would present, at the very least, an embarrassment. It is analogous to the cases discussed at the beginning of the chapter where, even if you are not aware that you are being monitored, harm is done, because you are diminished as a person and a free agent.

EXISTING PRIVACY LEGISLATION

Existing privacy legislation includes:

- *Fair Credit Reporting Act of 1971* (15 U.S.C. 1681), amended in 1997: All credit agencies must make their records available to the person whose report it is; they must have established means for correcting faulty information; and they are to make the information available only to *authorized* inquirers.
- *Crime Control Act of 1973*: Any state information agency developed with federal funds must provide adequate security for the privacy of the information they store.
- *Family Educational Right and Privacy Act of 1974* (20 U.S.C. 1232g): Educational institutions must grant students and/or their parents access to student records, provide means for correcting any errors in the records, and make such information available only to authorized third parties.

- *Privacy Act of 1974* (5 U.S.C. 552a): Restricts the collection, use, and disclosure of personal information, and gives individuals the right to see and correct such information.

Senator Sam Ervin had felt that the legislation required the establishment of a Privacy Commission. The report of the Senate Committee on Government Operations (September 1974) stated:

> It is not enough to tell agencies to gather and keep only data for whatever they deem is in their intended use, and then to pit the individual against government, armed only with the power to inspect his file, and the right to challenge it in court if he has the resources and the will to do so.
>
> To leave the situation there is to shirk the duty of Congress to protect freedom from the incursions by the arbitrary exercise of the power of government and to provide for the fair and responsible use of such power. (U.S. Senate 1976: 9–12; in Burnham, 1983, p. 364)

- *Tax Reform Act of 1976* (26 U.S.C. 6103): Tax information must remain confidential, and not be released for nontax purposes. (However, there has been an ever-increasing list of exceptions to the release restriction since 1976.)
- *Right to Financial Privacy Act of 1978* (12 U.S.C. 3401): Establishes some privacy with regard to personal bank records, but provides means for federal agencies to access such records.
- *Protection of Pupil Rights Act of 1978* (20 U.S.C. 1232h): Gives parents the right to examine educational materials being used in the schools, and prohibits intrusive psychological testing of students.
- *Privacy Protection Act of 1980* (42 U.S.C. 2000aa): Government agents may not conduct unannounced searches of news offices or files, if no crime is suspected of anyone.
- *Electronic Funds Transfer Act of 1980*: Customers must be notified of any third-party access to their accounts.
- *Debt Collection Act of 1982* (Public Law 97–365): Federal agencies must observe *due process* (of notification, etc.) before releasing bad debt data to credit bureaus.
- *Congressional Reports Elimination Act of 1983*: Eliminated the requirement under the Privacy Act for all agencies to republish all of their systems notices every year.

- *Cable Communications Policy Act of 1984* (Public Law 98–549): A cable subscriber must be informed of any personal data collected (and when), and the use and availability there will be of such information.[23]

 ## THE IMPORTANCE OF PRIVACY

Not only do all of these databases discussed have information on private citizens, which can be "matched," and from which patterns of behavior can be inferred, but there are the problems of *security* of the information (from parties who should not have access to it), whether *anyone* has a right to that data, and the *accuracy* of the information. We discussed security in Chapters 4, 5, and 6.

Rothfeder (1989) reports that a GAO survey made in 1990 of the Treasury Enforcement Communications Systems, Version II (TECS II) revealed errors in 59 percent of the records it examined. There is good reason to believe that the other computerized records (in the justice system, NCIC, voter records, credit bureaus, the IRS, the welfare system, and many more) are also filled with errors. Chapter 8 will discuss errors in computer systems.

Thus the problem becomes more than just one of an invasion of privacy; it is also one of "them" having lots of information on individual citizens, which "they" will use for various purposes to manipulate and tax those citizens—but much of that data is wrong (in small or in large ways).

There is an objection raised to the demand for privacy. It says that anyone who needs privacy must be planning to do something that he or she should not do, and so needs the protection of privacy to carry it out. We might call this the "ring of Gyges" objection. In Plato's *Republic*, Glaucon claimed that if the "just" individual and the "unjust" individual both had a ring of Gyges that would make them invisible at will, they would both behave exactly the same way (taking advantage of others for their own gain). Thus the objectors to demands for privacy say that anyone who would want the "cloak of invisibility" that privacy offers must be up to no good.[24]

It is true that privacy helps to protect the actions of the thief or the murderer or the terrorist. But it would be unfortunate to draw the conclusion that therefore no one should be allowed any privacy. Such a world has already been described by George Orwell and others, and it is not a world that anyone would want to live in.

Some can be immune to punishment without needing privacy, if they are sufficiently powerful. Not everyone who wants privacy is planning to do evil; you might, for example, want to plan a surprise birthday party for someone. And not everyone who is planning to do evil *needs* privacy; Hitler carried out much of his evil in full public view. Many criminals *want* the notoriety they feel they have earned. Think of examples of hackers like Kevin Mitnick, who seem to glory in the challenge and the recognition.

If we act on the assumption of a world where everyone is selfishly out for only personal gain, with no scruples, then we would seem to have no alternative to the society described in Hobbes' *Leviathan*. Then we could let a supercomputer like Colossus in the movie *Colossus: The Forbin Project* monitor all of our actions and punish misbehavior. But in such a world there would be no creativity, no flowering of the human spirit; we would all become cogs in a big machine, obediently doing what we are told by Colossus. Hopefully, this is not our world, and we do have the human right to exercise our choices.

In the Canadian report on *The Nature of Privacy* by the Privacy and Computer Task Force, the following insightful statement is made:

> If we go about observing a man's conduct against his will the consequence of such observation is that either the man's conduct is altered or his perception of himself as a moral agent is altered. The notion of altering conduct or self-perception against the will of the moral agent is offensive to our sense of human dignity. If, through a monitoring device, we are able to regulate or indeed to follow the conduct of a person it is obvious that we are in effect compromising his responsibility as a chooser of projects in the world, thereby delimiting or influencing the kinds of choices that we make available to the doer. (Weisstaub and Gotlieb, 1973, p. 46)

It is clear that, in order to be a moral agent, in order to be *responsible* for what we do, we must be in control of our own choices, we must be autonomous. If you are constantly monitored in everything you do, that monitoring will affect your behavior. It is sort of like the Heisenberg Uncertainty Principle in physics; when you try to measure something, you disturb what it is you are trying to measure, and so you do not get a true reading.

The real choices you make are internal, and you need to know that they are truly your own choices (not determined by some external pressure or other). You cannot have that assurance if everything you do is public. If it is, you will always wonder, did I just do that because Dad was watching me? Because I was afraid of being punished if I didn't do it? Then it is not really *my* choice.

Augustine pointed out that it is better to have choice than not to have it, even though that means you may make some bad choices. Similarly, it is better to have privacy than not to have it, even if sometimes others (and even you) misuse it. If we do not have it, just as if we do not truly have choice, we are not fully human, and we cannot fulfill our human potential (which Aristotle would say is to *choose* the life of understanding, which is a very private thing, though we may choose to share it).

■ ENDNOTES

1. In the first chapter of *Technologies of Freedom*, entitled "A Shadow Darkens," Ithiel de Sola Pool wrote: "Electronic modes of communication . . . are moving to center stage. The new communication technologies have not inherited all the legal immunities that were won for the old. When wires, radio waves, satellites, and computers became major vehicles of discourse, regulation seemed to be a technical necessity. And so, as speech increasingly flows over those electronic media, the five-century growth of an unabridged right of citizens to speak without controls may be endangered" (p. 1). We should be deeply concerned about anything that threatens our right to freedom of speech or our privacy. These are not the same, but we may require privacy to protect our freedom of thought and speech.

2. Charles F. Fried, *An Anatomy of Values* (Cambridge, MA: Harvard University Press, 1970), p. 9.

3. G. Marx, "I'll Be Watching You: The New Surveillance," *Dissent* (Winter 1985), 26.

4. "Sellers of Government Data Thrive," *New York Times*, 26 December 1991, sec. D, p. 2.

5. *Software Engineering Notes* 15, 1 (January 1990), 4.

6. *Software Engineering Notes* 16, 4 (October 1991), 8.

7. *Software Engineering Notes* 16, 4 (October 1991), 12.

8. *Software Engineering Notes* 16, 4 (October 1991), 11–12.

9. *Software Engineering Notes* 17, 1 (January 1992), 6–7.

10. "Police Computers Used for Improper Tasks," *New York Times*, 1 November 1992, sec. 1, p. 38.

11. Stephen Barr, "Probe Finds IRS Workers Were 'Browsing' in Files," *Washington Post*, 3 August 1993, sec. A, p. 1.

12. Scott Wallace, "The Computerized Patient Record," *Byte* (May 1994), 67–75; Sheri Alpert, "Smart Cards, Smarter Policy," *Hastings Center Report* (November–December 1993), 13–23.

13. 94th Congress, 2nd Session, *Legislative History of the Privacy Act of 1974*, 759. In Eaton, 1986, p. 152.

14. The interested reader is referred to the articles by John Markoff, "Wrestling Over the Key to the Codes," and Steven Levy, "Cypherpunks vs. Uncle Sam: Battle of the Clipper Chip."

15. *The CSPR Newsletter*, 11, no. 4 and 12, no. 1 (Winter 1994), 23.

16. Mitch Betts, "Computer Matching Nabs Double-Dippers," *Computerworld* 28, 16 (April 28, 1994), 90.

17. Section 7, Supreme Court Decision in appeal 1997.

18. Neil King Jr. and Ted Bridis, "FBI's System to Covertly Search E-Mail Raises Privacy, Legal Issues," *Wall Street Journal*, 11 July 2000, p. A3.

19. Ibid.

20. Dennie Van Tassel, "Daily Surveillance Sheet, 1989, from a Nationwide Data Bank." In Dennie L. Van Tassel and Cynthia L. Van Tassel, eds. *The Compleat Computer*, 2nd ed. (Chicago: SRA, 1983), pp. 216–17.

21. Mitch Betts, "Driver Privacy on the Way?", *Computerworld* (February 28, 1994), 29.

22. Brandeis was to serve as an Associate Justice of the Supreme Court from 1916 to 1939.

23. The main source of this list of legislation affecting privacy was Kenneth C. Laudon, *Dossier Society* (N.Y.: Columbia University Press, 1986).

24. There is another side to the story of the ring of Gyges, as you may recall. Socrates says that the truly just individual will behave the same way with or without the ring. One is truly just from within, not because of external sanctions. Kant would tie it to *intentions*. Two individuals may do the same thing that we view as a just act (such as helping a little old lady across the street), but one does it from ulterior motives (hoping to be remembered in her will) while the other does it from Kant's pure duty—just because it is the right thing to do. Only the second person's act has moral worth. Its worth arose because the person acted autonomously (governing her own actions), *and* acted from a good will. However, she may well value her privacy, and not want her act spread over the newspaper headlines.

■ SHORT ESSAY QUESTIONS

1. Computers are used now to monitor the rate of work of various employees (such as those doing keyboard work on the computer, those taking computerized airline reservations, the number and length of stops by truckers, and the like). Discuss briefly whether these constitute invasions of privacy, or are just legitimate management efficiency strategies.

2. Investigate just how private the information on you as a college student is. Who has access to that information, and how easy is it for them to get it? Are all those who have access legitimately entitled to have such access? What about outside agencies coming to campus to get information about you? Just how easy is it for them to obtain whatever data they want?

3. Many colleges now operate with a computerized record-keeping package (several companies market such packages), accessible from administrative terminals on the campus. But anything accessible by an administrative terminal is potentially accessible from a student terminal as well. Check into what protections against such illicit access are available on your local system. Given what we saw about computer intruders in the previous chapter, it should be clear that such protections can often be circumvented. What serious invasions of privacy could occur if an unauthorized person gained access to those records? How serious would they be? Are there other potential problems (such as tampering with grades) that could occur? Discuss.

4. Examine carefully the text of the Privacy Act of 1974 (5 U.S.C. 552a) and see whether you think it really has the weaknesses and loopholes that Sam Ervin feared it had. In *Dossier Society* (1986, pp. 374–75), Kenneth Laudon mentions some principal weaknesses of the Privacy Act; discuss these.

5. Examine the articles by Alpert (1993) and Wallace (1994) and discuss the problems of the privacy of computerized medical records.

■ LONG ESSAY QUESTIONS

1. Discuss how the "cashless society," in which everything must be paid for by some kind of credit card, constitutes a threat to individual privacy. Go beyond Van Tassel's imaginative story (Van Tassel and Van Tassell, *The Compleat Computer,* Chicago: SRA, 1983), pp. 216–17. Does such a society create occasions for discrimination and unfair distribution of access to the goods of the society?

2. Read Joseph W. Eaton's book *Card-Carrying Americans* (1986) and critically analyze the arguments presented there, both pro and con, regarding the proposal to have universal identification cards in the United States. (See also www.aclu.org/features/National_ID_Feature.html).

3. Judith Jarvis Thompson, in her article "The Right to Privacy" (in Schoeman, 1984), uses some clever examples to try to make a case that privacy is not a single concept, but rather a "cluster" of other concepts (such as rights to life, to property, to freedom from libel), and so it is not a fundamental property at all, but a *derivative* property. Analyze her arguments critically, and then either propose a defense of her position or argue against it, using examples and analogies as necessary.

4. Though Kant does not mention privacy in the *Foundations of the Metaphysics of Morals*, make a case for the necessity of privacy based on his concept of autonomy as necessary to morality, and his notion of the Kingdom of Ends.

5. In *The Right and the Good* (1930), W. D. Ross claims that Kantian ethics, for example, does not deal adequately with the problems of *conflicts* of duties. He proposes instead a system in which all *actual* duties may have exceptions. But there are still *prima facie* ("on first look," "on the face of it") duties, ones which would be actual duties *if* other moral duties did not interfere. There are thus *prima facie* duties which one should try to fulfill. These include, for Ross: (1) fidelity (keeping promises); (2) rectifying wrongs (pay-back); (3) gratitude; (4) beneficence (making things better for others); (5) not doing harm; (6) justice (distributing the goods); (7) self-improvement (a duty to self). These duties are, in a sense, *conditional*; they can be overridden if stronger considerations prevail. However, he gives us no rankings of prima facie duties. To decide which to follow in a case of conflict, he is much like Aristotle—the *moral individual* will "see" the right thing to do. ("The decision rests with perception.") Try to make some sense of Ross's position (as expounded in *The Right and the Good*) and apply it to the problem of privacy—better to uphold it or let it go since it protects criminals and terrorists?

■ REFERENCES AND RECOMMENDED READINGS

Alpert, Sheri. "Smart Cards, Smarter Policy: Medical Records, Privacy, and Health Care Reform." *Hastings Center Report* (Hastings-on-Hudson), November-December 1993, pp. 13–23.

Baird, Robert M., Reagan Ramsower, and Stuart E. Rosenbaum, eds. *Cyberethics: Social and Moral Issues in the Computer Age*. Amherst, NY: Prometheus, 2000.

Branscomb, Lewis M., and Anne M. Branscomb. "To Tap or Not to Tap." *Communications of the ACM* 36, 3 (March 1993), 36–37; see also Rotenberg (1992), Rivest (1993), and Marx (1993).

Brown, Geoffrey. *The Information Game: Ethical Issues in a Microchip World*. Atlantic Highlands, NJ: Humanities Press, 1990, chs. 3, 5, and 6.

Burnham, David. *The Rise of the Computer State: The Threat to Our Freedoms, Our Ethics, and Our Democratic Process*. Foreword by Walter Cronkite. New York: Random House, 1983.

Center for Philosophy and Public Policy. "Privacy in the Computer Age." *Philosophy and Public Policy* 4, 3 (Fall 1984), 1–5.

Computer Matching and Privacy Protection Act of 1986: Hearing Before the Subcommittee on Oversight of Government Management of the Committee on Governmental Affairs, United States Senate (99th Congress). September 16, 1986. Washington, DC: Government Printing Office, 1986.

Cotton, Paul. "Confidentiality: A Sacred Trust Under Siege." *Medical World News* (March 27, 1989), 55–60.

Dejoie, Roy, George Fowler, and David Paradice, eds. *Ethical Issues in Information Systems*. Boston: Boyd & Fraser, 1991.

Diffie, Whitfield, and Susan Landau. *Privacy on the Line: The Politics of Wiretapping and Encryption*. Cambridge, MA: MIT Press, 1998.

Eaton, Joseph W. *Card-Carrying Americans: Privacy, Security, and the National ID Card Debate*. Totowa, NJ: Rowman and Littlefield, 1986.

Ermann, M. David, Mary B. Williams, and Claudio Gutierrez, eds. *Computers, Ethics, and Society*. New York: Oxford University Press, 1990, chs. 4, 5, 10, 11, 12.

Flaherty, David. *Protecting Privacy in Surveillance Societies*. Chapel Hill, NC: University of North Carolina Press, 1989.

Forester, Tom, and Perry Morrison. *Computer Ethics: Cautionary Tales and Ethical Dilemmas in Computing*. 2nd ed. Cambridge, MA: MIT Press, 1994, ch. 6.

Freedman, Warren. *The Right of Privacy in the Computer Age*. New York: Quorum Books, 1987.

GAO. "Government Computers and Privacy." GAO/IMTEC–90–70BR. Washington, DC: U.S. General Accounting Office, 1990.

Garfinkel, Simson. *Database Nation: The Death of Privacy in the 21st Century.* Sebastopol, CA: O'Reilly, 2000.

Gellman, H. S. *Electronic Banking Systems and Their Effects on Privacy: A Study by the Privacy and Computer Task Force.* Department of Communications/Department of Justice, Canada.

Godwin, Mike. *CyberRights: Defending Free Speech in the Digital Age.* New York: Random House\Times Books, 1998.

Gould, Carol C., ed. *The Information Web: Ethical and Social Implications of Computer Networking.* Boulder, CO: Westview Press, 1989, chs. 1–5.

Hunter, Larry. "Public Image." *Whole Earth Review* (December 1984–January 1985), 32–40.

Ippolito, Milo. "Three Women Sue over Hidden Camera in Restroom of Firm." *Atlanta Journal-Constitution,* 14 June 2001, p. XJ1.

Johnson, Deborah G. *Computer Ethics.* 2nd ed. Englewood Cliffs, NJ: Prentice-Hall, 1994, ch. 5.

Johnson, Deborah G., and Helen Nissenbaum, eds. *Computers, Ethics, and Social Values.* Englewood Cliffs, NJ: Prentice-Hall, 1995.

Johnson, Deborah G., and John W. Snapper, eds. *Ethical Issues in the Use of Computers.* Belmont, CA: Wadsworth, 1985, part 3.

Jordan, F. J. E. *Privacy, Computer Data Banks, Communications, and the Constitution: A Study by the Privacy and Computer Task Force.* Department of Communications/Department of Justice, Canada.

Kant, Immanuel. *Foundations of the Metaphysics of Morals.* 1785.

Kimball, Peter. *The File.* San Diego, CA: Harcourt Brace Jovanovich, 1983.

Lacayo, Richard. "Nowhere to Hide." *Time* (November 11, 1991), pp. 34–40.

Langford, Duncan, ed. *Internet Ethics.* New York: St. Martin's Press, 2000.

Larson, Erik. *The Naked Consumer: How Our Private Lives Become Public Commodities.* New York: Holt, 1992.

Laudon, Kenneth C. *Dossier Society: Value Choices in the Design of National Information Systems.* New York: Columbia University Press, 1986.

Lewis, Peter H. "Censors Become a Force on Cyberspace Frontier." *New York Times,* 29 June 1994, pp. A1, D5.

Levy, Steven. "The Cypherpunks vs. Uncle Sam: The Battle of the Clipper Chip." *New York Times Magazine,* 12 June 1994, pp. 44–51, 60, 70.

Lin, Daniel, and Michael C. Loui. "Taking the Byte Out of Cookies: Privacy, Content, and the Web." *Computers & Society* (June 1998), 39–51.

Maner, Walter. "Unique Ethical Problems in Information Technology." *Science and Engineering Ethics* 2,2 (1996), 137–154.

Markoff, John. "Europe's Plans to Protect Privacy Worry Business." *New York Times*, 11 April 1991, pp. A1, D6.

Markoff, John. "Wrestling Over the Key to the Codes." *New York Times*, 9 May 1993, sec. 3, p. 9.

Marx, Gary T. "I'll Be Watching You: The New Surveillance." *Dissent* (Winter 1985), 26–34.

Marx, Gary T. "To Tap or Not to Tap." *Communications of the ACM* 36, 3 (March 1993), 41; see also Branscomb and Branscomb (1993), Rotenberg (1993), and Rivest (1993).

Miller, Arthur. "Computers and Privacy." In Dejoie et al. (1991), pp. 118–133.

Miller, Michael. "Lawmakers Begin to Heed Calls to Protect Privacy and Civil Liberties as Computer Usage Explodes." *Wall Street Journal*, 11 April 1991, p. A16.

Mitchum, Carl, and Alois Huning, eds. *Philosophy and Technology II: Information Technology and Computers in Theory and Practice.* Dordrecht, Netherlands: D. Reidel, 1986.

Moshowitz, Abbe. *Conquest of Will: Information Processing in Human Affairs.* Reading, MA: Addison-Wesley, 1976.

Perrolle, Judith A. *Computers and Social Change: Information, Property, and Power.* Belmont, CA: Wadsworth, 1987.

Pool, Ithiel de Sola. *Technologies of Freedom: On Free Speech in an Electronic Age.* Cambridge, MA: The Belknap Press of Harvard University Press, 1983.

Privacy Commissioner of Canada. *The Privacy Act.* Ottawa, Ontario: Minister of Supply and Services Canada, 1987.

Rachels, James. "Why Privacy Is Important." *Philosophy and Public Affairs* 4, 4 (Summer 1975), 323–33. Also in Johnson and Snapper (1985), in Dejoie et al. (1991), and in Schoeman (1984).

Rivest, Ronald L. "To Tap or Not to Tap." *Communications of the ACM* 36, 3 (March 1993), 39–40; see also Branscomb and Branscomb (1993), Rotenberg (1993), and Marx (1985).

Rosen, Jeffrey. "A Victory for Privacy." *Wall Street Journal*, 18 June 2001, p. A18f.

Ross, W. D. *The Right and the Good.* Oxford, England: Clarendon Press, 1930.

Roszak, Theodore. *The Cult of Information.* New York: Pantheon, 1986, chs. 8, 9.

Rotenberg, Marc. "Protecting Privacy" ("Inside RISKS" Column). *Communications of the ACM* 35, 4 (April 1992), 164.

Rotenberg, Marc. "To Tap or Not to Tap." *Communications of the ACM* 36, 3 (March 1993), 36–39; see also Branscomb and Branscomb (1993), Rivest (1993), and Marx (1985).

Rothfeder, Jeffrey. "Is Nothing Private? Computers Hold Lots of Data on You—And There Are Few Limits on Its Use." (Cover Story) *Business Week* (September 4, 1989), 74–82.

Rothfeder, Jeffrey. *Privacy for Sale: How Computerization Has Made Everyone's Private Life an Open Secret.* New York: Simon & Schuster, 1992.

Rule, James B. "Where Does It End? The Public Invasion of Privacy." *Commonweal* (February 14, 1992), 14–16.

Savage, John E., Susan Magidson, and Alex M. Stein. *The Mystical Machine: Issues and Ideas in Computing.* Reading, MA: Addison-Wesley, 1986, ch. 14.

Schoeman, Ferdinand David, ed. *Philosophical Dimensions of Privacy: An Anthology.* Cambridge, England: Cambridge University Press, 1984.

Shaffer, Jeffrey. "Watch the Watchers." *Christian Science Monitor,* 7 September 2001, p. 11.

Shattuck, John, and Richard Kusserow. "Computer Matching: *Should It Be Banned?*" *Communications of the ACM* 27, 6 (June 1984), 537–45.

Shattuck, John, and Muriel Morisey Spence. "The Dangers of Information Control." *Technology Review* (April 1988), 62–73.

Simons, G. L. *Privacy in the Computer Age.* Manchester, England: National Computing Centre, 1982.

Software Engineering Notes.

Spinello, Richard A., and Herman T. Tavani, eds. *Readings in Cyberethics.* Sudbury, MA: Jones and Bartlett, 2001.

Thompson, Judith Jarvis. "The Right to Privacy." In Schoeman (1984), pp. 272–89.

Tocqueville, Alexis de. *Democracy in America.* Ed. Richard D. Heffner. New York: Mentor/NAL, 1956.

Tuerkheimer, Frank M. "The Underpinnings of Privacy Protection." *Communications of the ACM* 36, 8 (August 1993), 69–73.

Turkle, Sherry. *Life on the Screen: Identity in the Age of the Internet.* New York: Simon & Schuster, 1995.

Van Tassel, Dennie L., and Cynthia L. Van Tassel, eds. *The Compleat Computer.* 2nd ed. Chicago: SRA, 1983.

Wallace, Scott. "The Computerized Patient Record." *Byte* (May 1994), 67–75.

Warren, Samuel D., and Louis D. Brandeis. "The Right to Privacy." *Harvard Law Review* 4, 5 (December 15, 1890), 193–220. Also in Schoeman (1984, pp. 75–103), and in Johnson and Snapper (1985, pp. 172–83).

Ware, Willis. "Information Systems Security and Privacy." *Communications of the ACM* 27, 4 (April 1984), 315–21.

Weisstaub, D. N., and C. C. Gottlieb. *The Nature of Privacy: A Study by the Privacy and Computer Task Force.* Department of Communications/Department of Justice, Canada, 1973.

Winner, Langdon. "Just Me and My Machine: The New Solipsism." *Whole Earth Review* (December 1984–January 1985), 29.

8

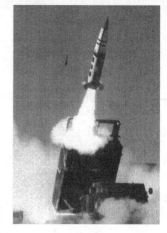

Errors and Reliability

*T*he existence of computers and the sophisticated programs that are run on them to carry out different important tasks raises new problems, in the sense that there are now many more ways for things to go wrong. These new problems, and the various ways in which computers have impacted the modern workplace (the subject of Chapter 9), suggest questions of *responsibility*. When something goes wrong, we generally want to know who was at *fault*, both to assign blame and to ensure that the problem does not happen again. If the trail leads to a computer, what are we to do then? This suggests two issues: (1) who (at bottom) is *responsible* for computer-related errors? and (2) are there some areas in which we *should not* rely on computers?

This chapter will examine the nature of "computer errors," a number of examples of recent serious computer errors, and the question of computer reliability. Chapter 9 will examine the impact (both positive and negative) of computers on the world of work, and Chapter 10 will look at the responsibilities of the computer professional regarding these problems.

 ERRORS

An error in a computer program is commonly referred to as a **bug**. The first use of this term in the computing field seems to have originated with a team on which Captain Grace M. Hopper was working. She describes the experience:

> In 1945, while working in a World War I–vintage non–air-conditioned building on a hot, humid summer day, the computer stopped. We searched for the problem and found a failing relay—one of the big signal relays. Inside, we found a

moth that had been beaten to death. We pulled it out with tweezers and taped it to the log book. From then on, when the officer came in to ask if we were accomplishing anything, we told him we were "debugging" the computer.[1]

The moth is preserved for posterity in the Naval Museum in Dahlgren, Virginia. It appears there taped to a copy of Grace Hopper's log book of September 9, 1945, as a piece of computing history.

A recent article points out that the moth found by Grace Hopper and her team at Harvard was not the reason that computer errors are called bugs to this day. The term was used as early as 1889 to refer to a defective fault. "The Pall Mall Gazette (March 11, 1889) reports 'Mr. Edison . . . had been up the two previous nights discovering a "bug" in his phonograph.'"[2]

There are two kinds of problems that can occur with computer programs. The first is that something goes wrong with the electrical system or the power supply or the like and causes a system failure. In some cases, the system may simply have "died," and this certainly can cause a problem if it is supposed to be continuously monitoring something, such as patients in a hospital or the status of a nuclear reactor. In these cases, the system being out of commission for a period of time can create a serious difficulty.

In other cases, the system failure actually causes damage to the computer itself, so that stored information (programs and data) is destroyed. This can happen in a disk "crash," when the read head gets too close to the disk (usually due to some sort of particle, like dust or smoke, that gets in between them) and wipes out what is stored on the disk. An electrical power surge can also destroy information stored, or damage computer components, and so it is wise to have a good surge protector on the electrical connection for your system.

These physical problems happen rarely, but the loss of time and/or information can be quite damaging. It is wise to protect against such occurrences. Continuous monitoring systems should have backups, such as a backup generator or a battery-powered power supply, and the capability for the computer system to switch over smoothly to such a system. There should also be a backup computer system, in case the system itself fails (a backup should be a system that has all the programs and information of the original). In the case of other computer installations, they should have good surge protectors and it is always wise to have backup copies of any important programs and data. Thus *redundancy* is the key to protecting the operations.

The second type of computer problem is more subtle, more difficult to notice and correct, and it can often cause considerable damage before it is corrected. This is an error either in the storage of information or in a program itself. The first such type of error might be just a bit (a binary piece of information) changing value (from 0 to 1 or from 1 to 0), which would alter the value stored or an instruction in a program.

Many systems have **parity checks** to detect such occurrences. For example, when information is written to magnetic tape, it is usually written in 6-bit or 8-bit "chunks" (or *bytes*). An additional bit (a "parity bit") can be added to give the string either **odd** or **even parity**. Parity refers to the number of 1s in a string; if the parity bit that is added is to give **odd** parity, it should make the number of bits that are 1s in the string odd. So if a 6-bit string 010101 is written to tape, a parity bit of 0 would be added to give it odd parity. If the 6-bit string were 111111, a parity bit of 1 would be added to give it odd parity. Then "parity checks" could be run on the tape periodically to be sure that it still has odd parity. If it does not, at least you would know that the information has gone bad, though you won't know exactly *which* bit changed value. It would take two bits changing value for such an error to go undetected, and the probability of this is very low. A more sophisticated system of parity bits could also be used for very important data (the work in this area is called "error-correcting codes").

The last, and most significant, problem with computer programs is that of **program error**. If the problem is not a physical one, of a bit changing value, it is more often that of an incorrectly written program, or using the wrong equation, or not taking into account special conditions that can occur. Though these are often referred to as **computer errors**, they are really **programmer errors** or, in some cases, **design errors**. In the latter case, the model that is programmed into the system may be incorrect—that is, it does not accurately model the real world.

If you get a billing error from the electric company or the phone company, they will often claim it is a *computer error* (and then you have to hope that the computer will fix it). But in most such cases, the computer has not done anything different than it was programmed to do, and the error (or the oversight) was the programmer's, or that of the person entering data to the system. In either case, they are *human* errors, not computer errors. The programmer errors are the serious "bugs" that were not found when the program was being written, since they are not errors in the *form* of the program (which would be caught by the compiler or assembler), but in the *logic* of the program, or even just simple transpositions in numerical values.

SOME NOTEWORTHY COMPUTER-RELATED ERRORS

We discuss many computer errors and computer frauds under other chapter designations in this book, such as computers and the military, artificial intelligence, hacking, piracy, and computer crime. In addition to those problems or risks,[3] here is a small selection of some of the more interesting computer errors in other areas.

Defense

An article in the April 18, 1992, issue of *New Scientist* was entitled "Patriot: The Missile That Failed." The original claims for the Patriot missiles used in the Gulf War were that they were 100 percent effective (according to General Norman Schwarzkopf), and then that they successfully intercepted 45 of the 47 Scud missiles they tried to shoot down. On February 15, 1991, President Bush said "Patriot is forty-one for forty-two." Then the estimate was reduced to 24 hits out of 85 attempts, and finally to an estimate of 10 percent hits. Steve Hildreth of the Congressional Research Service said that he was only convinced that one Scud warhead was actually destroyed by a Patriot missile. Tom Postol, a professor of science, technology, and national-security policy at M.I.T., was one of the first (and the most persistent) to question publicly the overblown estimates. Postol testified before a congressional committee about the Patriot capabilities, and made enemies in the Army, the government, and Raytheon.[4]

Postol pointed out how the Patriot had been originally designed to deal with *aircraft*, not with missiles, and that the modifications had been inadequate to deal with the new job. In fact, he said that a Patriot confronted with a Scud was not only incapable of downing it, but may have increased "the net level of ground damage relative to the case of no defense" (Hersh, 1994, p. 88). Scuds travel faster than the aircraft Patriots were originally designed for, and they tend to break up when they reenter the atmosphere, making an effective cloud of decoys around the warhead that serves to confuse the Patriot. One report said, "One software bug could have directed the Patriot to attempt to intercept an incoming missile at a point below ground. In one case this bug may have caused a Patriot to turn back and dive into the ground."[5]

Another problem that was discovered had to do with the Patriot's internal clock, a device that predicts when a Scud will appear next. The fact that the registers used in the Patriot control program were only twenty-four bits long creates a loss of precision that has an increasing effect the longer the system is running. The Israelis had noticed this and had alerted the Americans, who indicated that the system would not be run long enough to matter. However, the systems in the Gulf War were run for 100 hours, creating a "range-gate shift" of 678 meters. One Scud that was *not* intercepted impacted a U.S. position killing twenty-eight American servicemen at Dhahran. Postol remarked, "The problems that Patriot had intercepting primitive threats like a Scud underscores how difficult a set of tasks confront S.D.I. . . . We have still not solved any of the fundamental problems that have always confronted strategic-missile defenses" (Hersh, 1994, p. 89).

The Iran 655 Airbus was shot down by missiles from the USS Vincennes, killing 290 civilians, probably due to a combination of human error and a defective computer interface.[6] It has been pointed out that the tests of the system, to be used on battleships, were run in a cornfield![7] During the Falklands War, a British helicopter was shot down (all four aboard died) by a Sea Dart missile from the British destroyer Cardiff, which mistook it for an Argentine helicopter.[8] The test of the first Tomahawk missile failed because its program had been erased;[9] the second Tomahawk test failed because of a dropped bit in the program that caused the system to abort.[10]

A half-billion dollar computer designed to control British Air Defenses and scheduled to go on-line in 1987 wasn't ready ten years later due to serious bugs. The officials of the consortium (representing Hughes, Marconi, and Siemens) that developed the computer told Parliament that "We get wrong answers sometimes and the bugs have to be tracked down and sorted out. Secondly, from time to time it crashes. What this means is the equivalent of a nervous breakdown. It becomes confused with the information and goes wrong."[11] Would *you* want that system running the defenses of *your* country when the consortium finally brought it online?

A terrifying scenario is conjured up by the following report that was excerpted from the *Hartford Courant* (October 9, 1993):

> The Soviet military constructed a surefire system for retaliating against a U.S. nuclear strike without direct human involvement, and it could be activated today, a private U.S. expert on nuclear command systems said Friday. The expert, Bruce Blair, said that once the system is activated by senior Russian military officials, it could automatically send hundreds of nuclear-tipped missiles hurtling towards the United States. The system would be triggered if automatic sensors—which Blair said may be subject to error—detected a disruption of key

military communication links, as well as seismic disturbances, and flashes
caused by nuclear detonations inside Russia.[12]

Shades of the Doomsday Device in *Dr. Strangelove: Or How I Learned to Stop Worrying and Love the Bomb,* a movie directed by Stanley Kubrick in 1964. If you have not seen the movie, do so. It is recommended viewing for anyone living in the nuclear age, even though the "Cold War" is supposedly over. *Fail-Safe* (another 1964 movie) is also highly recommended.

An Associated Press article that appeared in the *San Francisco Chronicle* on May 26, 1992, claimed that at least $7.7 billion (out of a total of $29 billion spent to that point) on the Strategic Defense Initiative (SDI)—"Star Wars"—went for projects that "never got off the ground" and were deemed "unneeded, unworkable, or unaffordable." These included a surveillance satellite to track hostile missiles; a ground-based laser "to zap missiles in flight" by bouncing the lasers off mirrors positioned in space; a nuclear-bomb-powered X-ray laser weapon; and a pop-up probe to distinguish missile warheads from decoys.[13] The risks associated with SDI and its more recent incarnation, the Ballistic Missile Defense Organization (BMDO), are discussed in Chapter 11.

For a revealing description of a number of systems (both military and commercial) that were delivered very late, or not delivered at all, see Peter G. Neumann, "System Development Woes" (1993).[14] In addition, see examples in *Aviation Week & Space Technology* in 1989. A sample of reported delays included Boeing's years of delay in the $3.7-billion Peace Shield for Saudi Arabia due to hardware and software problems, the new Air Force satellite control system five years behind schedule, and the long-overdue upgrade of two North American Aerospace Defense Command (NORAD) computers that would be delayed another seven or eight years and cost an additional $207 million due to software problems.

The Aegis missile cruiser USS Yorktown had a systems failure off the Virginia coast in September 1997, due to a divide-by-zero error that the software did not protect against. The zero was apparently due to a data-entry error. The ship was dead in the water for almost three hours.[15]

Space Exploration

There have been many computer-related problems arising in the space program. For a more complete catalogue of these, see the *Software Engineering Notes* Index under "Space."[16] A few of the more notable cases include a launch-computer synchronization problem in the first space shuttle Columbia launch, called by Jack Garman "the bug heard 'round the world";[17] the launch failure of the Mariner 1 due to one incorrect symbol (a hyphen for a minus);[18] the Mariner 18 mission was aborted due to a missing NOT in its program;[19] a splashdown error of 100 miles for the Gemini V because the program had failed to take into account the revolution of the earth around the sun;[20] and the destruction of an $18.5 million rocket in the Atlas-Agena program due to a missing symbol in the program.[21]

One Hubble "trouble" with the telescope sent up to get clearer pictures of other spatial bodies was a programming error that shut the telescope down on December 9, 1991, due to "a 'fluke' buried undiscovered in its millions of lines of computer code."[22]

The Landsat 6 satellite, launched October 5, 1993, has been declared missing. The cause is attributed to either its having gotten into an "improper orbit," or being in the correct orbit but unable to communicate, since instead of tracking Landsat 6 the system was tracking a hunk of space junk. The spacecraft cost $228,000,000.[23]

Commercial Airlines

A scenario postulated by Pulitzer-Prize-winning writer Seymour M. Hersh in his book *The Target Is Destroyed* (1986) argues that the Korean Airlines Flight 007 disaster—in which the plane, with 269 people on board, inadvertently flew over Soviet air space and was shot down with all aboard killed—suggests that the problem was overreliance on the part of the crew in the plane's automatic inertial navigation guidance system (INS).[24]

In 1988, the Airbus A320 was the first plane certified to use a computer-controlled "fly-by-wire" system, where electrical wiring connects the pilot's command column to the plane's surfaces. Thus, all operations of the plane, including control of the lights and flushing the toilet, must go through a computer "filter,"[25] (Jacky, 1991, p. 619). An Air France Airbus A320 crashed at an airshow and three people were killed; doubts concerning the computer system creating a speeding up of the engines, a power loss prior to landing, and steering problems during taxiing have arisen, but the official ruling is pilot error.[26] An Indian Airlines A320 crashed 1,000 feet short of the runway, killing 97 people.[27] "Air India ran an ad in the *Wall Street Journal*; they're trying to sell all their purchased A320s and sublease their leased A320s."[28]

British Airways reported ten incidents in one month (January 1992) where software errors forced planes into sudden changes of speed and direction.[29]

Medical Risks

One of the most publicized computer-related errors in the medical area involved the million-dollar Therac–25, a computer-controlled *linear accelerator* radiation machine, manufactured by Atomic Energy of Canada, Ltd. (AECL). Five occurrences of an error ("Malfunction 54") left two patients dead and three others badly injured, due to overdoses of radiation. In one case where the patient died, it was estimated that he had received a dose of radiation 100 times that which was appropriate. A software error was responsible for these tragedies, which did not take into account the possibility that an operator might mistakenly select X-ray mode, and then switch to electron mode; the machine should have reduced the beam intensity for electron-mode (direct) treatment, and it did not (Jacky, 1991, pp. 612–15).

Over a ten-year period, more than a thousand people in Britain got the wrong cancer treatment (this time radiation treatments that were up to 35 percent *less* than prescribed) due to a program error.[30] Only 447 of the patients involved were still alive, suggesting that the low survival rate could well correlate with inadequate treatment.[31]

Robot Errors and Robots as Threats

The newspaper *Weekly World News*[32] provides some interesting, though perhaps exaggerated, stories of robots gone haywire. On July 10, 1984, it reported the story of a 58-year old Chinese man (Chin Soo Ying) who, in the 1950s, built an AI system (based on ideas from the early British Colossus computer) and taught it to express words of love and emotion. As the story goes, in the early 1980s he built a new machine, and the old system electrocuted him! The man's wife was sure that the machine had killed him out of jealousy, and then committed suicide. The *WWN* title of the story was "Jealous Computer Zaps its Creator."[33]

On March 14, 1989, *Weekly World News* carried a story titled "Computer Charged with Murder After Frying Chess Champ." The story claimed that in a Soviet chess championship, human player Nikolai Gudkov was up three games to none over his supercomputer chess opponent M2–11 when the machine sent a lethal dose of electricity to the metal chess board surface at the beginning of the fourth game. The story further went on to say that the computer would be put on trial (would it take the witness stand? how would it be punished, if found guilty?). The chief investigator Alexei Shainev supposedly said, "It might sound ridiculous to bring a machine to trial for murder. But a machine that can solve problems and think faster than any human must be held accountable for its actions."[34] This story may be an exaggeration or a misrepresentation, but it does raise problems that may well pose themselves with artificially intelligent machines in the future. We will discuss this further in the chapter on artificial intelligence and expert systems.

On the more serious side, a Japanese mechanic was killed by a malfunctioning Kawasaki robot,[35] and there were at least four (and possibly as many as nineteen) more robot-related deaths in Japan reported within the next year, some of which might possibly have been caused by stray electromagnetic radiation accidentally triggering an action in the robot.[36]

In Michigan, a man working on an auto assembly line was killed by a computer-controlled piece of die-casting machinery.[37] The problem of who is responsible in situations like these will be discussed in Chapter 10, which discusses professional responsibility, and in Chapter 12, which discusses artificial intelligence and expert systems. What is clear is that if the (now) old saw that "the computer did it" or "it was the computer's fault" continues to be accepted, and the buck stops at the computer, those who design such computer systems will not be inclined to take any more care than they are currently, and in many cases they will let profit and turning out a product as fast as possible be their only guiding principles.

We should evaluate the motives of such computer designers from an ethical standpoint. If monetary gain is their sole motivation, then there is something missing from their perspective. Money is just a means—to what end? To be rich? (Isn't this just a means?) Why be rich? (To be happy?) But is happiness to be found in cold coins and dry dollars? What of friendship, knowledge, beauty, health? And what of their obligations to those who are their customers? If not out of human sympathy, one should at least honor an implicit contract with those they serve.

A UPI report on October 10, 1992, indicated that Stanford University Hospital had discontinued use of its robotic transport devices for delivering supplies, records, and food, because one of the systems malfunctioned, veered off course, and tumbled down a flight of stairs.[38] (Images of the ED–209 "enforcement droid" in the movie *Robocop* falling down stairs come vividly to mind.)

Road & Track (November 1993) reported that an empty Saab automated factory apparently "jump-started itself," assembled 24 cars, and rolled them off the assembly line to crash into the wall of the factory.

Nuclear Energy Threats

A computer software error released thousands of liters of radioactive water, escaping as steam, at the Bruce nuclear station in Ontario, Canada, in early 1990. If the accident had gone much further, it could have contaminated the entire reactor complex.[39]

The *Gazette* in Cedar Rapids reported on August 21, 1992, that a signal from a nearby walkie-talkie seems to have triggered a shutdown of the Palo nuclear power plant.[40] It is frightening to think that random electronic transmissions can unpredictably affect the operation of sensitive and potentially dangerous nuclear facilities.

Computerized Translation

The advent of powerful computers brought an early period of euphoria where proponents thought that the computers would soon be able to do *anything* that humans could do, and more—and better and faster as well. One of the early areas touted as a "natural" for computers was that of machine translation of natural language. The early enthusiasm was soon dampened because of the difficulties with handling the nuances and ambiguities of natural language, something that a human does naturally by attending to context, but which was missed by purely syntactical systems such as computer programs.

Two of the early stories about the failures of "machine translation" are as follows: "Out of sight, out of mind" was translated as "blind idiot." In another system that was set up to translate English to Russian and Russian to English, "The spirit indeed is willing, but the flesh is weak" (Matthew xxvi, 41), was translated from English into Russian, and then (by the computer) back from Russian into English. The resulting retranslation reputedly was "The vodka is strong, but the meat is rotten."

Some more recent examples of failures of machine translation were provided by *Software Engineering Notes*. An automatic translation system named Systran—used to convert French into English in 1989—committed the following *faux pas*: the Commission President Jacques Delors asked in French to address a committee, and Systran translated this as his request to "expose himself to the committee." In addition, the French phrase *nous avions*, which in the context it was used was intended as "we had," was translated by Systran as "us airplanes."[41]

A report of the translation of a seventeenth century Japanese haiku poem by Basho, beautifully rendered by Daniel C. Buchanan as

Into the old pond
A frog suddenly plunges
The sound of water

was translated by the computer as

Sound of old pond
and water to
be crowded frog

No serious competition here, at least not yet (Impoco, 1988, p. 72).

Mistaken Identities

A Michigan man named Terry Dean Rogan was repeatedly listed (in error) in the National Crime Information Center (NCIC) system as wanted for robbery and murder. Another man, an escapee from prison, had been using Rogan's name. Rogan was arrested five times, beginning in October 1982, usually after he had been stopped on routine traffic checks; twice he was taken into custody at gunpoint, put in handcuffs, and taken to jail. In 1987, it was determined in a Los Angeles federal court that Rogan's constitutional rights had been violated by the city of Los Angeles, which failed "to properly train and supervise the officers in the constitutional protection aspects of using the crime center system and the necessity of adding more accurate information when it becomes available."[42] Rogan finally won his case, and settled for $55,000.[43]

Billing and Record-Keeping Errors

Since computers came onto the business scene, there have been stories of crazy bills that have originated in one computer system or another—phone bills in the millions of dollars, or a repeated bill for $0.00 which, when the recipient does not "pay" it, results in a slew of computerized requests for payment, threats of discontinued service, and threats of collection officers coming to the customer's door.

The August 14, 1990, issue of the *New York Times* reported on a "rogue computer" that was sending New Yorkers $19 million in bills for unpaid parking tickets that they had never received. A spokesperson for the city apparently claimed that they commit only $4 million yearly in errors, not $19 million! One victim, who does not have a driver's license and does not even know how to drive, received $4,152 in parking tickets and had his wages "attached" to pay the fines.[44]

Overwhelming phone bills are apparently not a thing of the past, even given today's much greater computer sophistication. In September 1990, a Chicago woman received a bill for $8,709,800.33 from Illinois Bell (the bill should have been $87.98). The woman said, "I only called my sister."[45]

In November 1990, a Cleveland woman received an electric bill from the Cleveland Electric Illuminating Company for $63 million (instead of the $63 she owed). The 76-year old woman remarked that it is a good thing that she is basically a calm person, or she could have had a heart attack or a stroke when she opened the bill. The electric company blamed it on a faulty entry error due to workers adjusting to a new system.[46]

However, sometimes the errors go in the other direction. From mid-February to the end of April in 1992, thousands of New Jersey Bell telephone customers were able to make long-distance calls without being billed for them, due to a "computer glitch." There were apparently about two million calls that were not billed.[47]

In what is viewed as a landmark decision, an English bank (Lloyds) that mistakenly bounced a number of checks from one of their clients, a couple running a meat firm, was ordered to pay more than 50,000 pounds in libel damages.[48] One would not normally think of an erroneously bounced check as libelous, but it *is* a reflection on the person's (or the firm's) credit, suggesting that it is unsound. This might easily affect the willingness of various constituencies to do business with the individual or company involved.

Not all accounting errors made by computerized systems are to the detriment of the recipient. According to a May 8, 1992, Associated Press report, a farmer in North Dakota who was expecting a check for $31 from the U.S. Agricultural Stabilization and Conservation Service actually received a check for $4,038,277.04! The head of the agency office in North Dakota said that "their computer program occasionally picks that particular amount and prints it out on something, although this is the first time it was printed on a check." (!) Apparently the farmer did not try to cash the check, and returned it to the agency the day after he received it.[49]

According to some Social Security Administration officials, close to 700,000 Social Security recipients had been underpaid since 1972, due to a computer error. The amount of unpaid benefits is estimated at $850,000,000 (the average amount per person about $1,500).[50]

Automatic Payments

Several cases have been reported of older people who have died in their homes without anyone knowing for many months. These people had all their financial transactions taken care of automatically by computer—their Social Security and pension checks were deposited automatically, and electric, gas, phone, and other bills were paid automatically, and so no one noticed that they were no longer alive. To the computer, everything kept on going just the same way as before.[51]

More "Dead Souls in the Computer"

Eugene Smith of Doylestown, Pennsylvania spent years trying to convince authorities that he was not dead. Apparently, his wallet was stolen in 1988; the thief accumulated numerous traffic violations and then was killed in a traffic accident, with Smith's wallet on him. In 1990, Smith was stopped by a police officer and told that the computer records showed that he was dead, and therefore he was not allowed to drive! Because he did not have a valid license (according to the state's computer records), he lost his job as a driver for a warehouse. When he finally got someone to go to bat for him and have the records corrected to show that he was alive, he still couldn't get a driver's license, because of all the unpaid traffic violations the thief had run up that were still on his record.[52]

The Associated Press reported on September 29, 1992, that for the three previous years residents of Hartford, Connecticut, had been excluded from federal grand jury pools because, due to an entry error in the wrong field, the 'd' in 'Hartford' had overflowed into a column designating status, and they were all considered dead.[53]

Military Dangers

In addition to the problems associated with battlefield computing systems (discussed in Chapter 11, which focuses on computers and the military), there have been a number of other difficulties that have arisen involving computers and military operations. One of these is HERO—Hazard of Electro-magmetic Radiation to Ordnance—where the electromagnetic radiation from various weapons systems can interfere with each other and with other systems, thus creating the possibility of downed aircraft, midair collisions, or accidental triggering of missiles or nuclear devices.[54]

"Surplus" Computers Sold with Sensitive Information Still in Them

There have been reported cases of "surplus" computers being sold at discount prices, some of which had belonged to the FBI, some of which had been used in the Gulf War, and so on, that the new owners have found to still contain top secret programs and files. This error, obviously a human oversight, points out the great vulnerability of sensitive systems to accidental access, not only through deliberate espionage, but through careless oversight.[55]

Miscellaneous Computer-Related Errors

The Pepsi-Cola Company had a promotional campaign in 1992 where "winning numbers" were written inside of bottle caps of Pepsi. Due to a "computer glitch," the big winning number that was to pay up to $38,000 was announced as "349," a number that appeared on roughly 500,000 bottlecaps. Pepsi offered $19 to each "winner" who made a claim, and thousands accepted this, but about 4000 sought action against Pepsi for fraud.[56]

On December 27, 1992, the computer system automatically (though inexplicably) unlocked all of the cell doors in a high-risk area in the new San Joaquin County Jail in California, releasing about 120 potentially dangerous inmates. Luckily, the area of these cells was isolated from other areas of the jail by doors that remained locked. The cause was attributed to a spurious signal from an encoded card that was to be used to open the doors in emergencies.[57]

On September 16, 1993, a computer bug in a new phone system left 12,000 customers in Hamburg, Germany, without phone service for 12 hours.[58] On January 15, 1990, the AT&T long-distance system "saturated" and was out of commission for 11 hours, due to a software error.

In September 1993, an entry error to the computerized Milan stock exchange, which indicated that the price of one of the best stocks in the Italian market (Generali) had dropped by about 12 percent, caused a temporary panic in the market. As the person commenting on this report noted, the software for a big system such as a stock market should have built in a check for values that are way out of line with previous values, and ask for a human double-check if they occur, before proceeding to post them.[59]

In November 1993, UPI reported that a committee of the Brazilian government investigating fraud in Brazil was stymied when the computer they were using to cross-check thousands of bank accounts, checks, and budget reports "froze up" and would not work. "The network ran out of processing resources, including memory, when trying to track down corruption in the government."[60] Perhaps this story points out a new application area for supercomputers.

The March 16, 1994, *Wall Street Journal* reported that a man named Davila entered the wrong transaction on his computer, typing in "buy" when he says he meant "sell" for a large block of Codelco stock (a state-owned Chilean company). Apparently his error cost the company at least $207 million (roughly 0.5 percent of Chile's Gross National Product). It is said that the Chileans have added a new word to their language—"davilar," which means "to botch things up miserably."[61]

In October 1996 in Boston, customers trying to use their ATM cards were told that their personal ID's were incorrect; when they reentered the ID's, the machine ate their cards. The link to the main ATM network was apparently broken.[62]

In March 1998, a staffer in then Vice President Al Gore's office hit the wrong icon and sent Senator Daniel Moynihan a congratulatory note on the birth of twins, when the best wishes should have been for his seventy-first birthday.[63]

Another issue besides errors that occur within computer systems is the system's reliability. To relate a personal incident, when our college library went over to a computerized card catalog, it made the decision to get rid of the old card catalog drawers. Twice within a two-week period, when I desperately needed to look up whether we had a few books I needed for working on this manuscript, I went to the library only to find out that the computerized system was down, and no one knew when it would be up again (someone was projecting it might be in three days!). Since the library had disposed of the old drawers of cards, there was no way to determine whether they had the books I needed. I suspect that some of my readers have had similar experiences. This is reflective of a tendency in our society to think that the new, faster, slicker computer systems will always do what we want them to do, and to forget to look carefully at the downside of computer errors and systems that crash. If the college had kept the old physical card catalog, it might not have been completely up to date, but it would have served as a useful backup in times of emergency.[64]

Two More Software Fiascos

In April 1994, the director of the California Department of Motor Vehicles said that the department spent $44 million over the last six years on a computer modernization project that has proved to be an unmitigated failure.[65] IBM sold a computerized fingerprinting system to a British police consortium in 1992, and is being sued because the system is said not to work.[66]

Y2K Bugs

There was great concern as the new millennium approached that there would be catastrophic computer failures—what were dubbed the year 2000, or Y2K, bugs. The problem was caused by the fact that the programmers writing programs a decade or two earlier had not taken into account the date change from one century to the next (most dates had been entered as MM/DD/YY, with the assumption that the two-digit year was prefaced by "19"). A lot of work was done writing patches to earlier code, and the transition to January 1, 2000, was generally pretty smooth, with a few minor glitches, and some that did not show up until a month to a year later. However, what could have been made a nonproblem by a little programmer foresight cost millions of dollars and many months to fix.

A few minor problems *did* occur, such as newborn babies being given birth certificates dated 1900, and a Nevada man who registered his car late being billed for $378,426.25 in interest due since 1900.[67]

Follow-up

The interested reader is referred to the regularly appearing sections in *Software Engineering Notes* (published quarterly) and the Risks column in *Communications of the ACM* (published monthly) for the latest snafus, laughable errors, and serious threats discovered in our increasingly computerized world.

 RELIABILITY

As we discussed briefly in the first section of this chapter, computer programs usually have errors ("bugs"). If you have ever written a computer program, even a short one, you are aware of this phenomenon. You write a program, and submit it to the compiler or the assembler. You think the program is perfect, but the computer spits out a whole list of **syntax errors**.

These can represent anything from a typing error (you entered FORAMT when you intended FORMAT), to the lack of an "END" statement, to a reference to a line number that does not exist, to the use of the wrong word for a command (for example, you asked it to PRINT but it only accepts the command WRITE). You fix all of these errors (though you find the cryptic messages from the compiler hard to decipher), the compiler unearths new errors that show up at this level, and the whole process must be repeated a few more times.

You finally have a program free of syntax errors, so you run it, and you find out that it goes into an infinite loop, or outputs meaningless results, or some other disaster. You now are dealing not with syntax errors but with *semantic*, or *logical*, errors. What you wrote in your program uses the programming language without any flaws in the form, but it does not make sense, or it does the wrong thing. An infinite loop occurs if you write something that is analogous to telling someone to "Do X forever"–for example, take the shampoo example of "apply shampoo, lather, rinse, repeat"; it is grammatically all right, but it sets up an impossible, unfulfillable task.

Other errors can occur if you simply solved your problem incorrectly, and so the algorithm you put into computer language will not work, or will give crazy results. You may also have made a typing error in a place that will not cause a syntax error message, but is wrong in your problem–for example, typing 1243 when you wanted 1234, or entering 1.0 E 6 (10^6), which stands for a million, when you meant a billion (1.0 E 9). Or you may have made a mistake in the mathematical formula you are using, such as entering a minus where there should have been a plus, which still gives a legal program language expression, or using the wrong formula for the job. These all represent program "bugs" that are much harder to detect, find, and correct.

Other program errors may exist on an even higher level. You may have typed everything correctly, used the right form of the mathematical equations, written no infinite loops, etc., but the model you are using is wrong for the application. For example, you are treating orbits as circular when in fact they are elliptical, or you are treating a system with simple billiard-ball mechanical laws when you should have been using quantum mechanics, etc. Thus your program will run, and will give you answers, but it does not fit the facts.

Another type of program "bug" that may not show up for a long time, but then can bring the system to its knees, is that of not taking special conditions into account. There are a number of examples in *Software Engineering Notes* and *Communications of the ACM* of programs that ran into difficulty when a value hit 32,768. On a computer with a 16-bit word size, the largest integer that can be stored is $2^{15} - 1$, or 32,767.[68]

If a program had to deal with customer numbers, or a calendar that counted days since the beginning of the century, when the count reached 32,768 (2^{15}) the location containing that value would **overflow**, causing unexpected results in the program. For example, a Washington, D.C., hospital had its computer system "collapse" on September 19, 1989, which is 32,768 days after January 1, 1900, and the Michigan Terminal System (MTS) crashed on November 16, 1989 (32,768 days after March 1, 1900). Peter G. Neumann, in his Inside Risks column in the *Communications of the ACM*, referred to this as an "unintentional time bomb." [69] Other calendar problems occur when an unprepared program runs into a leap year, but has no provision for inserting a date of February 29. [70]

Another such problem could occur if a value outside the expected range of values was entered (due, perhaps, to keyboard input error) that would cause an *overflow* or an *underflow* (though the latter is less likely). A program could run perfectly well on most data until a special condition was encountered on which it had not been tested. For example, imagine you are implementing the following simple "bubble sort" algorithm to sort numbers into descending order: Set a counter of switches made to zero. Go down the list checking adjacent pairs of values; if a pair is in the proper (descending) order, leave it alone; if not, interchange the two values and increase the switch counter by one (or just note that a switch has been made). When you come to the end of the list, check to see if any switches were made on this pass. If there were, repeat the procedure from the beginning. If no switches were made, the sort is complete.

The algorithm seems fine, and it should work, though more slowly than any more efficient sort procedures. The problem is in how you check for whether the two values are in the proper order. Well, you have a test for whether one value is greater than another (>, or .GT., or if the difference between first and second is positive, etc.), so you test the first against the second. If the first is greater than the second, you leave the pair alone; otherwise you switch. You write and check out the program on some lists of values, and it works fine. So you put it "into production," having it sort many lists for you. Things go along well until one day your program goes into an unexplained infinite loop. What happened? It hit a pair of values in a list that were *equal* (it had not had any lists like that before).

According to your test, if the first value wasn't greater than the second value, you switched the pair. Since the first value isn't greater when the values are equal, it switched them, counted a switch, and on each successive pass down the list it switched them again. Since for every pass in which *any* switches were made, you had to repeat the procedure, it goes on and on forever. Of course, all you have to do in the program is change the *greater than* test to a *greater than or equal to* test, and the sort will work correctly.

This is just one example of a program with a hidden bug that does not show up for some time because the programmer did not think the algorithm through well, and then failed to test the program under all conditions of lists it might encounter. There are countless ways in which a program can be wrong that may not show up until some time down the road, and its failure may then cause a system crash or some other disaster. Efforts to avoid this sort of occurrence include using structured programming methods, extensive testing of programs, and a method called program verification.

Program Verification

What is called *program verification* or *proving programs correct* is really a logical/mathematical way of proving "the relative consistency between the formal specifications of the program and the model in terms of which the program is formulated" (Smith, 1991, p. 1). Thus the verification process will show that the program "hangs together" consistently, but it will not give any information on whether there is a mistake in a mathematical formula, or whether the model used for the program has any relation at all to reality. Verification is effective only on rather short programs, and not usable on programs with millions of lines of program code.

Software Engineering

In the area of software development, much can be learned from the engineer's approach to problems (a sound knowledge of physical principles and mathematical techniques, combined with a touch of practical wisdom and a dash of creative genius), and this has given rise to the name *software engineering* for "the establishment and use of sound engineering principles in order to obtain economically software that is reliable and works on real machines."[71] A "software crisis" emerged in the 1970s, when the size of programs needed to solve the new problems seemed to have gotten beyond the control of the system designers. A new approach to large-scale problems that required 100,000 to a million lines was needed, to ensure quality and accuracy. Grady Booch indicated a need for such programs to be modifiable, efficient, reliable, understandable, timely, inexpensive, reusable, responsive, and transportable.[72] Not much to ask of a million-line program!

The programming language Ada (named after Ada, Lady Lovelace) was backed by the U.S. Department of Defense, which planned to make it the required "language of choice" on all government military contracts. There are some problems inherent in the complexity of the language itself that make it a possible source of serious programming errors. Charles Anthony Richard ("Tony") Hoare, a computer scientist of significant stature had the following to say about the Ada language in a 1981 talk entitled "The Emperor's Old Clothes":

> I knew that it would be impossible to write a wholly reliable compiler for a language of this complexity and impossible to write a wholly reliable program when the correctness of each part of the program depends on checking that every other part of the program has avoided all the traps and pitfalls of the language. . . . Do not allow the language in its present state to be used in applications where reliability is critical, i.e., nuclear power stations, cruise missiles, early warning systems, anti-ballistic missile defense systems. The next rocket to go astray as a result of a programming language error may not be an exploratory space rocket on a harmless trip to Venus; it may be a nuclear warhead exploding over one of our own cities.[73]

The point of the Ada story is that computer professionals should choose their tools carefully. A language that may be favored by military customers because of their desire for standardization and secrecy may not turn out to be the best or safest choice, and the professional should be willing to stand up to a client and be ready to explain why the choice is wrong. In 1964, IBM introduced the language PL/I (for "Programming Language I") in an effort to incorporate, and thus replace, FORTRAN, COBOL, and Algol. It turned out to be too large and unwieldy, "since the subtle and unpredictable interactions among the various features of PL/I meant that, practically, programmers had to be aware of the entire language. . . . The result [was] inevitably a language so large as to be unmanageable and too complicated to be mastered by most programmers."[74] In *A Short Introduction to the Art of Programming*, E. W. Dijkstra was said to have referred to PL/I as a "fatal disease." PL/I fell into disuse, though FORTRAN and COBOL remained, and Pascal emerged as a new language with a beautiful simplicity.

Engineers have a wide range of reusable *tools* at their disposal, from slide rules to mathematical techniques such as calculus and statistical analysis. These tools are mastered and then used over and over again. The good software designer should also develop reusable tools, generally in the form of subprograms that can be used in many applications, such as sort routines and averaging. These routines should be as general as possible; for example, a sort should not be written just to sort a list of length 100 items, but a list of any length specified to the routine. Such routines should be tested well, and have the capability to handle user errors without crashing.

Program Testing

All programs, whether designed for personal use or to customer specifications, or to be marketed to the public in general, should be as error-free as possible. After removing all the syntax errors, the programmer should "desk-check" the routine to see that it actually does what was intended. Then it should be run on a varied set of test data, including *illegal* values, to be sure the program handles them adequately, and does not fail or give erroneous results.

Structured Walkthroughs   Often it is very difficult to find your own errors. That is why when you write a paper, it is best to have someone else check it for any remaining errors, since you may read right past them (after all, *you* know what you *meant*). Similarly, the best way to find the errors in a program is to have someone else or, even better, a team, "walk through" the code looking for errors or ways to make it more efficient, and even to design the data to test it thoroughly (you as the programmer might inadvertently give it easy data to handle, subconsciously not wanting to see it fail). Such a team approach is referred to as a *structured walkthrough*. It is effective in program testing, and it also guarantees that more than one person understands the program so that if the original designer disappears from the scene, the secrets of the program do not also disappear. Such precautions will also make it easier for a number of different people to *maintain* the program—to remove any new bugs that are found and to modify it to fit changing needs.

All of this makes good, practical business sense. Yet in reality there is often a sense of urgency to get a job done, which means that the programmer or the company may not take the extra time for thorough testing. Thus a defective product can go into the market, or to the defense department to control missile guidance systems. This is where professional responsibility should come in; the computer professional should recognize his responsibility to colleagues and company *and* to the purchaser of the system and, in some cases of "risk-critical" software, to humanity. The responsible computer professional (and company) should be aware of the potential for error, and the possibly devastating effects of some errors.

When All Is Said and Done

In an article entitled "The Limits of Software Reliability," Ronald L. Enfield cites some statistics estimating the number of errors in a typical large software system, which are quite disturbing:

Number of lines of code: 1,000,000

Number of faults in the initial software (2% of the total, based on a widely reported average): 20,000

Faults remaining after testing (assuming that 90% of the faults are found and fixed): 2,000

Number of failures per year (10% of the faults, based on experience): 200

Faults corrected after failures: 200

Remaining faults: 1,800

Lines of code added or changed per year in routine maintenance (estimated as 10% per year): 100,000

Number of faults added to the system (2% of new code): 2,000

Number of new faults remaining after debugging new code (assuming 90% of new faults removed): 200

Number of faults not discovered in previous year: 1,800

Total number of faults: 2,000

Expected failure rate per year (based on prior failure assumption): 200
(Enfield, 1987, pp. 40, 42)

As the article points out, not all failures are catastrophic, and may only create an unexplained blip on a screen at times, but it would be pure foolishness to blithely assume that all results from such a program are always flawless. I was once told by a development editor that if one were a perfectionist, then publishing was the wrong place to be. It would seem that the same rule holds as well for the software industry.

 OBSERVATION

Someone has to take responsibility to protect against errors. Who, most reasonably, should that be? Those who design computer systems and write programs for them have a moral responsibility to those who will use them. Something is *promised*—the ability to do something wonderful using the computer. The promise should be backed up by good intentions and competent technology. The times of "let the buyer beware" were the times of a

Roman Empire that self-destructed. Some potential errors may seem trivial (such as whether columns come out properly aligned in a word-processing program), but even these *matter* to the user who expects what has been promised; other potential errors could result in large-scale destruction of society. What goods should we be striving for? Computers are at best a *means*, not an end in themselves (though some aficionados seem to treat them that way). The important question is, how can computers and reliable programs better human life, for the individual and for society?

■ ENDNOTES

1. Quoted in *Computerworld* (November 16, 1981).

2. Fred R. Shapiro, "The First Bug: Exposing the Myth," *Byte* 19, 4 (April 1994), p. 308.

3. *Risks*, as they are designated by Peter G. Neumann in his fascinating reports in *Software Engineering Notes*—"Risks to the Public in Computers and Related Systems"—and in the Risks column in *Communications of the ACM* by Peter Neumann and others.

4. The discussion in this section on the Patriot missiles has been drawn from *SEN* 17, 2 (April 1992), pp. 4–5; *SEN* 17, 3 (July 1992), pp. 16–17; and Seymour M. Hersh, "Missile Wars," *New Yorker* (September 26, 1994), pp. 86–90.

5. *Software Engineering Notes* (*SEN*) 17, 2 (April 1992), 4.

6. *SEN* 13, 4 (October 1988), 3.

7. Tom Forester and Perry Morrison, *Computer Ethics: Cautionary Tales*, 2nd ed. (Cambridge, MA: MIT, 1994), p. 108.

8. *SEN* 12, 1 (January 1987), 3.

9. *SEN* 11, 2 (April 1986), 3.

10. *SEN* 12, 1 (January 1987), 3.

11. *SEN* 15, 5 (October 1990), 16–17.

12. *SEN* 19, 1 (January 1994), 10.

13. *SEN* 17, 4 (October 1992), 13.

14. Peter G. Neumann, "System Development Woes," *Communications of the ACM* 36, no. 10 (October 1993), 146.

15. *SEN* 24, 1 (January 1999), 31.

16. *SEN* 16, 1 (January 1991), 2.

17. *SEN* 6, 5 (October 1981), 3–10.

18. *SEN* 14, 5 (July 1989); see also Paul Ceruzzi, *Beyond the Limits—Flight Enters the Computer Age* (Cambridge, MA: MIT, 1989), appendix.

19. *SEN* 5, 2 (April 1980), 4.

20. *SEN* 9, 1 (January 1984), 3–4.

21. *SEN* 10, 5 (October 1985), 10–11. The Ariane 5 rocket explosion was caused by computer error (*SEN* 21, 5 (September 1996), 15).

22. *SEN* 17, 1 (January 1992), 3.

23. *SEN* 19, 1 (January 1994), 10.

24. *SEN* 12, 1 (January 1987), 5.

25. Robert D. Dorsett, "Risks in Aviation" (Inside Risks Column), *Communications of the ACM* 37, 1 (January 1994), 154.

26. *SEN* 14, 2 (October 1988), 3.

27. *SEN* 15, 2 (April 1990), 20–21; *SEN* 15, 3 (July 1990), 15–16.

28. *SEN* 15, 5 (October 1990), 16.

29. *SEN* 17, 3 (July 1992), 18–19.

30. *SEN* 19, 1 (January 1994), 3.

31. Forester and Morrison, p. 105.

32. *WWN* seems to have some similarities to the *National Enquirer* in its selection and presentation of news items.

33. This story was repeated in *SEN* 10, 1 (January 1985), and also mentioned in *SEN* 14, 5 (July 1989), 7, in their discussion of the next story we cover in the text (perhaps to put *WWN* reports in perspective).

34. *SEN* 14, 5 (July 1989), 7–8.

35. *SEN* 10, 1 (January 1985), 8.

36. *SEN* 11, 1 (January 1986), 7–9; *SEN* 12, 3 (July 1985), 7–8.

37. *SEN* 10, 2 (April 1985), 5.

38. *SEN* 18, 1 (January 1993), 7.

39. *SEN* 15, 2 (April 1990), 3–4.

40. *SEN* 18, 1 (January 1993), 12.

41. *SEN* 15, 1 (January 1990), 7.

42. *SEN* 12,4 (October 1987), 9.

43. *SEN* 13, 2 (April 1988), 11.

44. *SEN* 15, 5 (October 1990), 5.

45. *SEN* 16, 1 (January 1991), 16.

46. *SEN* 16, 1 (January 1991), 16–17; the original story by Sabrina Eaton appeared in the Cleveland *Plain Dealer*.

47. *SEN* 17, 4 (October 1992), 7.

48. *SEN* 18, 1 (January 1993), 13.

49. *SEN* 17, 3 (July 1992), 2.

50. *SEN* 22, 1 (January 1997), 20.

51. For example, see *SEN* 16, 2 (April 1991), 11, "Inhabitant of Amsterdam Lies Dead for Half a Year"; *SEN* 19, 1 (January 1994), 2, which reports of an elderly woman in Stockholm, Sweden, who lay dead for three years (!) before she was found.

52. *SEN* 17, 4 (October 1992), 3.

53. *SEN* 18, 1 (January 1993), 7.

54. See *SEN* 16, 2 (April 1991), 18.

55. For example, see *SEN* 16, 3 (July 1991), 6.

56. *SEN* 17, 4 (October 1992), 4.

57. *SEN* 18, 2 (April 1993), 4. This is similar to the incident discussed earlier where a walkie-talkie signal shut down a nuclear plant. In both, a random electronic emission could have potentially disastrous effects.

58. *SEN* 19, 1 (January 1994), 3.

59. *SEN* 19, 1 (January 1994), 5.

60. *SEN* 19, 1 (January 1994), 4.

61. *SEN* 19, 3 (July 1994), 5.

62. *SEN* 22, 1 (January 1997), 21.

63. *SEN* 22, 1 (January 1997), 23.

64. Nicholson Baker writes in "Discards" of the great loss of tradition with the extermination of the card catalogs across the country. He speaks of "the national paroxysm of short-sightedness and anti-intellectualism"; he cites the assessment of Helen Parish, a historian specializing in the sixteenth century, that it is "in a class with the burning of the library at Alexandria." Much wonderful information that was included on the original cards is thrown out when they are transferred to a database; the databases are "full of new errors, much harder to browse efficiently, are less rich in crossreferences and subject headings, lack local character, do not group related titles and authors together particularly well, and are in many cases stripped of whole classes of historical information (e.g., the original price of the book, the acquisition date, its original cataloging date, its accession number, the original cataloguer's own initials, the record of any copies that have been withdrawn, and whether it was a gift or a purchase) that existed free, using up no disk space or computer-room electricity, requiring no pricey software updates or daily backups or hardware service calls." *New Yorker* (April 4, 1994), pp. 64–86.

65. Carl Ingram, "DMV Spent $44 Million on Failed Project," *Los Angeles Times*, 27 April 1994, p. A3.

66. "U.K. Police Sue IBM Over Alleged Failure of Fingerprint System," *Wall Street Journal*, 31 March 1995, p. B8.

67. *SEN* 25, 3 (May 2000), 19.

68. One bit is used for the sign of the integer, and the largest value that can be stored in a system where the number of symbols is s in a string of length n is $s^n - 1$; for example, the largest decimal (base 10) integer that can be stored in four columns is $10^4 - 1$, or 9999).

69. Peter G. Neumann, "The Clock Grows at Midnight," *Communications of the ACM* 34, 1 (January 1991), 170.

70. This is usually a fairly simple matter to program for, except that the rules get more complicated for leap years if you have to deal with years divisible by 100. A year divisible by 100 is only a leap year if it is *also* divisible by 400. Furthermore, years divisible by 4,000 are not leap years.

71. Fritz Bauer, "Software Engineering," *Information Processing* 71 (Amsterdam, Netherlands: North-Holland, 1972), p. 530.

72. Gary Booch, *Software Engineering and Ada* (Redwood City, CA: Benjamin Cummings, 1987).

73. C. Hoare, "The Emperor's Old Clothes," *Communications of the ACM* 24, 2 (February 1981), 82–83.

74. Bruce J. MacLennan, *Principles of Programming Languages*, 2nd ed. (New York: Holt, Rinehart, Winston, 1987), 176.

■ SHORT ESSAY QUESTIONS

1. Obviously it is not just computers that make errors; humans make errors as well. In fact, most of the time what is called a "computer error" is really traceable to a human error, usually a programming or a design error. What are the usual ways of handling human errors? Take a human example of error in which *responsibility* is traced and assigned; what happens to the human found responsible? Now draw a parallel between your case and one in which "computer error" is said to occur. How can (or should) responsibility be assigned in this case, and how should the responsible party be treated?

2. Discuss briefly why the technique of program verification does not guarantee that the program will not have errors in its application to the real world. Discuss how such "verification" (of real-world viability) would have to be carried out.

3. Examine a complex macroeconometric theory like the "Wharton Model" (from the revered business program at the University of Pennsylvania), how it employs thousands of variables simultaneously (which is only possible using a computer), and how well its results match with reality.

■ LONG ESSAY QUESTIONS

1. Given the discussion of program reliability, does it look as if large, complex programs (say, from 100,000 to a million lines or more) will *ever* be reliable? Discuss critically. If the answer is "no," then what would you recommend regarding large programs? That people should stop writing them? That they should *never* be used in "safety-critical" applications? Or might there be some way to still use the large programs, if lots of safety traps are built in? Does there need to be some special training or at least "consciousness-raising" for those who write such software so that they are sensitive to the potential risks and try to program to prevent them? This is a rather open-ended question, and it will take some careful and imaginative thinking on your part. (There is an area called "safety engineering"; does it seem that the principles in that area could be carried over into the writing of safety-critical computer programs?)

2. Why do you suppose that computers have such difficulties in translating natural language texts? Writing on this topic involves looking carefully into distinctions between *syntax* and *semantics*, examining the ambiguity present in natural languages, and how humans make use of *context* in resolving such ambiguities. Why would it be difficult to program a computer to do this? Has anyone (say, Noam Chomsky, in *Aspects of the Theory of Syntax* [ch. 4], or in *Cartesian Linguistics*; or anyone following Chomsky who is advocating the computational theory of mind) argued that semantics is reducible to syntax? Could a good case be made for this? In that case, could the problems of computer translation be solved?

3. List as many reasons as you can *not to trust* computers, and as many reasons as you can think of *to* trust them. On balance, what does this tell you about information from computers?

■ REFERENCES AND RECOMMENDED READINGS

Brooks, Frederick P., Jr. *The Mythical Man-Month: Essays on Software Engineering.* Reading, MA: Addison-Wesley, 1979.

Brown, Geoffrey. *The Information Game: Ethical Issues in a Microchip World.* Atlantic Highlands, NJ: Humanities Press, 1990, ch. 4.

Computer Crime and Computer Security: Hearing Before the Subcommittee on Crime, U.S. House of Representatives, May 23, 1985. Washington, DC: Government Printing Office, 1986.

Crenshaw, Albert B. "When a Computer Error Renders You a Deadbeat." Washington *Post* (National Weekly Edition), 1–7 November 1993, 17–18.

Dejoie, Roy, George Fowler, and David Paradice, eds. *Ethical Issues in Information Systems.* Boston, MA: Boyd & Fraser, 1991, ch. 2.

DeLanda, Manuel. *War in the Age of Intelligent Machines.* New York: Zone Books, 1991.

Dunlop, Charles, and Rob Kling, eds. *Computerization and Controversy: Value Conflicts and Social Choices.* Boston: Academic Press, 1991, part VI: Security and Reliability.

Enfield, Ronald L. "The Limits of Software Reliability." *Technology Review* (April 1987), 36–43.

Ford, Daniel F. *The Button: The Pentagon's Strategic Command and Control System.* New York: Simon & Schuster, 1985.

Forester, Tom, and Perry Morrison. *Computer Ethics: Cautionary Tales and Ethical Dilemmas in Computing.* 2nd ed. Cambridge, MA: MIT Press, 1994, ch. 5.

Hersh, Seymour M. "Missile Wars." *New Yorker* (September 26, 1994), 86–99.

Hoare, C. A. R. "The Emperor's Old Clothes." *Communications of the ACM* 24, 2 (February 1981), 75–83.

Impoco, Jim (in Tokyo). "Computers That To Translate Good Enough." *U.S. News & World Report* (December 5, 1988), 72.

"Inside Risks Forum" columns in *Communications of the ACM*. (Always found on the last inside page of the issue.)

Jacky, Jonathan. "Safety-Critical Computing: Hazards, Practices, Standards, and Regulation." In Dunlop and Kling, 612–31.

Johnson, Deborah G. *Computer Ethics*. 2nd ed. Englewood Cliffs, NJ: Prentice-Hall, 1994, ch. 7.

Laudon, Kenneth C. "Data Quality and Due Process in Large Interorganizational Record Systems." *Communications of the ACM* 29, 1 (January 1986), 4–11.

Lee, Leonard. "Computers Out of Control." *Byte* (February 1992), 344.

Neumann, Peter G. "Expecting the Unexpected Mayday!" *Communications of the ACM* 34, 5 (May 1991), 128.

Neumann, Peter G. "Survivable Systems." *Communications of the ACM* 35, 5 (May 1992), 130.

Neumann, Peter G. "Aggravation by Computer: Life, Death, and Taxes." *Communications of the ACM* 35, 7 (July 1992), 122.

Neumann, Peter G. "Accidental Financial Losses." *Communications of the ACM* 35, 9 (September 1992), 142.

Neumann, Peter G. "Avoiding Weak Links." *Communications of the ACM* 35, 12 (December 1992), 146.

Neumann, Peter G. "System Development Woes." *Communications of the ACM* 36, 10 (October 1993), 146.

Peterson, I. *Fatal Defect: Why Computers Fail*. New York: Random House, 1995.

Shapiro, Fred R. "The First Bug: Exposing the Myth." *Byte* 19, 4 (April 1994), 308.

Smith, Brian Cantwell. *Limits of Correctness in Computers*. (Presented at a Symposium on Unintentional Nuclear War at the Fifth Congress of the International Physicians for the Prevention of Nuclear War, Budapest, Hungary, June 28–July 1, 1985.) Stanford, CA: Center for the Study of Language and Information, 1985. Reprinted in Dunlop and Kling, 632–46.

Software Engineering Notes.

Spinello, Richard A. *Ethical Aspects of Information Technology*. Englewood Cliffs, NJ: Prentice-Hall, 1995, ch. 4.

Wagner, Peter. "Hit the Wrong Key, Become a Verb. . ." *SEN* 19, 3 (July 1994), 5.

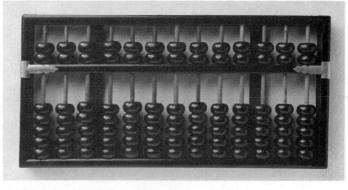

Chapter 9

The Computer World Of Work

 THE CONTROL REVOLUTION

In an excellent book, *The Control Revolution: Technological and Economic Origins of the Information Society,* James R. Beniger describes how our world has turned from an agrarian to an industrial to an information and control society, and gives us a perspective on how we got to where we find ourselves today. He begins by asking, "For the economies of at least a half-dozen countries, the processing of information has begun to overshadow the processing of matter and energy. But why? Among the multitude of things that human beings value, why should it be information . . . that has come to dominate the world's largest and most advanced economies?" (Beniger, 1986, p. 5). He notes that Alvin Toffler added to the two earlier revolutions (agricultural and industrial) a "Third Wave": "We are engaged in building a remarkable new civilization from the ground up; . . . the Third Wave will sweep across history and complete itself in a few decades" (Toffler, 1980, p. 26).

Within the Control Revolution, Beniger notes the development of virtually all of the basic communications technologies within a century—photography and telegraphy (1830s), rotary power printing (1840s), typewriter (1860s), transatlantic cable (1866), telephone (1876), motion pictures (1894), wireless telegraphy (1895), magnetic tape recording (1899), radio (1906), and television (1923)—followed by the development of computers. He uses *control* to imply two essential elements: *influence* of one agent over another (resulting in changed behavior) and *purpose*.

A **feedback system** involves communicating influence from the controller to the controlled and reporting results of the action in the reverse direction. Norbert Wiener took great interest in natural and humanmade feedback systems in a book entitled *Cybernetics*. A simple feedback system is the body sweating in the heat to cool off. An analogous humanmade feedback system is the thermostat in your home; when the temperature drops below a certain set desired level, a signal is sent for the heating system to be turned on. Computer chips have brought feedback control to many areas, including cars and kitchens.

Beniger (1986, p. 9) observes that "technology defines the limits on what a society *can* do." He points out that the Neolithic Revolution followed the refinement of stone tools and the domestication of plants and animals; the Communication Revolution resulted from technical improvements in ships and navigational equipment; the Industrial Revolution began a century earlier with increased use of coal and steam power and new machinery for manufacture of textiles and the like; and the Control Revolution resulted from innovations in information processing technology. So the technology creates the framework within which a society develops and changes.

Emile Durkheim noted in 1893 that industrialization tends to break down the barriers that isolate markets, thus widening the distribution of goods and services to include far-flung markets. This, he points out, disrupts the market equilibrium, since there is no longer any direct communication between the producer and the consumer. The crisis of control results in a breakdown of standards of behavior, largely due to the lack of human interaction. "The producer can no longer embrace the market in a glance, nor even in thought. He can no longer see limits since it is, so to speak, limitless. Accordingly, production becomes unbridled and unregulated. It can only trust to chance . . . . From this come the crises which periodically disturb economic functions" (Durkheim [1893], 1933, pp. 369–70).

The impact of the "Information Society" can be seen, explains Beniger, by looking at its effect on the segment of the U.S. economy involved with the "production and distribution of knowledge," involving industries in five major areas: education, research and development, communications media, information machines, and information services. Measures in these areas indicate that they comprised 29 percent of the Gross National Product (GNP) and 31 percent of the workforce in 1958 (a doubling over ten years before), 42 percent of the labor force by 1960, 46.4 percent by 1970, and 46.6 percent by 1980. In contrast, agriculture, which had represented 87.2 percent of the labor force in 1800, and 35.3 percent in 1900, was down to 2.1 percent in 1980 (Beniger, 1986, pp. 21–222).

Simon Nora and Alain Minc, in *The Computerization of Society: A Report to the President of France* (1978), likened the growing interconnection of information-processing, communication, and control technologies throughout the world to an alteration in the "entire nervous system of social organization," and introduced the term *telematics* for the phenomenon. If this analogy is pursued, it makes each of us individual neurons in this great interconnected network. On many models, the individual neuron knows little or nothing about what the whole system is doing;[1] it has its own simple job to perform in a narrow area. We should keep this model in mind when we look at some of the concerns raised about the new information society.

Evolution of Systems

According to Beniger, living systems have thus far evolved four levels of programmable structures and programs: life (genetic programming in DNA), the brain (cultural learning by imitation), bureaucracy (organizations with decision rules), and technology (mechanical and electronic processors with algorithms) (Beniger, p. 112). Not all species that are social have brains (e.g., sponges), and not all species that have brains are social. Of the million or more animal species that currently exist, several tens of thousands are social, and about twelve thousand (the birds and the mammals) have relatively well-developed brains. Brains and sociality overlap in a few thousand species, roughly ten times the overlap number to be expected by pure chance.[2]

In an appendix entitled "What Is Life? An Information Perspective," Beniger asks how we recognize a living organism. There is a tendency to cite some physical constituent of organic matter (e.g., protoplasm), but reputable scientists now discuss the possibility of life on other planets that may have a radically different chemical base than our own. In *The Life Puzzle* (1971), the molecular chemist Alexander Graham Cairns-Smith even speculates that our own earliest ancestors might not have been based on organic molecules at all, but on tiny mineral crystals capable of self-replication. When we program computers sent into deep space to look for life, what do we program them to look for? Many biologists simply list a number of properties they consider to be most basic to life. The most common six cited are (1) **organization** (essential to which is *homeostasis*—the maintenance of a relatively stable internal environment); (2) **metabolism and growth** through destruction and reconstruction of organic material; (3) **responsiveness** to stimuli; (4) **adaptability**, including the ability to learn; (5) **reproduction**; and (6) **evolution** through natural selection, involving the continual readjustment to environmental variation and change (Beniger, 1986, pp. 105–9). Are we still evolving?

Three Functions of DNA.   Beniger continues, "Even in living systems that have evolved brains, culture, and control technologies, most control remains programmed at the genetic level. . .. All living systems maintain control through three genetic processes—replication, regulation, and reproduction" (Beniger, 1986, p. 112). These correspond to three control dimensions:

1. **Existence** (through *replication* of programming for distributed control): With perhaps a quadrillion cells in the human body, how do they come to achieve the coherence of a single organism? By virtually identical programming, replies Beniger.
2. **Experience** through *regulation* of physical processes via *feedback* (adaptive control by DNA through the manipulation of only twenty different amino acids): "As in the design of new computers, natural selection had to decide which functions to build into the hardware (programmable structure), which to program into the firmware (the genome), and which—in the case of the higher vertebrates—to leave to subsequent development in software (culture)" (Beniger, 1986, p. 115).
3. **Evolution** (becoming) through *reproduction* of programming in new entities (a kind of "gene-shuffling" down generations). "Only at the levels of brains, culture, and control technology has evolution enabled some species to partially *short-circuit* the relatively slower process of reprogramming through natural selection" (Beniger, 1986, p. 118).

Through information processing, great strides have been made and can be made by humans. Just as it was our brains that allowed us to survive as a species, by extending mental capacities to learn and process information (by the use of computers), we can evolve much more rapidly. But this raises two questions: (1) Evolve toward what? (it is crucial here to be purposive and to choose worthwhile goals); and (2) Are computers just another set of tools that humans have constructed to manipulate the world, or are computers themselves the next step in the evolution of intelligence? We will examine the latter question in Chapter 12.

"Evolve toward *what*?" is the question of ethical interest. If evolution is just another deterministic process rolling us along in its wake, then there is no point in discussion. If, however, we *do* have choice and some power to change things, then we can have an effect on the direction human futures take. Ethics presupposes such freedom to choose; the question is, what kinds of ends should we seek? Suggestions can be found in the hierarchy of goods in Chapter 3—friendship, knowledge, health, acquaintance with beauty, and the rest. The choices lie in the means to achieve such ends, and the recognition of what ends are worthwhile. So, even though Aristotle pointed out that we do not choose ends, only means, there *is* a choice that needs to be made—the choice to look hard to find the valuable ends, and not have our perception clouded by things like wealth.

A related question, in our modern technological age, is whether we should choose to genetically alter ourselves to achieve certain ends. One example would be the question we discussed earlier: What if we could reduce human size, over two generations, to half what it is now, for an environmental benefit? Another one, which sounds like science fiction, is what if we could "map" our brain patterns onto a computer, and so extend our mental lives? (See Hans Moravec, 1988, and Daniel C. Dennett, 1978.)

The Industrial Revolution Crisis of Control

Beniger begins by saying:

> Throughout all previous history material goods had moved down roadways and canals with the speed of draft animals; for centuries they had moved across the seas at the whim of the winds. Suddenly, in a matter of decades, goods began to move faster than even the winds themselves, reliably and in mounting volume, through factories, across continents, and around the world. For the first time in history, by the mid-nineteenth century the social processing of material flows threatened to exceed in both volume and speed the system's capacity to contain them. Thus was born the crisis of control, one that would eventually reach, by the end of the century, [all] levels of America's material economy. (Beniger, 1986, p. 219)

Problems included a safety crisis with the railroads, inability to keep track of goods distributed in a huge maze of warehouses, and the struggles of those producing basic needed materials (such as iron, copper, and glass) to keep up competitive rates of production. In the 1880s, reports Beniger, the crisis reached goods that are consumed, such as flour, soap, grain, cigarettes; the United States was producing twice as much as it needed, so other markets had to be found.

Observers of the overproduction phenomenon at the end of the nineteenth century predicted that it would cause further exploitation of underdeveloped nations. Rich industrial nations such as England, Holland, France, and Germany "moved into" underdeveloped nations, primarily in Asia and

Africa, and "took control." They claimed to be bringing culture to the uncultured and religion to the heathen, but primarily they were establishing markets to which they could export their excess industrial goods.

The three problems that arose were safety, the inability to keep track of goods that were widely distributed, and an ever-increasing demand for speed in production. All of these problems are prominent in the information society, as we shall soon see.

The industrial explosion gave rise to a need for better information technology. Manufacturers wanted to communicate information about their products to the buying public, and they needed information on the preferences of their buyers. Thus a revolution that began with coal and steam ended with "innovation at a most fundamental level of technology—that of information processing and communication," and ushered in the next revolution, that in information processing (Beniger, 1986, p. 287).

Data Processing and an Information Bureaucracy

Beniger traces the evolution of information-processing devices at the end of the industrial revolution, from the typewriter (1873), the stock ticker (1870), messenger news services (1882), and press clipping services (1883), to the keyboard calculator (1887), Hollerith's punch-card tabulator (1889), and the desk telephone (1886) (Beniger, 1986, pp. 390–91). Beniger traces the connection between information hardware development and the growth of bureaucracy:

> The idea that information processing and computing hardware might be used to enhance bureaucratic control appears to have emerged only gradually during the transition phase of the Control Revolution. Initial impetus came largely from government bureaucracies. First applications were to statistical compilation and aggregate analysis during the 1870s and 1880s and to larger-scale data processing beginning in the 1890s. Only in the late 1910s and 1920s did bureaucracies begin to realize that processed numerical data might be used to process information more generally and thereby strengthen the control maintained by the entire bureaucratic structure. (Beniger, 1986, p. 408)

Thus information was coming to be considered a commodity, one that could be processed by a machine. The government bureaucracies moved from mere statistics to using information to control people through fingerprinting, personal income tax (begun in 1913), draft psychological screening (begun in 1919), keeping track of employment, and the Social Security Act in 1935

(Beniger, 1986, p. 408). We have already seen how much of this information control has affected our privacy.

The strong connection between economics and information seems to account for the amazing growth of the new information industries. Of course, people still need *things*—food, houses, clothing, shoes, toothpaste—but a whole new industry has arisen to advertise different brands for the consumer to buy and to keep track of what has been bought. On top of this, information itself has become a commodity. Mailing lists are sold from one source to another, so the latter can distribute its advertising where it will be most effective. Information as embodied in books has always been a commodity—we wish to learn (both abstract and practical things), and to be entertained. The entertainment business itself, which is primarily based on the transmission of information in plays, movies, musical performances, videos, novels, and the like, has grown at an amazing rate. Entertainers (movie stars, musical talents, and sports figures) get paid huge salaries because the information about what they do keeps us amused. Technical information is also a commodity, one often sold and occasionally stolen.

James R. Beniger has brought us up to the present, showing us some aspects of what came before, and given us some things to think about. Now we need to examine just what information is, how it can be measured and sold, and what effect all of this has on the workers of today and tomorrow.

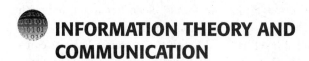

INFORMATION THEORY AND COMMUNICATION

W. Ross Ashby, in *An Introduction to Cybernetics*, said that cybernetics might be defined as "the study of systems that are open to energy but closed to information and control." Since we live in a time of cybernetic systems, and they will dominate our future, it is important to understand what they can and cannot do. It is also crucial to understand the nature of information in our "information society."

Somewhat like Augustine's famous musings on time (*Confessions*, Book XI), we might say when we wonder "What is information?" that if no one asks us, we know well enough. However, if we are asked what it is and try to explain, we are baffled. We do not want a definition so broad that information seems to encompass *everything*, because the concept would make no meaningful distinctions and would be useless. Is information knowledge? But, then, is all knowledge information? (Perhaps not common knowledge, since it does not inform us of anything new?) Is all information knowledge? Perhaps not, since the reading of today's temperature, which is informative and not previously known, may not really qualify as knowledge in some important sense. Are errors, lies, emotions, sex appeal, and sickness information? What about tautologies (like "A is A" or Gertrude Stein's "A rose is a rose")? What about ambiguous expressions, such as my coffee cup from a local FM classical music station, which says "I'm a classic lover"? What sort of information do they convey, and how?

Claude Shannon and Warren Weaver worried about a scientific definition of information—one that could indicate how it could be *measured*, like a good scientific quantity such as temperature—in order to build on it a scientific theory of communication. Shannon and Weaver (1963, pp. 95–97) identified three major levels of problems in communication: the technical, semantic, and effectiveness levels.

Levels of Problems in Communication

Shannon and Weaver's three levels are:

1. *Technical.* The problem here is simply how to communicate a message in the presence of noise. Communication by telephone is a good example here, since you have probably tried to carry on a conversation on a line with static. Another example would be my trying to communicate to my young daughter the message that she should clean her room, but with food in my mouth. The message does not arrive clearly.

2. *Semantic.* The technical level has to do with the syntactic level of communication—that is, whether or not the physical message was transmitted accurately. The semantic level, however, deals with the *meaning* of the message. If the message is received accurately, does the receiver understand what it means? If it is in a foreign language, or contains ambiguity, or is just very difficult (say something in higher math or physics), it may not be understood.

   A very serious example comes from July in 1945, at the end of World War II. The Allies sent Japan the Potsdam Ultimatum which told them to cease fighting "or else." The Japanese cabinet replied with a single word, which phonetically is "mokusatsu." It means, in Japanese, either to ignore or to reserve judgment. The Allies took it to mean that the Japanese were *ignoring* the ultimatum, and the result was the Allied bombing of Hiroshima and Nagasaki. A less serious example would be my still trying to get my daughter to clean her room by asking her "Do you want to clean your room?", to which she might reply, simply, "No." I've failed to make my message understood because of the way I phrased it.

3. *Effectiveness.* The third level in communication arises when the message has been transmitted accurately and its meaning has been understood. The question still remains though: Will the message achieve the desired result? Does a work of art or music produce the desired effect on the perceiver? Does a threat of war succeed in getting the nation threatened to cease its human rights violations? Or again, on the less serious side, if I tell my daughter that if she doesn't clean her room, I will cut off her allowance, will the room be cleaned?

Shannon and Weaver, after this analysis, determined that the only level that a science of communication can deal with is the first one, that of the accurate transmission of a message from sender to receiver, in the presence of noise. Shannon says that the "semantic aspects of communication are irrelevant to the engineering problem" (Shannon and Weaver, 1963, p. 3). One way an accurate transmission can be achieved is to reduce the noise; another is to repeat the message several times. Since the English language is 50 percent redundant, one most often does not have to repeat oneself in a noisy phone conversation, since the missing word or phrase may be obvious from the context. This redundancy in the language takes the place of simple repetition.

The measure of information is tied to its "surprise" value; the most information is conveyed by a message that is totally unexpected. In a system using a set of symbols to convey information, the optimum setup is if each symbol is equally likely (or unlikely). In an area where it rains a lot, the message "Rain" on the weather report is not very surprising. However, the message "Sunny" or "Tornado" will be much more unexpected, and so much more informative.[3]

 # THE INFORMATION WORKPLACE

Many people who several generations ago would have been making a living by planting and harvesting crops are now hard at work indoors in front of computer terminals, manipulating data. For them, manual labor has turned into mental labor. Some of it may be very challenging and exciting, but unfortunately much of it is boring data entry that dulls the mind and psyche.

Marx and Engels wrote of the importance of controlling the **means of production** in society. They argued that these should not be in the hands of a few, who profit from the hard work of the rest; rather, they felt that the means of production should be held in common for the good of all. In any society, the modes of production affect the way the society is shaped. If there are great advances in transportation and industry, the society will become one defined by significant industrial output and distribution. Countries with good methods of agriculture and sufficient fertile land can feed their people well. In 1850, Ludwig Feuerbach noted that to improve a nation one should give it better food, not speeches. The great advances in the information industry have changed the way much of the world today does business.

Entertainment today revolves largely around motion pictures and television, media unknown a hundred years ago. Many of the kinds of work engaged in today were also unknown a few years ago. What you do in your work and the way in which you spend your leisure time affect your life greatly, and shape many of the choices you make.

If, in our work, we are becoming more and more dependent on machines (in particular, computers), are we losing much of our own creativity? Or are we using computers to free us from menial tasks to do more creative and interesting things, as inventors of calculating devices like Leibniz, Pascal, and Babbage had envisioned? With the advent of inexpensive hand calculators, few bother to remember or even learn how to do simple calculations by hand any more. How many other skills will we forget because we have turned the work over to machines? One does not have to engage in doomsday scenarios to see that someone should retain the knowledge of how these things are done. If we retain the fundamental knowledge, we can always rebuild machines if we want them; however, if we keep the machines and let the knowledge slip away, what happens if the machines are no longer here, or cease to work for us?

In her extensive study *In the Age of the Smart Machine* (1984), Shoshana Zuboff writes: "In its capacity as an automating technology, information technology has a vast potential to displace the human presence. Its implications as an informating technology, on the other hand, are not well understood" (p. 10). She emphasizes that dependence on human skills is decreasing as computerization increases. Furthermore, some of the computer operations are so complex that no human being can track them (for example, the calculations for weather prediction, or the details that went into the computer proof of the Four-Color Theorem, discussed in Chapter 12). Advancing technology has displaced many human workers, and made many of those who remain mere appendages of the machines (recall Charlie Chaplin caught up in the cogwheels of a huge machine in *Modern Times*). The ascendance of machines turns many humans into *inferior* machines.

Marx had a good point in noting that human beings need creative and productive work to feel fully human, a part of the *species being*—a concept that, for Marx, represented the human capacity to choose, judge, and create. A human is a *needy* being, but also a *social* being. *Species life* is productive, life creating more life. A human, in exercising this creativity, becomes more than just one person; she represents, thought Marx, the *universal* human, the entire species. If that creative work is taken away from humans, or if they are forced (by economic pressures) to do work that they hate for a good portion of their lives, of course they will be alienated and angry. This is a real problem for today's society, when much work has become of this degrading kind. With machines doing much of the *interesting* work, many humans are reduced to just feeding material or data into those machines.

However, if automation is used wisely, it could increase the productivity of a nation while lessening the need for human labor, and truly free humans for more creative endeavors. This is a challenge both to technology and to education. Marshall McLuhan wrote, in "Automation: Learning a Living": "Paradoxically, automation makes liberal education mandatory." He goes on to say that humans are released from servitude to become "nomadic gatherers of knowledge," and that "the social and educational patterns latent in automation are those of self-employment and artistic autonomy."[4]

As individuals and as part of our society, we face important choices here: Will we passively become, paradoxically, tools of the machines, or will we assert our autonomy to use them for the improvement of the human condition and the environment, at the same time freeing ourselves for more creative achievement?

We must not, at such an important juncture, suffer what Arthur C. Clarke terms failures "of nerve" or "of imagination."[5] A failure of nerve would be to claim that something cannot be done—for example, humans flying. In our situation, a failure of nerve might be to say that working conditions and unemployment cannot be improved significantly, that they "go with the territory." A failure of imagination would be to dismiss as pure fiction or magic the idea of humans walking on the moon, or manning submarines, or the like. For our concerns here, a failure of imagination would be to pooh-pooh the idea of computerized robots as doctors, or as lawyers, or even politicians. If we get past such barriers, then our imaginations need to carry us to what new possibilities are open for humans. This is a crucial social question that cannot be separated from ethics: What duties do we owe to ourselves and future generations in this regard?

The required emphasis on improved and universalized education is unavoidable. We then face the age-old question, as Plato did, about what this education should be. Education must not be merely to accumulate *facts* (*information*); it should be to achieve **understanding**. Butchvarov explains the difference as follows:

> Another way of explaining the difference between information and understanding would be to say that to seek information is to attempt to determine which of two given and clearly understood contradictory propositions is true, while to seek understanding is to attempt to discover, formulate, or become clear about a pair of contradictory propositions such that one of them may be seen to be true. But what is obviously more fundamental and, I suggest, of far greater *intrinsic* value is the discovery of the pair of propositions, or the coming to grasp them more clearly, not the seeing of the truth of one of them, which may or may not follow. For this reason I shall often apply the term "understanding" to the grasp of the propositions even when neither of them is (yet) seen to be true. The former is a cognitive achievement independent of, but presupposed by, the latter. Without it the seeing cannot take place. Without understanding there can be no information. (Butchvarov, 1989, p. 99)

To apply Butchvarov's analysis to our investigation of computer ethics, we use the following example: We wish to know whether the concept "thinking" applies to computers. The two contradictory propositions Butchvarov refers to then would be "Computers *can* think" and "Computers *cannot* think." The attempt to resolve this problem, as we shall discuss in Chapter 12, does not merely involve the gathering of *information* about the characteristics of computers to see if the property "thinking" is one of them, or even a comparison of them with the list of characteristics of something that does think. We find, on facing this question, that the concept "think" is not sufficiently clear. We need to do considerable further work both on our *understanding* of the concept "think" and on our list of the possible characteristics of computers. The *understanding* raises the question, formulates the two propositions, and undertakes the conceptual clarification necessary to an answer.

In the sort of education that is needed for the future, it is *understanding* that must be developed; secondarily, the ways in which to acquire information to resolve the questions raised by understanding must also be taught. With respect to *moral* education, the discovery of the important questions is key. Students must learn to ask, with respect to fundamental ethical issues, not "How do I *feel* about this?" or "What does my society say about this?" (see Chapters 1 and 2), but "What *reasons* can I provide for deciding this issue one way or the other?" (see Chapter 3). These reasons should be based on the most solid ground we can provide. Some grounds we have examined include Kantian universalizable maxims, utilitarian calculations, virtue ethics, and appealing to the hierarchy of goods. We want to be able to provide the best possible reasons for our moral choices, in order to justify them to ourselves and to convince others as well that this is the *right* course of action.

Loss of Jobs, or Just Relocation?

When the Industrial Revolution was in its infancy, workers smashed the machines that they felt would be taking away their jobs. Today, similar acts of aggression are directed against computers (like shooting them, or demagnetizing tapes or disks), but this is more often because of anger against some "computer error" like repetitive overbilling than for loss of jobs. The occasional disgruntled employee may plant a "logic bomb" that will go off and wipe out files a month after he was fired, but on the whole there has not evolved any large-scale guerrilla attack on computers. Yet the advent of computers in many, if not most, workplaces has changed them considerably.

There are many positive effects: the improved billing and inventory system for Sam's Lumber Yard, the ease of correcting letters and documents for many secretaries, the speeded-up operation of the IRS (which could not handle all the returns it faces now without the aid of computers) and the Post Office. But even these are not purely positive; they have their negative side as well. Computerization in the typical office has reduced the need for filing clerks and some secretaries, and whatever lone secretary remains may be confronted with the tiring monotony of looking at a computer screen.

There are also negative aspects. Tax returns keep getting more complex. The IRS might have to simplify its tax process if it did not depend so heavily on computers, and then not so many people might have to take their returns to paid preparers. Another problem is that of IRS employees "browsing" through the returns of friends, families, or celebrities.[6] The Post Office tries to speed mail delivery by automatic handling of mail, but the machines do not read handwritten envelopes well, and so they may be processed even more slowly than before. One wonders whether the two warehouses discovered in Washington, DC, full of undelivered mail contained mostly handwritten envelopes that the machines refused to process.

In a time when such wonders of technology should be making our lives easier, it seems that we are working harder. Americans seem to be working longer hours than they did 25 years ago, and having considerably less leisure time (see Juliet Schor, *The Overworked American*). This might be accounted for by pure greed, but it is more likely that many workers are finding themselves in lower-paying jobs and so are working overtime or holding two jobs to make ends meet. It could also reflect the effect of the faster pace of computers demanding more of the workers, who have to put in extra work time just to keep up with the machines.

A robot is said to pay for itself in five years. If this is true, for long-term jobs the robot is very attractive to management. A robot does not get ill, go on strike, ask for a raise, or even go on coffee breaks. How can a human worker compete effectively with that? James Albus, a leading robotics expert, argues that more work can always be created for both humans and robots, and that the real problem is figuring out how the wealth created by the new technology can be distributed to those who need it. "If this were done, markets would explode, demand would increase, and there would be plenty of work for all able-bodied humans, plus as many robots as we could build."[7]

Albus also has some interesting suggestions as to how this healthier economy might be accomplished through the creation of a National Mutual Fund and mandatory savings that would make all citizens stockholders in the national economy.[8] One is reminded of a speech by actor Ned Beatty in the 1976 movie *Network*:

> The world is a college of corporations, inexorably determined by the immutable laws of business. The world is a business. . . . Our children will live to see that perfect world, in which there's no war or famine, oppression or brutality. One vast and ecumenical holding company for whom all men will work to serve a common profit, in which all men will hold a share of stock—all necessities provided, all anxieties tranquilized, all boredom amused. (Chayefsky, 1976)

Albus certainly does not suffer from a failure of imagination. He says "I believe we have it within our power to create an everyperson's aristocracy based on robot labor."[9]

Yet so far there has been significant job displacement due to automation in industry and computerization in offices. The big question is whether there are new jobs awaiting those people whose work has been taken over by a machine. Other jobs in the United States have been lost to cheaper foreign labor. Workers are let go and companies move part of their operations to Asia. For data entry work, there has been a big trend toward sending the work "offshore," often to Third World countries.

Changes like these can be seen throughout industry. People who worked at certain kinds of jobs for years, such as file clerks or those taking inventory, are finding that those jobs are no longer available. So it is a question of where they can go from here. Some undertake retraining and move on to better, more interesting and higher-paying jobs. But there are not many of these that are directly connected to computers. There are not many positions needed for those skilled in operating systems, computer architecture, and automata theory. There is not a huge demand for highly skilled programmers, since most people use prepackaged programs that computerize common jobs. A decreasing number of older male employees are remaining in the workforce when their jobs become obsolete (Carnoy, 2000, p. 8).

The evidence is that many of the displaced workers go to lower-paying jobs, primarily in service industries (like fast-food operations, for which business is booming). But even those may be threatened by automation. A recent article describes Pizzabot, a robotic arm developed at Carnegie Mellon's Center for Human Service Robotics, that prepares pizzas. In its first day at work, Pizzabot prepared 50 pizzas in a time of under four minutes per pizza.[10] Waseda University in Japan is building a series of robots called WABOTs to perform service-oriented jobs; I recall reading at least 15 years ago about a robot bartender in Buffalo, New York.

Frederick W. Taylor (1856–1915) pioneered "scientific management" and the efficient use of assembly lines. Taylorism places the skill in the production process, not the worker. A worker that thinks too much may disrupt operations. Many workers today are being put into jobs of this kind, a condition called **deskilling**. Some experts argue that management today embraces Taylorism, while others hold out hope that wise management and imagination will open up a whole new realm of job opportunities.[11]

The Spanish philosopher Ortega y Gasset, writing in 1930 prior to the Spanish Civil War, argued for the need for standards and described the evils of "idiot specialization." The specialist sees only one small part of the world and has no idea of how that part ties in with the rest. The specialist becomes so caught up with one small project or area of interest that the rest of the world is shut out, ignored. Ortega y Gasset argues on behalf of the "life of effort" that has a sense of history and takes as much as possible into account in acting and making choices.

Early twentieth century architect R. Buckminster Fuller wrote:

> If the great design of the universe had wished man to be a specialist, man would have been designed with one eye and a microscope attached to it which he could not unfasten. All the living species except human beings are specialists. . . . [Man] is the most generally adaptable [of living species] but only by virtue of his one unique faculty—his mind. (Cited in Toffler, 1972, p. 301)

Our minds are what make us adaptable to new situations; they account for our survival with weak bodies. As many thinkers have pointed out, the best life for a human being is one that makes the best use of our unique capability to think—but we should not think too narrowly. We may develop special activities we are particularly good at, but it should not be at the expense of losing touch with the rest of the world. We are part of a family, a town, a society, a nation, a world, a universe, and we should be aware of all of those connections and our responsibilities in them, as well as the benefits they bring us. If new technology shifts the emphasis of what humans are needed to do, then *we* should see that the shift is upward, to new and more creative endeavors, not downward to becoming less than human. Education is a key to this, and a commitment of the resources of society to broaden human development.

The End of Work? In the provocative book *The End of Work* (1996), Jeremy Rifkin points out that global unemployment is now at the highest level since the Great Depression in the 1930s: "more than 800 million human beings are now unemployed or underemployed in the world" (p. xv). As Rifkin draws out the details, it starts to look as if things are only going to get worse. The claims that the new technology was not just going to replace old jobs but create new ones seem not to be materializing. As the United States experiences a recession in 2001, we hear of more and more large lay-offs by major corporations, with no indication of where the people will go. A proposal to extend the time period when one may receive unemployment compensation from 26 weeks to 39 weeks does not solve the real problem— that of what the displaced worker is going to do *after* the unemployment compensation runs out. Perhaps the government could take the money it plans to put into welfare and tax cuts and use it to create *jobs* for people, analogous to FDR's WPA. Surely there is much work that needs to be done in the country, in rebuilding, in improving security, even in providing homes at reasonable cost for those who need them.

Even as we witness large industrial shrinkage, we see at the same time that humans are being replaced in the oldest profession—farming—by expert systems and improved machinery. There is even an automated process for shearing sheep (Rifkin, 1996, p. 116). Rifkin speaks of bioengineering techniques (he makes reference to Michael Fox's *Superpigs and Wondercorn*) that will eventually replace traditional farmers. Just one example involves the growing of the vanilla bean. Madagascar, which produces 70 percent of the world crop, has 700,000 peasant farmers who rely on growing vanilla for their livelihood. "Now, the new gene-splicing technologies allow researchers to produce commercial volumes of vanilla in laboratory vats—by isolating the gene that codes for the vanilla protein and cloning it in a bacterial bath— eliminating the bean, the plant, the soil, the cultivation, and the farmer"

(Rifkin, 1996, p. 124). And, as he points out, vanilla is only the beginning. What will become of all the people in countries that have relied primarily on farming to live, when food production is carried on without them?

As there becomes less work to be done by humans, what will happen in general? If it were Marx's ideal society, the machines would produce enough for everyone to be comfortable, and free people up to be creative. We are far from such a point, however. One way to handle less work is to spread it around more evenly, as has already been done in Europe. In Italy, trade unions marched under the slogan, "Work Less, and Everyone Works" (Rifkin, 1996, p. 224). Surely a tradeoff of income for free time would be desirable. Some employers are already offering, and employees are negotiating for, reduced work weeks at reduced pay. This could turn out to be beneficial not only to individuals, but to society as a whole. In the delightful movie *Dave* (1993), Dave (the substitute president) puts forward a proposal that the government will provide a job for everyone who wants one—not a bad idea!

"Technostress"?

In 1984 Craig Brod wrote a book called *Technostress: The Human Cost of the Computer Revolution*. As a psychotherapist, his interest in this area was aroused when a man, a programmer for a bank, came to him for help complaining of "feeling down and depleted," and that he was having marital problems because his wife did not make a good "peripheral"(!). (Brod, 1984, p. xi). Though the man said he really liked his work, Brod unearthed problems in the work itself that contributed to the programmer's problems—what he labelled *technostress*. Brod says that he found that workers "were beginning to internalize the standards by which the computer works: accelerated time, a desire for perfection, yes-no patterns of thinking. These internalized standards combined to reduce the ability of a person to perform creatively or to relate to others in a loving way" (Brod, 1984, p. xii). He found evidence of technostress not only in computer workers such as programmers but also in the computer *users*, especially young people who spent a great deal of time with their computers and computer games.

Brod sees two categories of people with technostress: those who have "computer phobia," and react very negatively to having anything to do with a computer; and those who overidentify with computers, adopting "a mindset that mirrors the computer itself" (Brod, 1984, p. 17). Those in the first group run away from the new technology or are miserable if they are forced to confront it; those in the second group, Brod fears, are becoming dehumanized by working too closely with the machine. He also fears that the computer, with its capability for simulation, has put too much distance between us and the real world (Brod, 1984, p. 9). One very serious aspect of this is that video games and "war game" simulations run for the government both glorify war and victory and depersonalize killing to mere numbers, the accumulation of points toward a "win."

The speeded-up world of the computer demands speeded-up performance from those who work with it. Brod notes that "a minimum of 80,000 keystrokes an hour is expected of the average VDT operator, as compared to 30,000 keystrokes expected of the average typist" (Brod, 1984, p. 40). As we all know, when we are pressured to do something in a great hurry we are more inclined to make mistakes. If these mistakes are detected, they make the job situation worse; if they are not detected, they may do damage somewhere down the line, in a customer's incorrect bill or in the data that controls a nuclear power plant.

One can quickly become obsolete in the computer world, where new technologies are constantly supplanting older ones. Older engineers may not have the background for the new technology, and are soon passed by and passed over. Job security may be threatened, or one may be, at age 50, pressured to go back to school.

Brod also fears that the computer age will signal the end of romance in our time. Not only are there the effects mentioned earlier of the computer worker coming to think and act more like a machine, and expect fast responses and yes-no logic, but also many wives have become "computer widows," since their husbands spend much of their time when they *are* home working on a home computer or on a modem link to the office computer. Presumably, there are "computer widowers" as well.

"Technomalady"?

There are many illnesses, psychosomatic and physical, that can be attributed to working with computers. Brod speaks of those with computer anxiety who exhibit headaches, nausea, irritability, and nightmares (Brod, 1984, p. 16) at the mere idea of having to deal with computers. Many who do work with computers develop eyestrain, headaches, neck pains, dizziness, or muscle problems (like tendonitis or carpal tunnel syndrome) in their hands, arms, or backs. There is concern that spending too much time in front of a video display terminal might cause sterility in men or cause women to experience difficulties during pregnancy.[12]

Forester and Morrison report that "the Office of Technology Assessment (OTA) has estimated that stress-related illnesses cost businesses between $50 billion and $75 billion per year."[13] Change creates stress, and there are many changes in the new workplaces that some established workers find unappealing. Working on the same form day after day and month after month, feeding a computer program that does most of the interesting work, can readily lead a worker to severe boredom and job-avoidance. It is easy to wake up in the morning sick with a headache if you hate to go to work.[14] If job-related absences and stress-related occupational disease claims are a growing factor in the modern office or industry, it certainly is to the industry's benefit to try to improve the working conditions. A simple appeal to their naked self-interest should bring about change, even if appeals to moral obligation do not.

Health concerns should be addressed by management, as should various ways to improve physical working conditions (for example, *ergonomics*— movable keyboards, shields that reduce glare, etc.). The Computer Professionals for Social Responsibility (CPSR) devoted its Summer 1994 issue to articles on "participatory design," where both management and employees work together on such problems and in making business decisions.

Job Monitoring

Management has always wanted to keep track of how well its workers are working. This has taken the form of supervisors, whose only job is to observe what work others are doing, and of the hiring of "efficiency experts" to suggest ways in which workers can be made more productive. These experts do "time-and-motion" studies, and suggest new configurations of machines and keyboards in the workplace, and so on. Recently, a more subtle form of monitoring has become available to management—the computer itself can readily give reports on its rate of use. Computer monitoring can include reports on the number of keystrokes per hour, amount of "downtime," number of corrections made, and so forth. Computers can also be used to report on phone usage, length of calls, and the like, for workers whose jobs involve communication by telephone. The Office of Technology Assessment, in a report to Congress, estimates that 25 percent to 30 percent of clerical workers in the United States are monitored by computers.[15]

A programmer's efficiency can be monitored by the number of lines of new code written per week, the number of trial runs before all the "bugs" are found, etc. People taking airline reservations can be monitored as to how long they spend on each call, and how many reservations they make per hour. A trucker may have a computer device in his truck which records his average gas mileage and how many stops he has made.[16] Some managers actually tape or listen in on employees' phone calls, read their electronic mail, and tap into what they are doing at their computer terminals.

A number of new software programs have been introduced, like PC Sentry, Direct Access, Peek and Spy (!), and Close-Up LAN, which can tell the user (the manager or supervisor) how long a computer was used, what files were accessed, and what programs were installed or deleted. Some programs are used to measure typing speed and time spent away from the terminal. Often managers do not tell their employees that they are under such supervision, and some of the software packages brag about the secrecy in which they can operate. An ad for Close-Up LAN reads, "You decide to look in on Sue's computer screen. . . . Sue won't even know you are there! . . . All from the comfort of your chair." [17]

Labor unions and privacy and health advocate groups are very concerned about these practices. A House Subcommittee in 1992 estimated that as many as 26 million American office workers were being monitored through their own computers. The software manufacturers claimed (to the subcommittee) that the snooping aspect of the software is rarely used.[18] A *MacWorld* survey in 1993 reported that 60 percent of companies that electronically eavesdrop on their employees conceal the activity. A new program called Proxy lets managers see what is being typed on eight different employee terminals at once; however, Proxy signals users when they are being monitored, or if the manager is taking control of their computers. The article on Proxy begins with "Employees who write love letters on office personal computers, beware. It's getting easier for the boss to look over your shoulder." [19] A recent Reuters report (July 10, 2001) says that the Privacy Foundation has determined that more than one-third of employees who use e-mail and the Web at work are routinely monitored.

Studies by the Communications Workers of America and other similar organizations report that workers who are monitored experience higher levels of stress, depression, and fatigue. In May 1993, Senator Paul Simon (D–Ill.) introduced the Privacy for Consumers and Workers Act, which would require a "right to know" for monitoring to take place, and require that companies inform their employees that their e-mail is being monitored (Nelson, 1994, p. 135).

Companies resist notifying employees of the surveillance, saying that would defeat the purpose of the exercise.[20] The companies say that they have a right to monitor the work because they own the computers on which the employees work. A worker named Alana Shoars sued Epson America for firing her after she protested Epson's reading the employees' electronic mail. The Federal Electronic Privacy Act of 1986 protects the privacy of e-mail messages sent through public networks like CompuServe and MCI Mail, but it does not cover internal systems within a company.[21]

There are two issues here. The first is whether secretive surveillance is either legal or ethical. The second is whether a company has the right to monitor its employees so closely, just because it owns the equipment.[22] If such surveillance is to be part of the job package, then it seems it should be explained up front as a condition of employment so that employees know what they are getting into. The general effects of such monitoring have been negative, making employees nervous and more error-prone. It sets a bad tone for the office, one of "Big Brother" from Orwell's *1984*, or the boss in Charlie Chaplin's *Modern Times* who *observed* Charlie's bathroom break and told him to get back to work. (Apparently, a software package came out in 1997 that has a database of 45,000 websites that are categorized as "productive," "unproductive," or "neutral," and is used to monitor employee Web browsing; it is called LittleBrother!) Keystroke or other activity monitoring also only measures work *quantitatively,* not *qualitatively.* It seems to emphasize the worker as only an appendage of the machine.

It is good for humans to have *autonomy*; close surveillance and control of an employee's every move stifles this. Humans need the satisfaction of achieving knowledge, of accomplishing creative work. The purpose of society (government) should be to allow such human growth to occur, to secure individual life, health, and freedom. Thus the government should take a dim view of activities of corporations that infringe the basic *rights* of its citizens, which are tied to the fundamental human *goods.*

Women in the Computer Workplace

In the job displacements that are occurring due to automation and computerization, more women's jobs are being affected than those of men. Though more and more women have been entering the workforce in the past several years, either as part-time or full-time workers, the majority of these women have been employed in lower-level jobs. The positions of secretary, file clerk, and other office jobs are held primarily by women ("pink collar jobs"). Women in the workplace generally face inequities in position, salary, and promotion.[23]

Any married working woman feels the effect of the "marriage tax," the fact that when filing a joint (or a "married, filing separately") tax return, her salary is essentially added on to the top of her husband's income, and so is taxed at the highest level without benefit of the graduated structure of the tax table. Of course, the husband in a working couple feels the pinch as well, and it seems inequitable, since couples who just live together are not similarly penalized. For example, a couple who jointly made $120,000 in 2000 (let us say they each made $60,000) and who have no dependents and claim just the standard tax deduction,[24] would pay $24,306.50 in federal tax. If they both could file as single, though, they would each pay $11,575, or a total of $23,150. This $1156.50 difference is the "marriage tax," which penalizes married couples who both work. This is an inequity continued by a large portion of the (mostly male) Congress who apparently feel that married women should not work outside the home.

Women workers are those most harmed by the dehumanization of the workplace and the monitoring of work as they hold the majority of the positions affected: low-level data entry, record-keeping, reservations, and secretarial work. It is also in such positions, and in assembly line work, particularly in the garment industry, that women feel the effects of being kept away from contact with other human beings and doing mechanical work that requires no creativity and gives no satisfaction. In a study of terminal users (70 percent of whom were women), workers indicated experiencing much greater levels of stress than nonterminal users, citing frustration in their work, too fast a work pace, feeling hurried and the pressures of not enough personnel, and protesting "unreasonable demands for efficiency."[25]

There has been considerable emphasis in recent writings in feminist philosophy on an ethics of *caring*.[26] Women are said to be more concerned with nurturing individual growth and well-being than with Kantian universalizable rational moral principles, which criticism has pointed out may lack content. This outreach to others is not satisfied by jobs that isolate women from other people in the workplace, or that involve them with dry data and statistics for which they can see no human worth. Thus the best jobs for women in the information era, according to this view, are not those that just involve entering or massaging data, or building large financial or military systems, but rather those that use the computer's capability to better the human condition.

Women should have equal employment opportunities, and they should receive "equal pay for equal work," but in fact this still is not the case. Women have tended to cluster in certain kinds of jobs—office workers and secretaries, nurses, librarians, elementary and secondary school teachers, and social workers. They are beginning to make inroads in the fields of medicine, college teaching, and law. It is often thought that women do not have the aptitude for the "hard sciences" and mathematics, and so there is still a shortage of women in those areas. Yet this seems to be a matter of socialization, not a matter of ability. If the prejudices can be overcome, the field of computer technology opens up great professional opportunities for women. After all, recall that the first programmer—Ada—was a woman.

The Grace Hopper Celebration of Women in Computing was held in Washington, DC, in 1994 to highlight the accomplishments of women in the computing field and to look to the future. It was noted that "the percentage of women entering the computing field is declining, and the conference was conceived as one way of reversing that trend by increasing the visibility of women in computing, to the general public and especially to young women who have not yet made a career choice." [27]

There are not many jobs for those who improve computer design and operating systems, but these jobs provide valuable contributions in which women can be involved. There are many jobs that make effective use of computers to solve problems that were hitherto unsolved, or to deal with new problems. The potential of computers in this area, used for human betterment rather than for defense or destruction, is only beginning to be tapped. But the education for such work cannot be just a narrow specialization (in computer technology or any other narrowly defined field), but a broad liberal perspective on human history, needs, and potential. There is a need for education in computer proficiency as well, but only a wider perspective will yield any great advances of benefit to humanity in general.

Does Gender Matter in Computing? Increasingly the question of gender has arisen with regard to the computing field. It remains a field that does not attract many women to the workplace or to undergraduate and graduate programs. Why? It certainly is not a matter of natural aptitude. It may still be that, even in today's more liberated workplace, females are socialized more to areas other than machines, mathematics, and computers. I read that there was a "talking Barbie" doll a few years ago who said "Math is hard!" as one of her canned locutions; I also heard that Mattel changed this feature, under pressure from women's organizations. It may have something to do with women being more social, and working on a computer all day is a lonely profession. Yet it can be challenging and rewarding as well.

There have been many studies (largely surveys) that claim to show that women have different attitudes regarding ethical issues than do men. The baseline study is that of Carol Gilligan, whose *In a Different Voice* (1982) contrasted the nurturing characteristics of women with the more aggressive nature of men. Her studies reflected that, in response to ethical questions, males were more inclined to think in terms of *rights* whereas the women looked to compromise and continuing relationships with others. Women's views on privacy and power may well be different from those of men. Women may have more concerns about certain types of invasions of privacy (say, with pornography on the Web) than men, and be more sensitive to misuses of power (as in monopolistic grabs for an entire market share).

The evidence is that almost all hackers (especially the young, destructive ones) are males. This is not just due to the fact that there are more males than females involved with computers, since the proportions are far from even. It may be that, due to the interconnected feelings of women, as part of a network of relationships, the impulse to do harm to someone else is just not compelling.

Judith Broadhurst suggests that there are nine factors that account for the fact that there are roughly half as many women online as men: (1) lack of time; (2) "the dollars don't make sense"—the money should be spent on something else more valuable, like one's kids; (3) "negative media"—not as much online to appeal to women's interests; (4) "the graphics-are-good fallacy"—women are more interested in getting information and making contacts than in fancy graphics; (5) "combat is not hospitable"—many online groups appear hostile and intimidating; (6) "technology's not a turn-on"—men tend to equate computer power with real power, whereas women are more interested in functionality; (7) the "geek chic" stereotype—an outdated impression of "computer nerds"; (8) "fear of an alien nation"—computers seem impersonal (but the idea of chat room "community" does appeal to women); (9) "misdirected marketing"— the online service providers haven't figured out how to attract women yet (and if they don't worry about it because "many more men are online," it will be a self-fulfilling prophecy). Broadhurst concludes: "No medium of communication and information since the telephone and television is likely to have such a profound impact on education, politics, and the way we live and work as this one. That's why it's so important that women— who are traditionally said to be more verbally adept and better communicators—help guide its direction rather than dismiss it as all hype and hoopla" (Broadhurst, 1997, pp. 153–56).

Increased Access for Disabled Workers

The computer is a marvelous tool for the disabled person. It allows the expression of creative ability or technical prowess to shine through, that might otherwise remain hidden. Researchers have created many devices that allow nonstandard access to computers, and are working on more innovations in this area. There are special terminals for the deaf, robotic arms that can be controlled by amputees, and voice synthesizers such as the Kurzweil reader for the blind computer user.[28] A company called Oxford Intelligent Machines has designed a system that allows disabled people to use a joystick, a roller ball, or a chin switch to access a computer for many applications. They are working on an integration of a robot arm with fingerlike "end effectors" with windowing software.[29]

Congress passed the Rehabilitation Act Amendments of 1986 (Public Law 99–506) to further clarify the intent of the Rehabilitation Act of 1973. The new law has a section (508) specific to electronic equipment accessibility. The General Services Administration developed guidelines for implementing Section 508 in the Federal Information Resources Management Regulation (FIRMR), which states:

> Federal agencies shall provide handicapped employees and non-handicapped employees equivalent access to electronic office equipment to the extent such needs are determined by the agency. . . and the required accessibility can be provided by industry. In providing equivalent access to electronic office equipment, agencies shall consider:
>
> i. Access to and use of the same data bases and application programs by handicapped and non-handicapped employees;
> ii. Utilization of enhancement capabilities for manipulating data (i.e., special peripherals) to attain equivalent end-results by handicapped and non-handicapped employees; and
> iii. Access to and use of equivalent communications capabilities by handicapped employees.[30]

The Americans with Disabilities Act (1990), fully implemented now, requires *all* employers of 15 or more employees (as well as all state and local government employers *of any size*) not to discriminate against a "qualified individual with a disability"; this applies to all areas of employment—job applications, hiring, compensation, advancement, job training, and benefits. The act begins by stating that 20 percent of Americans (an estimated 43 million) have disabilities. The Equal Employment Opportunity Commission (EEOC) administers the provisions of Title I of the act, and all complaints of discrimination should be filed with EEOC. The Justice Department is responsible for the enforcement of Title II of the act, relating to employees in state and local governments.

ADA requires that all employers covered by the act provide "reasonable accommodation" for workers with disabilities. This includes making work and other related facilities physically accessible, restructuring a job if necessary, providing work areas with necessary equipment to accommodate the disability, implementing part-time or modified work schedules, if desirable, making appropriate modifications of written materials (such as company policies, training manuals, examinations), and providing qualified readers or interpreters if necessary.[31]

These federal statutes will do much to enhance professional advancement for persons with disabilities, and are to be commended. This should create many more opportunities for the disabled, many of which will be related to the use of computers. The computer equipment industry will have to continue its research efforts in devices that will make this accessibility all the more possible.

TELECOMMUTING

Telecommuting, a term coined by Jack Nilles in the 1970s during the oil crisis,[32] also referred to as *remote work* or *home work*, refers to the ability of many workers to do their work at home rather than in an office. Writers have worked at home for a long time. But now, with the advent of personal computers, laptops, modems and communications networks, cellular phones, faxes, and the like, many people whose primary work is on a computer can do that work at home. As Margrethe Olson noted, it allows work patterns to be flexible in space and time.[33]

Thus, instead of people traveling to the work, the work can travel to them (and back again when finished) over communication networks. Alvin Toffler predicted that telecommuting would end alienation of workers because "they would become, in effect, independent entrepreneurs rather than classical employees—meaning, as it were, increased ownership of the 'means of production' by the worker" (Toffler, 1980, p. 205).

The benefits of telecommuting to the worker are obvious—no long and harrying commute to the office, setting your own work hours, working in a comfortable and familiar place, more time outside of work for home, family, and community. The disadvantages are less obvious, but real.

The LINK Resources Corporation reported that, in 1993, 7.6 million Americans in 5.8 million households were company employees working at least part-time at home during business hours. Of this total, 74 percent were knowledge/information workers, 13 percent were executives and managers, 12 percent were teachers, 11 percent were scientists, and 11 percent were business professionals (obviously there is some overlap in the categories here).[34] This total represented a 15 percent growth from the 6.6 million LINK found in 1992, and represents 6.1 percent of the adult workforce. This is in addition to (and distinct from) 12.2 million primarily self-employed home workers (including home businesses and freelance consultants and contractors), and 12.1 million part-time self-employed home workers. These categories do not include the many workers who take work home on evenings and weekends.

Recently, flexible telecommuting work programs have been developed at many banks, offices, and corporations.[35] One of the most impressive programs is at Bell Atlantic Corporation, which recently gave 16,000 of its managers in New Jersey, Virginia, West Virginia, Maryland, and Washington, D.C. the opportunity to work several days a week at home as telecommuters.[36] A network message from EDUPAGE indicated that AT&T is encouraging its employees to stay home on Tuesdays and do their work by telecommuting.[37] The Bank of Montreal set up its first "floating office" in 1991, where employees can work at a branch office, a client's location, or at home, using laptop computers. A report from University of California–Davis says that the bank is "realizing significant cost savings, improved customer service, and higher employee cooperation and morale."[38] Telecommuters work from prison in New York and California using the telephone for tasks such as answering inquiries for the Department of Motor Vehicles and taking airline reservations. (This upsets labor unions who feel these prison workers are taking jobs away from their union members.)[39] It would seem these inmates could also do telemarketing.

John Scully, chairman of Apple Computer, talked about how he got more work done on his sabbatical from the office, due to fewer distractions and increased productivity.[40] These are clear advantages for someone who is well-disciplined and self-motivated. If one can remove local distractions from the home office (which may be hard to do), then there will more peace and quiet than at a busy office, where there are always interruptions. Time is gained by not having to commute to work, which takes some people up to two hours a day, plus the time required to unwind once they get home. In addition, those working at home do not have to spend as much time getting dressed up.

For families with children, telecommuting means that a parent will be at home when children get home from school. Although it is probably unrealistic to expect to take care of young children at home and also do any serious amount of job-related work, a flexible time schedule does allow much more time to be spent with school-age children than would be possible with an office job. Workers may feel less stress in a home environment. They may actually enjoy the work, since they are in control.

There are a number of disadvantages to telecommuting. One of the major ones is that it creates a new class structure, since telecommuters clearly fall at present into two disparate groups. There are the managers, business executives, scientists, computer programmers and analysts, and the like (such as Scully), who find that they work very effectively at home, and make advances even more rapidly than they would if chained to the office.

The other group consists mainly of those who do data entry and secretarial work, which is lower level and so can be farmed out piecemeal; some of this is also done, as we have seen, in a global telecommuting workplace, sent to countries with lower pay scales. Many of these workers are paid by the hour or by the piece of work, and they have no benefits, no vacations, and no job security. They (like the prison inmates mentioned earlier) are often unrepresented by any labor union that would look out for their interests. They take the jobs because of the resulting flexibility in their lives, but they do not find their jobs satisfying and they are very poorly paid. The large majority of people in this category are women, who take the jobs that allow them to spend more time at home.

There is also a growing middle category of people who work at an office on a regular basis, say once a week or so, but telecommute the rest of the time. They hold down regular jobs, with benefits and a chance for advancement. For some, this works out well but, as Sue Shellenbarger says, others "wilt." Many find it very difficult to discipline themselves to concentrate on work at home; they are easily distracted by the many demands a home offers. Some suffer the "infinite time syndrome," where they waste more time than they work.[41] Parkinson's Law says that work will expand to fill the time available, and if there is no outside pressure to be efficient, one will not be efficient. Systems that monitor work at least would provide skeptical supervisors with a means of assessing work accomplished, but we have already seen the negative impact of such procedures.

Some workers complained that they gained weight working at home (too much temptation to snack), or started smoking again, or drank too much coffee.[42] There is also a concern among workers that they may not be thought about when the time comes for raises and promotions ("out of sight, out of mind"). Some people in the office are always skeptical about whether the telecommuters get anything done at home. There also may be a tendency for neighbors to drop in if they know someone is at home, to chat. They, too, doubt that you are really working. There is also the possibility that some workaholics may overwork themselves, since in a sense they never leave work—it is always there, in the home office, nagging. In our society, unfortunately, a woman working at home is taken less seriously than a man.[43]

Telecommuting does not appeal to everyone. Some workers want an excuse to get out of the house, to get dressed up, to interact with other people professionally. Not all jobs lend themselves to telecommuting (e.g., a surgeon, hospital orderly, classroom teacher, day care worker, or experimental nuclear physicist). In general, though, jobs connected with computers offer a broad range of possibilities for telecommuting, for those employers and employees who want to use them. An employer can use the telecommuting option as an attractive "carrot" to a potential employee. Management can benefit from improved recruiting, better retention, extended usefulness of retirees, increased productivity, and a significant savings in office space, thus saving on rent, upkeep, cleaning crews, and so forth.[44] One could even have a "virtual organization"[45] with no centralized office space, and with just about everything being done over communications networks. Schools in the 1970s introduced "classrooms without walls"; here we could have "companies without walls."

There is another significant benefit from telecommuting—less pollution from cars. The Clean Air Act of 1990, which took effect in November 1992, requires that companies in certain high-pollution metropolitan areas (like Los Angeles), that employ more than a small number of workers, ensure that fewer cars of their employees are on the roads. They encourage car-pooling and public transit, and many are coming to realize the benefits of making telecommuting arrangements for their employees. Extensive damage from two earthquakes in four years has alerted workers in Los Angeles to the possibility and the advantages of telecommuting. It is estimated that "in Los Angeles, for instance, 205 million vehicle miles of travel and 47,000 tons of pollutants could be eliminated annually if only 5 percent of the commuters telecommuted one day per week."[46] The San Francisco Bay area sponsors "Spare the Air" days.

Nilles claims that studies have shown a 20 percent reduction in worker turnover and a 10 percent to 15 percent increase in productivity among telecommuters. With a growth rate of 20 percent a year (a bit more optimistic than the 15 percent reported by LINK), Nilles projected between 24 or 25 million people telecommuting by the turn of the century (Sharpe, 1994, pp. 82, 86). The *Atlanta Journal-Constitution* (January 4, 2002) reported that 28.8 million American workers telecommute at least one day a week.

Some of the buildings in which people may work have bad air conditioning systems, asbestos in the walls, or other health hazards. There are various noxious fumes from copy machine fluids, cleaning fluids, and other sources. By staying at home to work, the telecommuter avoids all of these hazards, as well as avoids the dangers of driving many miles in rush-hour traffic.

An article in *Technology Review* described two reports from the Clinton administration, on reinventing government and the national infrastructure, that point to the use of information technology as a tool to increase productivity. However, there is a debate over the "productivity paradox," which claims that there is not an expected payoff correlating higher corporate profits with the estimated $1 trillion that corporate America has invested in information systems. However, Eric Brynjolfsson and graduate student Lorin Hitt, two researchers at MIT's Sloan School of Management, examined 380 *Fortune 500* companies and concluded that they have been making 50 cents profit on every dollar invested in information technology.

On the other side, Paul Strassman (former chief information officer for the Department of Defense) said that if the productivity effect were positive, it would show up in other aspects of the economy, and that it hasn't. Brynjolfsson says that there is an expected lag-time between such investments and results showing up on a broad economic scale. Perhaps the real payoff will come with increased use of information technology in a broader theater, such as in telecommuting. Providing more people with jobs they enjoy doing must be good for the economy in the long run, and telecommuting is also better for the environment.

It may well be that telecommuting, which has not been embraced by many companies yet, may begin to seem more attractive in the aftermath of the terrorist attacks in New York and Washington.

Changing Job Panorama

A new term is emerging when companies talk about their resources: *intellectual capital*—the knowledge and skills of their employees.[47] Clearly for many companies today, their major resource *is* intellectual capital; think, for example of the giant Microsoft, whose major product is a kind of "mindware," created from the knowledge base of its employees.

The February 26, 2001 issue of *Computerworld* included an article listing the top ten information technology jobs of 2001.[48] They are Web developer, database administrator, security analyst (becoming all the more important with the proliferation of attacks such as those discussed in Chapter 6), Unix administrator, e-commerce application developer, C++/object-oriented/Visual Basic developer, Java programmer, network engineer, PC technical support, and quality assurance tester. It is interesting to note how much online communication has influenced the demands of today's organizations.

 ## EMPLOYEES AND EMPLOYERS

There are countless issues that arise in any employment situation, and many of them take on some new aspects in a computerized workplace. These include loyalty (of employee to employer and vice versa), whistle-blowing, and the ownership of ideas.

Loyalty

Loyalty is akin to friendship. Friendship arises from what Hume referred to as our feeling of *sympathy* (or empathy) for other people. When we have a strong feeling of this kind toward someone we consider that person our friend. However, friendship can also have a *rational*, not *emotive*, basis. One could rationally *see* that a person is deserving of friendship and loyalty. Aristotle devoted Books VIII and IX of the *Nicomachean Ethics* (1155a) to friendship, a virtue "most necessary for our life." Aristotle continues that friendships may be for utility, or for pleasure, but the best, complete friendship is that between good people "similar in virtue" (*Nicomachean Ethics* 1156b 7). Friends spend time together, share, and want happiness for each other, and do not deliberately cause each other pain. We have duties or obligations to friends.[49]

Loyalty is also a strong feeling, or a strong rational conviction, which carries with it duty and obligation. One could imagine a similar division of types of loyalty to those Aristotle outlines for friendship: out of utility, for pleasure, or complete loyalty to what is intrinsically good. Loyalty out of utility would be generally what we would find in the employee/employer relationship. You are expected (or required as a condition of employment) to be "loyal" to your employer—not to divulge any of the company's secrets, to do your best work for the company, and so on.

Loyalty for pleasure, like friendship for pleasure, may be a tie made too quickly in the heat of emotion, but one that does not hold up to the test of time or to conflicting feelings. One may pledge undying loyalty to a romantic attachment, but the romance may fade, and with it, the feeling of loyalty.

So, for our analogy, the best, *complete* loyalty would come from the good aspects of your own nature and be directed toward someone or some principle that is intrinsically good and worthy of your fealty. Some candidates for this kind of loyalty have been considered to be family (e.g., motherhood), dear friend, country, or God.

Loyalty is a relationship between or among entities. A person (P) is loyal to someone or some thing or principle (S), so it is at least a two-part relationship. But it is really more complex than that. If you are loyal to S, you have an obligation to S, and that obligation means you will not betray that duty by following S' (not-S). If I am loyal to my lover, this means I will not run off with someone who is not my lover. If I am loyal to my country, and do my "duty to my country," this means that I will not betray my country's secrets to another country, or that I will die in battle fighting for my country rather than defect or just turn tail and run. Loyalty to God is generally thought to entail not disobeying God's rules, or giving one's life to God (as one who spreads God's word), rather than leading a life of pleasure that might tempt one away from God's path.

Loyalty implies that one will not betray that loyalty. The root of the word comes from the French word for law; in loyalty, one is bound not to break the obligation of loyalty in a way analogous to one's obligation not to break the law. If one does break the obligation of loyalty, there are presumably penalties to bear: loss of love, loss of employment, loss of country (through exile), loss of life, loss of God's love and protection. The lowest circle of Hell in Dante's *Inferno* is dedicated to those who commit "compound fraud"—they are the traitors to kin, to country, or to masters—and they receive the severest punishment, buried in ice and pelted with freezing rain, farthest away from love and warmth.

Loyalty involves promises, either explicit or implicit. You pledge to be faithful to your lover (perhaps even in a ceremony), or by being with your lover it is understood that you will (should) be faithful. One may be asked to sign a contract promising to be loyal (to your spouse, your company, or your country), in which the moral obligation also becomes a legal obligation. Or you may be understood to owe loyalty (to your family, or your friend, your college, or your country) simply by virtue of your relationship to the entity in question. In the *Crito*, Socrates refuses to take his friend's help to escape the death penalty laid on him by Athens by running to another city-state. His argument is, essentially, that by living in Athens all his life and accepting all the advantages of being an Athenian citizen, he has an *implicit* obligation (though he never signed any contract) to obey its laws, even when they work against him.

Loyalty may be unquestioning (as expected by the biblical God of Job and Abraham), or it may seek reasons for its basis (Socrates was always questioning everything). It may find its basis in feeling, or in a contract, or in tradition, or it may look to a "higher law." Antigone, in Sophocles' play, refuses to obey the law of Creon, the King of Thebes, to not bury her brother, who Creon considers a traitor, because of a higher obligation ("the law of the gods") to give the dead—especially loved ones—proper burial, lest their souls wander forever. Any conscientious objector believes that there is a higher law that current civil law violates and will act according to conscience—not to serve in an immoral war, or to challenge a rule of segregation, or not to support a government plan that is ill-advised and dangerous.

Thus there may be conflicts among loyalties, and this is where the difficult moral decisions come in. One's loyalty to a friend may conflict with loyalty to family, or loyalty to country may conflict with perceived loyalty to God, or loyalty to one's employer may conflict with broader loyalties to humanity. In such cases, one must weigh the strength of each loyalty, the reasons for making and keeping the obligation, and the penalties for betrayal.

George Fletcher distinguishes between minimal demands of loyalty, in which simply nonbetrayal is expected, and maximum loyalty ("Be One With Me").[50] Minimal loyalty might be that of a mere contract—for example, to pay a loan or to do certain things connected with a job. One is expected not to break the contract, but it is not a Faustian contract for one's soul. In a marriage contract, one is expected not to commit adultery.

If one begins to examine *why* one should not commit adultery, beyond the mere penalties for breaking the contract, one might get into the quandary young Evodius finds when discussing the matter with Augustine. Evodius wonders why adultery is evil, and surmises it is because he would not want anyone to commit adultery with *his* wife. Thus (a kind of golden rule), if he does not want it done to him, he should not do it to others. But Augustine asks, "What of the case where a man is perfectly willing to have another seduce his wife so that he can commit adultery with another's wife?" (A case of "Take my wife, please"—Henny Youngman.) Augustine then goes on to say that it is the lust in adultery that makes it innately evil.[51] But is even *this* the right reason? Adultery can harm your wife, and harm the friendship with your wife. It is also deceitful (what would Kant say?). The point here is perhaps that one should see clearly why, with good reasons, the loyalty commitment is one that should be made before making it. Then if conflicts arise, there is the reason why this obligation of loyalty was formed to hold it fast.

Fletcher's maximum kind of loyalty, "be one with me," occurs in deep love relationships, or in the rituals of patriotism or religion. A country or a person hopes to inspire this sort of loyalty; the devotee will then act out of self-love with regard to the country or person.

Loyalty in the professional world is at least of the minimum sort—a contractual obligation that should not be broken. Some companies may hope that it is stronger than this, that the loyal employee will feel a real bond with the company and its goals, and a few (as in the movie *The Firm*) may really expect a "be one with me" commitment. It is wise for the potential employee to read the contract carefully before signing, and to try to determine what, if any, implicit demands exist beyond the wording of the contract.

Since loyalty involves a relationship (between P and S, as we discussed), there is a tendency for P to think and talk in terms of "*my* S" (my family, my friend, my company, my country, my God), which implies a sense of closeness, of belonging. There is an unfortunate tendency for loyalty to go overboard into favoritism, as in cases where a relative is hired over someone more qualified, or a teacher gives the best grade to his daughter even though she is not the best student in the class. Considerations of justice quickly show that these applications of loyalty are inappropriate, beyond reasonable limits. A company may also exceed reasonable limits by expecting its employees to think and vote as the company does, never to differ with the company "line," to buy only company products in their area, never to leave the company.

Whistle-Blowing

Whistle-blowing occurs when an employee recognizes that his or her company is doing something illegal or immoral, and tries to do something about it. In the section on loyalty we discussed civil disobedience; whistle-blowing is a kind of "organizational disobedience."[52] The employee should probably start within the organization to try to change things, but often this only gets the employee fired. There are many instances of this, including air force analyst A. Ernest Fitzgerald, who revealed a $2 billion cost overrun on a transport project and other weapons systems. He was fired by the Department of Defense, but fought back through the legal system and in 1982 was reinstated to his original position (Chalk, 1988, p. 48).

In January 1986, all of the engineers for Morton Thiokol, as well as four other employees, recommended postponing the launch of the manned shuttle *Challenger*. NASA officials challenged the recommendation, and Thiokol management ignored its employees' recommendation to postpone. The result was that on January 28, 1986 the shuttle exploded 73 seconds after liftoff, killing the crew of seven people in the world's worst space flight disaster. Roger Boisjoly testified before a number of investigative agencies after the disaster. Morton Thiokol reassigned him; however, after severe criticism of this action, he was reinstated, but his responsibilities were radically changed. He was (in 1988) on long-term disability leave from the company, and sued both NASA and Morton Thiokol (Chalk, 1988, p. 54).

Another case is that of a whistle-blower who alleged that the Resolution Trust Company (RTC) was going easy on its savings and loan executives. The RTC copied the whistle-blower's files, and said that he had been working on personal matters during office hours.[53] The RTC claimed that "No federal worker, the government's legal specialists say, should assume that his or her constitutional right to privacy extends . . . into the federal workplace" (Barr, 1993, "Copying," p. 15).

David Parnas and other computer scientists publicly took a stand against the U.S. government's "Star Wars" project (SDI). Parnas resigned from an advisory panel that paid $1,000 a day, the SDIO Panel in Support of Battle Management, because he "consider[s] the use of nuclear weapons as a deterrent to be dangerous and immoral" (Parnas, 1987, p. 46). Parnas then took an active role against "Star Wars," writing a number of position papers against it.

Rosemary Chalk reports that at least 26 states have provided support for whistle-blowers by recognizing "public policy exceptions" to the tradition that an employer can fire without cause. The tradition was set by a Tennessee Supreme Court decision in 1884 (*Payne v. Western & Atlantic R.R. Co.*, 81 Tenn. 507), which stated: "[all employers] may dismiss their employees at will . . . for good cause, for no cause, or even for cause morally wrong, without being thereby guilty of moral wrong." It seems that the court reasoned that the employer–employee relationship is a voluntary arrangement between equals, for mutual benefit, which either can terminate at will (without cause). Of course, if the terms of a contract define conditions of termination, then the employer is bound by the terms of the contract.

For a whistle-blower who needs legal help in a grievance against an employer, the main resource center is the Government Authority Project (GAP) in Washington, DC (Chalk, 1988, p. 53). There is even an 800 number established for whistle-blowers. It is not clear, though, just how much legal support they actually get. A dissenting worker's view should be "sincerely held and in good faith, based on credible data or information, and related to the safe and adequate performance of the job" to be "worthy of legal protection" (Feliu, 1985, p. 3).

The issue in whistle-blowing is that your loyalty to your employer does not extend to supporting the company in illegal or immoral activities. When you were hired, presumably you did not sign a "blind loyalty" oath. In some classified work for the government, you must sign an oath not to reveal the contents of your mission (or project), and so this could presumably lead to a conflict if you felt the government project you were working on endangered humanity. Consider, for example, the action of the character played by Dustin Hoffman in the movie *Outbreak* (1995).

You feel some loyalty to your employer, generally; after all, the company helps pay your bills. But you did not agree to be a party to breaking the law or acting unethically. It seems that Butchvarov has already laid out the problem for us. Morality has to do with our relationships with others, and when we ask "Who are the others?" there are a number of different answers, ranging from lesser to greater breadth. We have a greater moral responsibility to the people in our nation, or to all of humanity, than we have to an unethical employer. The cost (professional, financial) to a whistle-blower could be great, but the moral personal loss incurred by just "going along with it" would be much greater.

Who Owns Your Ideas?

Another aspect of the loyalty issue is just how much loyalty should an employer reasonably expect, and how much control should the employer have over an employee's creative products? You go to work for company X, and you have followed all of the contract rules about nondisclosure, and so on. You have been working on something in your spare time that turns out to be a blockbuster innovation that you can patent and sell for great profit. Does your employer have any claim on your invention? The employer will probably want to claim that it does, and many cases like this have come up, in the computer area and elsewhere.

If you have been "hired to invent" something, or hired to work in a specific area of development for the company, then your employer has rights to any invention falling in the area in which you have been working for the company. A California District Court of Appeals defined an employer's "shop-right" to an employee's invention as occurring under the following conditions:

> Where an employee (1) during his hours of employment, (2) working with his employer's materials and appliances, (3) conceives and (4) perfects an invention for which he obtains a patent, he must accord his employer a non-exclusive right to practice the invention. (Lieberstein, p. 16)

However, if these conditions, or the "hired to invent" condition, do not hold, then it is not at all clear that an employer has a right to the employee's invention, and these cases get argued out in court. For example, Dr. J. Robert Cade invented Gatorade in the mid–1960s. At the time, he was employed at the University of Florida as an associate professor of medicine, and he had also done work funded by two government grants. Both the University of Florida and the Department of Health, Education, and Welfare claimed rights to Cade's discovery. The case was eventually settled out of court, but it raises difficult issues of ownership (Lieberstein, 1979, pp. 8–9). Would *anything* that a professor does while working for a university belong to the university? What if he worked on it in his spare time in his garage? And how much control does a government granting agency have over work done by the grantee, and for how long (past the grant period)?

The "hired to invent" condition seems too ambiguous in the case of computer programmer/analysts. Their job description may say that they are "hired to program" (on whatever problems may arise for the company). Does that then mean that the company owns *any* programs that they write in their spare time? This seems much too broad, and too much in the employer's favor. A person who has programming skills may use them in various ways, on the job and elsewhere. It would be like saying that if a man works as a carpenter for a company that builds houses, he may not use his ability to build a house for himself.

What about when an employee wants to leave a job, and go to another job or go into private business? Clearly, such an employee cannot leave with the company's customer/client mailing lists, or use or reveal their trade secrets. But the company cannot compel the employee to stay, and if there is not a noncompetition clause in the contract, it cannot prevent the employee from getting another job or setting up a business in the area; the courts apply a condition of *reasonableness* to this (Lieberstein, 1979, p. 55). In fact, companies often raid other companies to benefit from the experience employees have gained there. If one claims to only be using the *generic* knowledge gained at the first company—not specific company secrets—the new work cannot be prohibited. Yet suits arise where companies feel that their rights have been compromised.

In certain fields, such as engineering and computing, the best way for an employee to advance quickly is to job-hop, since each new position can provide raises and promotions that would not be available so quickly in the old position. Companies can combat this only by rewarding their valuable personnel as deserved, in order to keep them. If the job market gets tight, management then finds it can afford to keep the purse strings tight. Again, the employee is facing a situation where supply and demand determine the going rate for services.

It is clear that no one else can *own* the knowledge and skills that you have acquired. If as an employee you are careful not to step on any contractual toes, you should be perfectly free to seek gainful employment elsewhere if your current job is not to your taste. Just don't violate any trade secrecy agreements.

■ ENDNOTES

1. Some researchers working in artificial intelligence and the philosophy of mind take this view of the atomic building blocks of "mind." For example, see, Marvin Minsky, *The Society of Mind* (New York: Simon & Schuster, 1986), and Daniel C. Dennett, *Consciousness Explained* (Boston: Little Brown, 1991).

2. "The power of self-nutrition...is the originative power, the possession of which leads us to speak of things as living" (Aristotle, *De Anima* 413a-b).

3. Shannon performed a simple experiment of approximations to English, constructed by random choices of symbols. A zero-level approximation would contain the most information, since each letter (including the space) is assumed to be equally likely, and so the maximum information is conveyed. This yields 4.76 ($\log_2 27$) bits of information per character, but the simulation does not look at all like English or any other natural language. In the first-order approximation, he makes use of the relative frequency of the symbols in English (space most likely, then E, T, A, etc.), and if one Gestalts the text it *looks* like English, but there are very few entries that look like real words, and some impossible transitions, such as JK or QZ. This is said to convey four bits of information per character.

   The third-order approximation is simulated using *digram* information—that is, statistics on the occurrence of various letter pairs in English ('TH' is very common, for example). The information conveyed is said to be 3.1 bits per symbol, and it looks more like English, with an occasional short word (AT) or a word that is close to English (DEAMY) showing up. The fourth-order approximation incorporates *trigram* statistics, only has two bits of information per character, and looks even more like English (still few real words, though everything is pronounceable). Shannon then went on to use word frequencies and word transition frequencies in later simulations (Shannon and Weaver, pp. 13–14). The point here is to show the built-in redundancy of the English language, which helps aid communication (in English) in the presence of noise, but which is very inefficient (as a code) to convey maximum information in each symbol.

One can imagine a simple and efficient code to represent the various positions on a 64-square chess board. If you randomly pick a square on the board, I should be able to determine which square it is by asking you only 6 "yes-no" type questions. I will first ask "upper?" and then "left?", and then alternate these questions three times. A "yes" answer will be represented as a '1' and a "no" as a '0'. Each time you give me an answer, the part of the board I need to look at is reduced by half (this is a **binary search procedure** in two dimensions). The uppermost, leftmost square on the board will be represented by the code 111111 (you answered "yes" to all my questions), and the lower-right corner of the board will be represented by 000000. The second square from the left on the top row is 111110, and so on. The six-bit code, or "byte," gives complete information on the position of each square (2^6 is 64, the number of positions to be coded).

An "ideal language" for maximizing the communication of information would be one in which each symbol (there are, say, s of them) is equally likely. Then in a message of length n, there are s^n possible different versions, each equally (un)likely. The measure of the information produced by a process is called its *entropy*, H, and is a function of the relative probabilities of the symbols that will be generated. When each symbol has equal probability, the maximum entropy, 1, is achieved. If the probabilities of the symbols differ, the entropy measure is correspondingly less than the maximum of 1. Entropy H is

$$H = -K\sum p_i \log p_i$$

where K is a scaling constant, and the $p_i \log p_i$ are summed up for all the symbols in the system.

When Shannon has set up a numerical measure of information, he then can go on to study the information capacity of different noisy channels, and set a basis for the science of information. What is interesting here is the choice of entropy as the measure of information. In physics, entropy is a measure of the tendency (according to the Second Law of Thermodynamics) for physical systems to go from a state of higher order to one of lesser order. So in physics, entropy is a measure of the increasing chaos in a system.

Illustrative of these two different kinds of entropy is **Maxwell's demon**. The physicist Clerk Maxwell imagined the following "thought-experiment." There is a closed box with gases in it, where one side is hotter than the other. There is a partition between the two halves of the box, and a hole in the partition. If the partition is left open, and the whole system is kept closed to outside influences, the hotter (faster-moving) molecules will tend to distribute themselves to the cooler side, and the overall temperature of the box will eventually stabilize to a lower temperature throughout than was the initial temperature of the hotter side. This movement to a lower temperature is characteristic of physical entropy.

Maxwell then postulates a "demon" who is in the system. This demon stands at the partition, and when he sees a fast-moving gas molecule come toward the hole to the cooler side, he slams the partition closed. Similarly, if a faster-moving gas molecule from the cool side moves toward the hole, he opens the door to let it into the hotter side. Thus the demon takes *information* (about which molecules are fast or slow) and translates it into reversing the natural physical entropy, or disorder, of the system. Maxwell's demon serves as a model of how humans can use information to control certain destructive physical processes.

4. McLuhan is cited in Alvin Toffler, *The Futurists* (New York: Random House, 1972), pp. 71–72.

5. Arthur C. Clarke, "Hazards of Prophecy," in Toffler, 1972, pp. 133–50.

6. Stephen Barr, "Probe Finds IRS Workers Were 'Browsing' in Files," *Washington Post*, 3 August 1993, p. 1.

7. James S. Albus, "The Robot Revolution: An Interview with James Albus," *Communications of the ACM* (March 1983), p. 180.

8. James S. Albus, *Brains, Behavior, and Robotics* (Peterborough, NH: Byte Books, 1981), pp. 331–38.

9. Albus, 1983, p. 180.

10. "Taking a Byte Out of Pizza Prep Time," *Training and Development Journal* 45, 3 (March 1991), pp. 81–82.

11. Judith A. Perrolle, *Computers and Social Change* (Belmont, CA: Wadsworth, 1987), pp. 153–55. For a discussion of the position that workers are being deskilled, see Harry Braverman, *Labor and Monopoly Capital: The Degradation of Work in the Twentieth Century* (New York: Monthly Review Press, 1974); Mike Cooley, *Architect or Bee? The*

Human/Technology Relationship (Boston: South End Press, 1980); and Harley Shaiken, *Work Transformed: Automation and Labor in the Computer Age* (New York: Holt, Rinehart, and Winston, 1984). For the other side of the picture, see Daniel Bell, *The Coming of Post-Industrial Society* (New York: Basic Books, 1973); V. Giuliano, "The Mechanization of Office Work," *Scientific American* 247, 3 (September 1982), 148–65 [also in Ermann et al. (1997) and Dunlop and Kling (1991)]; and Larry Hirschhorn, *Beyond Mechanization: Work and Technology in a Postindustrial Age* (Cambridge, MA: MIT Press, 1984).

12. Perrolle, pp. 84–85; cf. Forester and Morrison, *Computer Ethics* (Cambridge, MA: MIT, 1994), p. 216.

13. Forester and Morrison, p. 208.

14. For more on modern job-related illnesses, see Barbara Garson, *The Electronic Sweatshop: How Computers Are Transforming the Office of the Future into the Factory of the Past* (New York: Simon and Schuster, 1988); and Robert Karasek and Tores Theorell, *Unhealthy Work: Stress, Productivity and the Reconstruction of Working Life* (New York: Basic Books, 1990).

15. *Federal Government Information Technology: Electronic Surveillance and Civil Liberties.* Office of Technology Assessment, U.S. Congress, Washington, DC, 1985.

16. Karen Nussbaum, "Computer Monitoring: A Threat to the Right to Privacy?", in DeJoie, Fowler, and Paradice, *Ethical Issues in Information Systems* (Boston: Boyd & Fraser, 1991), p. 136; cf. Rothfeder, p. 172.

17. Nussbaum, p. 136.

18. "Labor Letter: Computer Snooping," *Wall Street Journal*, 26 May 1992, p. A1.

19. John R. Wilke, "Technology: For Network Managers, Snooping Gets Easier," *Wall Street Journal*, 23 March 1992, p. B1.

20. Laurie Flynn, "PC Software Bosses Turn into Snoops," *Washington Post*, 28 June 1993, p. 21.

21. Glenn Rifkin, "Do Employees Have a Right to Electronic Privacy?" *New York Times*, 8 December 1991, sec. 3, p. 8.

22. See the discussion by Corey Nelson and Bonnie Brown, "Is E-mail Private or Public?", *Computerworld* 28, 26 (June 27, 1994), 135, 137.

23. Marie Richmond-Abbott reports in 1992 that "men who work in 'women's fields' still earn $1,200 more annually than women do on the average, and in male-dominated occupations, men's salaries exceed those of women by an average of $2,400. Segregation *within* professions may also mean different pay scales. Male computer specialists get $3,714 more than their female counterparts" (Richmond-Abbott, "Women Wage Earners," in Kourany et al., eds., *Feminist Philosophies* (Englewood Cliffs, NJ: Prentice-Hall, 1992, p. 141).

24. Note that the Standard Deduction for a married couple filing jointly in 2000 was $7,350, whereas for a single person it was $4,400 (or $8,800 for two single persons).

25. Gunilla Bradley, "Computers and Work Content—Work Load and Stress—Analyses and Women's Participation Strategies," in Olerup et al., *Women, Work and Computerization* (Amsterdam, Netherlands: North-Holland, 1985), p. 255.

26. For example, see: Nel Noddings, *Caring: A Feminine Approach to Ethics and Moral Education* (Berkeley, CA: University of California Press, 1984); Claudia Card, ed., *Feminist Ethics* (Lawrence, KS: University Press of Kansas, 1991); and Rosemarie Tong, *Feminine and Feminist Ethics* (Belmont, CA: Wadsworth, 1993). A related and influential discussion may be found in Carol Gilligan, *In a Different Voice: Psychological Theory and Women's Development* (Cambridge, MA: Harvard University Press, 1993).

27. *Software Engineering Notes* 19, 3 (July 1994), 14; see also *Communications of the ACM* 38, 1 (January 1995), an issue on women in computing.

28. Perrolle, pp. 85–86.

29. Max Glaskin, "Robot Helper for Disabled Workers," *New Scientist* 141 (February 22, 1994), 21.

30. "FIRMR Regulation," Regulation of Information Resources Management Service, General Services Administration, appearing in the *Federal Register* 53, 198 (October 13, 1988), 40066–40068. This material is available from the Clearinghouse on Computer Accommodation. For information on this issue, see Richard E. Ladner, "Computer Accessibility for Federal Workers with Disabilities: It's the Law," in Dejoie et al., pp. 202–9.

31. American Federation of Teachers, *ADA: Americans with Disabilities Act (American Federation of Teachers Executive Summary).* American Federation of Teachers, 555 New Jersey Avenue, NW, Washington, DC 20001 (202–879–4400).

32. J. M. Nilles, F. R. Carlson Jr., P. Gray, and G. J. Hanneman, *The Telecommunications-Transportation Tradeoff: Options for Tomorrow* (New York: Wiley, 1976).

33. Margrethe H. Olson, "Remote Office Work," *Communications of the ACM* 26, 3 (March 1983), 182.

34. *The 1994 Information Please Almanac* (Boston: Houghton Mifflin, 1994), p. 42.

35. For example, at Harris Bank, Chicago's fourth largest commercial bank—Kimetha Firpo, "Online Commuting: Big Benefits for Business and Employees," *PC World* 12, 5 (May 1994), 39–40. Travelers Insurance in Hartford, Connecticut, has had a telecommuting program since 1987 (Ross, "The Telecommuting Imperative," *PC World* 11, 9 (September 1993), p. 53).

36. "Bell Atlantic Gives Managers a Telecommuting Option," *New York Times*, 30 September 1992, sec. D, p. 5.

37. *Atlanta Journal-Constitution*, September 15, 1994 (cited in network message from EDUPAGE).

38. U.S. Department of Commerce, Technology Administration, *The Information Infrastructure: Reaching Society's Goals* (Washington, DC: U.S. Government Printing Office, 1994), p. 76.

39. *Wall Street Journal*, 22 July 1986, p. 1.

40. Nick Sullivan, "In Search of Productivity," *Home-Office Computing* 7, 9 (September 1989), 96.

41. Donna Minnick, "Infinite Time Syndrome," *Home-Office Computing* 12, 4 (April 1994), 86.

42. Olson, p. 187.

43. Sue Shellenbarger, "Home Work: I'm Still Here," *Wall Street Journal*, 16 December 1993, p. B1.

44. Gil E. Gordon and Marcia M. Kelly, *Telecommuting: How to Make It Work for You and Your Company* (Englewood Cliffs, NJ: Prentice-Hall, 1986).

45. Samuel E. Bleecker, "The Virtual Organization," *The Futurist* 28, 2 (March/April 1994), 9–14. The Environmental Protection Agency has a quarter-million-dollar pilot project in which companies in Washington, Denver, Houston, Los Angeles, and Philadelphia can get air pollution credits if they allow their employees to telecommute ("Credits for Telecommuting," *Washington Post*, 25 April 2001, p. E02).

46. Gary Ritter and Stan Thompson, "The Rise of Telecommuting and Virtual Transportation," *Transportation Quarterly* 48, 3 (Summer 1994), 239.

47. Christie Taylor, "Intellectual Capital," *Computerworld* 35, 11 (March 12, 2001), 51.

48. David S. Bernstein, "America's 10 Most Wanted," *Computerworld* 35, 9 (February 26, 2001), 40–41.

49. For a collection of some of the great writings on friendship (Aristotle, Plato, Cicero, etc.), see Michael Pakaluk, ed., *Other Selves: Philosophers on Friendship* (Indianapolis, IN: Hackett, 1991).

50. George P. Fletcher, *Loyalty* (New York: Oxford University Press, 1991), chs. 3, 4.

51. Augustine, *On the Free Choice of the Will*, trans. Anna S. Benjamin and L. H. Hackstaff (Indianapolis, IN: Bobbs-Merrill, 1964), Book One, ch. 3, 16–20 (pp. 7–8).

52. A phrase coined by James Otten in Flores, *Ethical Problems in Engineering* (Troy, NY: RPI, 1980), pp. 182–86.

53. It's not clear how they established that he was working on the files during office hours just from their existence.

■ SHORT ESSAY QUESTIONS

1. Look at Arthur C. Clarke's "Hazards of Prophecy" in Toffler, *The Futurists* (1972), and update it for the current more computerized society.

2. What job choice(s) are you contemplating as your life's work? How do computers impact that job area now, and how will they do so in the future?

3. Do you know of anyone suffering from "technostress"? If so, describe the job conditions and the person's reactions.

4. Do you think e-mail is a boon or a problem? Some have suggested that employees' work efficiency has gone down considerably since they connected to e-mail and the various services available on the Internet. Discuss (and perhaps compare workplace e-mail with its use on your college campus).

5. Clearly state the issue of employers eavesdropping on their workers. Discuss both the pros and cons, and arrive at a considered judgment regarding its justifiability.

6. Read the articles by Bonnie Brown and Corey Nelson on e-mail—public or private? Summarize their positions and comment critically on them. Is either right?

7. Discuss telecommuting from the employee's perspective and from the manager's viewpoint. Can you envision a near future with many of the downtown office buildings in our large cities largely empty due to telecommuting? Would this be good or bad?

8. State clearly what a *whistle-blower* is, and discuss the action from various ethical standpoints—Kantian, Utilitarian, virtue ethics, the goods view.

■ LONG ESSAY QUESTIONS

1. Consider carefully the question of "equal pay for equal worth." How is "equal worth" determined? By credentials? (Would that put in a discriminatory bias toward those who could afford a "better education"?) Note that this does not just mean equal pay for two people (regardless of race, creed, color, disability, or sex) doing the same job; what about two very different jobs—how do you determine if they are of equal worth? Use examples. Evaluate the claim made by some conservative economists that raising wages for women's work would cause uncontrollable inflation. Should the "dehumanizing" work we have described (e.g., data entry, assembly line work) receive higher wages because of its negative effects? Obviously in some ways it is much harder to do than a job someone enjoys, like teaching. Notice that the law of "supply-and-demand" often determines wages; in an ideal world, how would you fix this?

2. Examine the references given on feminist ethics. Describe briefly how this differs from the more traditional positions in ethics that we have examined. If feminist ethics were the guide, how should the workplaces of the future be changed?

3. Can nondiscrimination become "reverse discrimination"? Discuss critically the application of the rule that if a woman, a minority person, or a person with disability *is qualified for the job* (does that mean "can do the job"?), that person should be given preference in hiring? Can this lead to not hiring the person *best* qualified to do the job? What effects do you see of this in the computer industry?

4. Do some research into the Equal Rights Amendment (ERA) and why it failed. Were the reasons given for its defeat sound? Assess whether or not it would pass if it were brought up again today.

5. We began a discussion of education for the future in the section on the information workplace; we said that such education should emphasize understanding first, and then information-gathering and assessment second. Think seriously about what the structure and content of such an education for the future should be (not omitting *moral* education), and try to write a plan for such education. (Plato attempted this in the *Republic*; his primary goal was to create a society in which justice would naturally flourish.) What role would computers play in this education? Note that, if understanding is to be emphasized, rote learning by repetition, of the kind implemented by many computer-assisted-instruction (CAI) systems, would not help with this, though it might provide quick access to information.

6. Milton Friedman said that the only social responsibility of business is to increase its profits. Do you agree with this, based on the discussions of ethics we have had so far? How does it rate as a moral position, given various foundations for ethics we have discussed? If one were to claim that business has nothing to do with morality, how would you respond? Note that you have to take into account that a certain framework must exist in order for business/free enterprise to exist. Does this social framework require an ethical foundation? Why or why not?

7. Evaluate the proposal on telecommuting in NII–2 (73–86). (*National Information Infrastructure*, U.S. Government Printing Office)

■ REFERENCES AND RECOMMENDED READINGS

Adam, Alison. "Gender and Computer Ethics." *Computers & Society* (December 2000), 17–24.

Adam, Alison, and Jacqueline Ofori-Amanfo. "Does Gender Matter in Computer Ethics?" *Ethics and Information Technology* 2, 1 (2000), 37–47.

Agonito, Rosemary. *No More "Nice Girl": Power, Sexuality and Success in the Workplace.* Holbrook, MA: Bob Adams, 1993.

Albus, James S. *Brains, Behavior, and Robotics.* Peterborough, NH: Byte Books, 1981.

Albus, James S. "The Robot Revolution: An Interview with James Albus." *Communications of the ACM* (March 1983), 180.

Bailyn, Lotte. "Toward the Perfect Workplace?" *Communications of the ACM* 32, 4 (April 1989), 460–71.

Baron, Marcia. *The Moral Status of Loyalty.* Center for the Study of Ethics in the Professions. Dubuque, IA: Kendall/Hunt, 1984.

Barr, Stephen. "Copying of Whistle-Blower's Computer Files Stokes Bitter Dispute." *Washington Post*, 10 May 1993, sec. A, p. 15.

Barr, Stephen. "Probe Finds IRS Workers Were 'Browsing' in Files." *Washington Post*, 3 August 1993, sec. A, p. 1.

Beniger, James A. *The Control Revolution: Technological and Economic Origins of the Information Society.* Cambridge, MA: Harvard University Press, 1986.

Bleecker, Samuel E. "The Virtual Organization." *The Futurist* 28, 2 (March/April 1994), 9–14.

Bok, Sissela. "The Morality of Whistle-Blowing." In Ermann et al., pp. 70–78.

Booker, Ellis. "Work Escapes the Office." *Computerworld* 27, 27 (November 29, 1993), 33.

Broadhurst, Judith. "Gender Differences in Online Communication." In Ermann et al., 1997, pp. 152–57.

Brod, Craig. *Technostress: The Human Cost of the Computer Revolution.* Reading, MA: Addison-Wesley, 1984.

Brown, Bonnie. "Is E-mail Private or Public?—Companies Own E-Mail and Can Monitor It." *Computerworld* 28, 26 (June 27, 1994), 135, 137. Cf. Corey L. Nelson.

Brown, Carl. "Assistive Technology Computers and Persons with Disabilities." *Communications of the ACM* 35, 5 (May 1992), 36–45. Note especially the Product References (p. 40) and the Guide to Rehabilitation Organizations (p. 42) in this article.

Butchvarov, Panayot. *Skepticism in Ethics.* Bloomington, IN: Indiana University Press, 1989.

Cairns-Smith, A. G. (Alexander Graham). *The Life Puzzle.* Toronto: University of Toronto Press, 1971.

Campbell, Jeremy. *Grammatical Man: Information, Entropy, Language, and Life.* New York: Simon & Schuster, 1982.

Card, Claudia, ed. *Feminist Ethics.* Lawrence, KS: University Press of Kansas, 1991.

Carnoy, Martin. *Sustaining the Economy: Work, Family, and Community in the Information Age.* Cambridge, MA: Harvard University Press, 2000.

Chalk, Rosemary. "Making the World Safe for Whistle-Blowers." *Technology Review* (January 1988), 48–57.

Chayefsky, Paddy. *Network* (the movie). 1976.

Dejoie, Roy, George Fowler, and David Paradice, eds. *Ethical Issues in Information Systems.* Boston, MA: Boyd & Fraser, 1991.

Dennett, Daniel C. "Where Am I?" In *Brainstorms: Philosophical Essays on Mind and Psychology.* Montgomery, VT: Bradford Books, 1978, pp. 310–23.

Dunlop, Charles, and Rob Kling, eds. *Computerization and Controversy: Value Conflicts and Social Choices.* Boston, MA: Academic Press, 1991, Part III.

Durkheim, Emile. *Division of Labor in Society.* Translated by George Simpson. New York: Free Press, [1893] 1933.

Ermann, M. David, Mary B. Williams, and Claudio Gutierrez, eds. *Computers, Ethics, and Society.* 2nd ed. New York: Oxford University Press, 1997, chs. 11, 16–23.

Feliu, Alfred G. "The Role of the Law in Protecting Scientific and Technical Dissent." *IEEE Technology and Society Magazine* (June 1985), 3–10.

Feulner, Terry, and Brian H. Kleiner. "When Robots Are the Answer." *Personnel Journal* 65, 2 (February 1986), 44–47.

Finley, Michael. "Telecommuting's Not Always a Trip." *Washington Post,* 28 June 1993, sec. WBIZ, p. 27.

Fisher, Lawrence M. "Quakes Four Years Apart Show How Far Telecommuting Has Come." *New York Times,* 13 February 1994, sec. 3, p. 10.

Fleming, Lis. *The One-Minute Commuter: How to Keep Your Job and Stay at Home Telecommuting.* Davis, CA: Acacia Books, 1989.

Fletcher, George P. *Loyalty: An Essay on the Morality of Relationships.* New York: Oxford University Press, 1993.

Flores, Albert, ed. *Ethical Problems in Engineering.* 2nd ed. Troy, NY: RPI Center for the Study of the Human Dimensions, 1980.

Flynn, Laurie. "PC Software Bosses Turn into Snoops." *Washington Post,* 28 June 1993, sec. WBIZ, p. 21.

Forester, Tom, and Perry Morrison. *Computer Ethics: Cautionary Tales and Ethical Dilemmas in Computing.* 2nd ed. Cambridge, MA: MIT Press, 1994, ch. 8.

Gilligan, Carol. *In a Different Voice: Psychological Theory and Women's Development.* Cambridge, MA: Harvard University Press, 1982.

Glenert, Ephraim P., and Bryant W. York. "Computers and People with Disabilities." *Communications of the ACM* 35, 5 (May 1992), 32–35.

Gordon, Gil E., and Marcia M. Kelly. *Telecommuting: How to Make It Work for You and Your Company.* Englewood Cliffs, NJ: Prentice-Hall, 1986.

Irving, R. H., C. A. Higgins, and F. R. Safayeni. "Computerized Performance Monitoring Systems: Use and Abuse." *Communications of the ACM* 29, 8 (August 1986), 794–801.

Johnson, Deborah G. *Ethical Issues in Engineering.* Englewood Cliffs, NJ: Prentice-Hall, 1991.

Joyner, Tammy. "Business Still Gets Done As Snow Falls: Teleworkers Don't Have Commutes." *Atlanta Journal-Constitution,* 4 January 2002, p. F1.

Kourany, Janet A., James P. Sterba, and Rosemarie Tong, eds. *Feminist Philosophies: Problems, Theories, and Applications.* Englewood Cliffs, NJ: Prentice-Hall, 1992; see "The World of Work" section.

"Labor Letter: Computer Snooping." *Wall Street Journal,* 26 May 1992, sec. A, p. 1.

Lieberstein, Stanley H. *Who Owns What Is in Your Head? Trade Secrets and the Mobile Employee.* New York: Hawthorn, 1979.

Miller, Jerry, and the Business Intelligence Braintrust. *Millennium Intelligence: Understanding and Conducting Competitive Intelligence in the Digital Age.* Medford, NJ: Cyber Age Books, 2000.

Minsky, Marvin. *The Society of Mind.* New York: Simon and Schuster, 1986.

Moravec, Hans. *Mind Children: The Future of Robot and Human Intelligence.* Cambridge, MA: Harvard University Press, 1988.

Nelson, Corey L. "Is E-mail Private or Public? Employers Have No Right to Snoop Through Mail." *Computerworld* 28, 26 (June 27, 1994), 135, 137; cf. Brown (1994).

Nussbaum, Karen. "Computer Monitoring: A Threat to the Right to Privacy?" In Dejoie, Fowler, and Paradice, 1991, 134–39.

Olerup, Agneta, Leslie Schneider, and Elsbeth Monod, eds. *Women, Work and Computerization: Opportunities and Disadvantages (Proceedings of the IFIP WG 9.1 First Working Conference on Women, Work and Computerization, Riva del Sole, Italy, September 17–21, 1984).* Amsterdam, Netherlands: North-Holland, 1985.

Olson, Margrethe H. "Remote Office Work: Changing Work Patterns in Space and Time." *Communications of the ACM* 26, 3 (March 1983), 182–87.

Ortega y Gasset, José. *The Revolt of the Masses.* New York: Norton [1932], 1960.

Pacelle, Mitchell. "Vanishing Offices: To Trim Their Costs, Some Companies Cut Space for Employees." *Wall Street Journal,* 4 June 1993, sec. A, p. 1.

Parker, Donn B., Susan Swope, and Bruce N. Baker. *Ethical Conflicts in Computer Science, Technology, and Business.* Wellesley, MA: QED Information Sciences, 1990. Though this collection of scenarios does not give any guidance on ethical standards by which these moral dilemmas may be solved, it does present a number of hypothetical cases that relate to the workplace, and solicits the opinions of people selected for their concern for ethics in the computer field. Scenarios of particular interest to this chapter include ignoring fraud (p. 37), installing an inadequate system (p. 41), accepting a grant on a possibly unachievable program (p. 45), ignoring voting machine malfunctions (p. 60), taking a personal program to a new job (p. 81), the ownership of software developed at a university (p. 83), copying software for a client (p. 89), and diverting research funds (p. 132).

Parnas, David Lorge. "SDI: A Violation of Professional Responsibility." *Abacus* 4, 2 (Winter 1987), 46–52.

Patton, Phil. "The Virtual Office Becomes Reality." *New York Times,* 28 October 1993, sec. C, p. 1.

Perrolle, Judith A. *Computers and Social Change: Information, Property, and Power.* Belmont, CA: Wadsworth, 1987.

Pool, Ithiel de Sola. *Technologies of Freedom: On Free Speech in an Electronic Age.* Cambridge, MA: Belknap Press of Harvard University Press, 1983.

Richmond-Abbott, Marie. "Women Wage Earners." In Kourany et al., 1992, 135–48.

Rifkin, Glenn. "Do Employees Have a Right to Electronic Privacy?" *New York Times,* 8 December 1991, sec. 3, p. 8.

Rifkin, Jeremy. *The End of Work: The Decline of the Global Labor Force and the Dawn of the Post-Market Era.* New York: Putnam, 1996.

Ritter, Gary, and Stan Thompson. "The Rise of Telecommuting and Virtual Transportation." *Transportation Quarterly* 48, 3 (Summer 1994), 235–248.

Ross, Randy. "The Telecommuting Imperative." *PC World* 11, 9 (September 1993), 52–55.

Roszak, Theodore. *The Cult of Information: The Folklore of Computers and the True Art of Thinking.* New York: Pantheon Books, 1986.

Rothfeder, Jeffrey. *Privacy for Sale: How Computerization Has Made Everyone's Private Life an Open Secret.* New York: Simon & Schuster, 1992.

Savage, John E., Susan Magidson, and Alex M. Stein. *The Mystical Machine: Issues and Ideas in Computing.* Reading, MA: Addison-Wesley, 1986, ch. 13.

Schepp, Brad. *The Telecommuter's Handbook: How to Work for a Salary Without Ever Leaving the House.* New York: Pharos Books, 1990.

Schor, Juliet. *The Overworked American.* New York: Basic Books, 1990.

Shannon, Claude, and Warren Weaver. *The Mathematical Theory of Communication.* Urbana, IL: University of Illinois Press, 1963.

Shapiro, Anna. "Where Will All the People Go?" *Nation* 242, 9 (March 8, 1986), 268–70.

Sharpe, Patricia. "Workforce Revolution." *Self* 16, 2 (February 1994), 82–86.

Shellenbarger, Sue. "Work & Family: Working at Home to Clean the Air." *Wall Street Journal*, 19 October 1992, sec. B, p. 1.

Shellenbarger, Sue. "Home Work: Some Thrive, But Many Wilt Working at Home." *Wall Street Journal*, 14 December 1993, sec. B, p. 3.

Shellenbarger, Sue. "Home Work: I'm Still Here. Home Workers Worry They're Invisible." *Wall Street Journal*, 16 December 1993, sec. B, p.1.

Spinello, Richard A. *Ethical Aspects of Information Technology.* Englewood Cliffs, NJ: Prentice-Hall, 1995, chs. 4, 5.

Spinello, Richard A., and Herman T. Tavani, eds. *Readings in Cyberethics.* Sudbury, MA: Jones and Bartlett, 2001.

"Taking a Byte out of Pizza Prep Time." *Training and Development Journal* 45, 3 (March 1991), 81–82.

Toffler, Alvin, ed. *The Futurists.* New York: Random House, 1972.

Toffler, Alvin. *The Third Wave.* New York: William Morrow, 1980.

Tong, Rosemarie. *Feminist Thought: A Comprehensive Introduction.* Boulder, CO: Westview Press, 1989.

U.S. Department of Commerce, Technology Administration. *The Information Infrastructure: Reaching Society's Goals.* Washington, DC: Government Printing Office, 1994.

Unger, Stephen H. *Controlling Technology: Ethics and the Responsible Engineer.* New York: Holt, Rinehart, and Winston, 1982.

Waldrop, M. Mitchell. *Man-Made Minds: The Promise of Artificial Intelligence.* New York: Walker and Company, 1987, ch. 10.

Weijers, Thea, Rob Meijer, and Erno Spoelman. "Telework Remains 'Made to Measure'." *Futures* 24, 10 (December 1992), 1048–55.

Weiner, Norbert. *Cybernetics: Or Control and Communication in the Animal and the Machine.* Cambridge, MA: MIT Press, 1961.

Wessel, Milton. *Freedom's Edge: The Computer Threat to Society.* Reading, MA: Addison-Wesley, 1974.

Wilke, John R. "Technology: For Network Managers, Snooping Gets Easier." *Wall Street Journal,* 23 March 1992, sec. B, p. 1.

Winner, Langdon. "Just Me and My Machine: The New Solipsism." *Whole Earth Review* (December 1984–January 1985), 29.

Young, Jae-Bok. "Ranks of Telecommuters Grow." *Christian Science Monitor,* 25 February 1993, p. 7.

Zuboff, Shoshana. *In the Age of the Smart Machine: The Future of Work and Power.* New York: Basic Books, 1984.

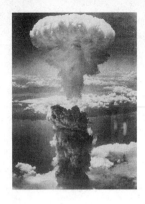

Chapter 10

Responsibility, Liability, Law, and Professional Ethics

 ## RESPONSIBILITY

The root of the word 'responsibility' is 'response', so we should examine just what questions responsibility responds to. They include: "Who did this?", "Who is in charge?", "What should I do in this case?", "Why should I do X (or not do Y)?", "Why did agent A do action Z?", and so on.

J. R. Lucas analyzes the question "Why did you do it?" into three component parts—*you*, *do*, and *it* (Lucas, 1993, pp. 6–8). With respect to the *you* part, the only problem may be that the question is addressed to the wrong person. In such a case, I reply, "Don't ask *me*," or perhaps more specifically, "Don't ask *me*, ask *Joe*." Then the responsibility is Joe's, not mine. With respect to the *do* part of the question, the action may have been mine, but it may have been one that I could not help—I might have been brainwashed to do it by the enemy (as in the movie *The Manchurian Candidate*). Or, as I held a knife in my hand, a stronger person might have forced me to stab someone. In such cases, the responsibility lies with the brainwasher, or the strong person who controlled the stabbing, not with me. The last part of the question relates to *it*: did I *cause* "it," and is the "it" you name a proper description of the action? If I voted for the best candidate in the election, and you describe my action as treason, the act has not been accurately characterized, and so I cannot be said to be responsible for (that is, guilty of) treason.

On the other hand, if "Why did you do it?" is correctly addressed to me as the agent who did *it*, if the *doing* was indeed within my control, and if the *it* you describe is indeed a fair characterization of the action, then I may be said to have been responsible for the action (and deserve the appropriate blame, or praise, as the case may be).

We have a commonsense view of what it is to be a "responsible person." Lucas characterizes this as follows:

> A responsible person is one who can be left in charge, who can be relied on to cope, who will not slope off, leaving the job undone, or switch off, leaving the business unattended to. So long as a responsible person is responsible, you can sleep easy, knowing that no extra vigilance on your part is called for, and that he will see to it that all goes well. (Lucas, p. 11)

We want those we work with, those who work for us, and those who control our lives to some extent (such as employers or the government) all to be responsible persons. If we have such hopes or expectations of others, we should be responsible ourselves. This is a kind of Kantian universalized principle, though it might also be justified on Utilitarian grounds—practically, if I am not responsible in my actions toward others, they may well feel I do not fall within the realm of their responsibility.

Free will, as we discussed in Part One, is an essential presupposition of an ethical system. It is also, obviously, a necessary condition for attributing responsibility. Thus, any position (say, materialism or the computational theory of mind) that reduces choice, value, and mental activity in general to some physical or calculational basis destroys freedom and eliminates responsibility. If we were not free and responsible, there would have been no point in writing this book. I should just have written a scientific tome describing some features of computer systems. But these systems impact on human lives, and in those lives choice, value, and responsibility play major roles. If they did not, the lives would cease to be human and they would cease to have value, because value is one of the notions that a materialism does not explain.

Thus, much as Kant does, we will pursue our discussion of responsibility among those who are involved in creating, using, and maintaining computer systems, with all of their attendant contributions and disadvantages. At least to this point, the responsibility and choice still falls to the humans working with the systems. Perhaps in the future we will also need to deal with the choices and responsibilities of artificially intelligent computer systems. This will be discussed in Chapter 12. Lucas suggests that there is a Modern Samaritan parable: "The first passer-by is not a priest but a social worker, who goes over and, on seeing the man who fell among thieves, says, 'My goodness, the person who did that is in need of professional help'" (Lucas, 1993, p. 103, fn. 12). Just what do we mean by *professional help*? Generally this is help that one *pays for*; the psychiatrist in the movie *Love at First Bite* says, "If you don't pay for it, you won't get cured." The help is given by someone designated as a professional. *Professionals* tend to be considered members of groups that have specific advanced training and degrees, and are certified, by taking a test and/or by approval of a qualified group of their peers, as being expert or at least proficient in their field—law, medicine, engineering, nursing, cosmetology, accounting, and so on.

If, within the realm of being a professional, one makes some claim(s) to be able to help someone (to get well, for example) or to construct something (such as a building or a bridge), then that person is *responsible* for doing what was claimed. If they do *not* fulfill their claim or contract or agreement, then they are *liable* for having failed. They may be held liable by a court of law, or by a professional group of their peers. In any case, their being held accountable is for the protection of those with whom they make agreements.

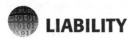 ## LIABILITY

Liability is a more *legal* notion than responsibility; that is, it not only deals with whoever is responsible for something happening (or not getting done), but it also sets punishments for the breach of responsibility; it refers to being *bound by law*. Thus, if X is deemed a crime or misdemeanor, the question then is not only who committed X, but whether the person (or organization) that committed X is *liable* for the damages that resulted and must *pay* in some way—in money, or loss of position, or prison, or death, or some combination of the former penalties.

There are generally two conditions involved in legal *criminal* liability: (1) a **causality condition** (did agent A *cause* X to occur?); and (2) a **condition of intention** (*mens rea*, or literally the thought or understanding of the accused A). Neither of these is easy to establish. Causality is clear in a few cases, such as one billiard ball hitting another, or A being seen by ten witnesses stabbing someone to death.[1]

Direct causation is difficult to observe or prove, especially if there is a *chain* of events between the act of agent A and the effect X that represents harm of some kind. If I hit someone with my car, I have directly caused any injuries sustained. If I throw a ball that breaks a light controlling an electronic eye to hold a dog in check, and the dog gets free, jumps into a parked car, releases the hand brake, and the car rolls down the hill to hit and injure someone, then I am the initiator of the sequence of causes, but no one may know that (even me), and it may be judged that the dog inadvertently caused the accident.

If I shoot and kill someone with a gun, I am liable under the law for the harm, and subject to punishment, perhaps even death. If I design a gun that is sold, or if I am a merchant who legally sells a gun, and the person who buys the gun commits murder with it, I am (under current law) not considered liable for the murder, because I designed or sold a legal tool under legal conditions. Yet I hold a share in the responsibility (if not the liability) for the murder, since I had a hand in making it possible. I have contributed to the very existence of guns, whose clear purpose is to cause harm.

Similar questions arise with issues of liability involving computers. If I commit a crime with my computer (such as theft), then I am liable for the crime. If I design or sell a computer (which is a tool) and the person who legally buys it uses it to commit a crime, am I liable? It would seem not, in analogy to the gun example. Yet we saw that class action suit charges were brought against IBM for providing the computers used in the Equity Funding scandal. Once again this seems to indicate the need for the law to catch up with technology.

If the computer I design and build is used in a successful crime, it would at least seem that I share the responsibility for the act, since without my computer it could not have been committed. Yet computers have so much potential for good uses; if a human chooses to put it to an evil use, am I as the builder *responsible* for the evil choice he made? It would seem not, any more so than if I am an apple-grower (which is generally for the public good, promoting health), and someone uses one of the apples bought from me to kill a man by jamming the apple down his throat. However, if I design and market software that, though it has an innocent-sounding name like "Barney," is really a tool for breaking into other people's personal computers and company networks, it would seem that I share in the responsibility when a buyer uses it to do just that.

There is a line of thought that says if I hadn't designed or sold the computer (or the gun), someone else would have, so I might as well, since I am not breaking any law in doing so. But if I am creating or selling something (like a gun, or destructive software) that has the potential to do harm, am I not responsible to an extent for what evil is done with it? My *distance* (physically) from the actual harm does not remove me from the causal chain. But such distant connections are often difficult to prove in a court of law, or the legal system is only concerned with the *immediate* (or *proximate*) cause.

The other condition, *intention*, is even more difficult to prove. Who knows what someone else is (or was) thinking? Some people are good actors, who can feign grief, anger, and the like. Yet there are ways in which the legal system is satisfied that intent has been demonstrated—for example, finding notes in the accused's handwriting planning the crime, or the like. If damages have occurred, and causality can be proved, but not intent, then the penalty is less harsh. For example, Robert T. Morris Jr. was judged not to have intended the Internet Worm to cause the damage it created, and thus received a reasonably light sentence. In many criminal cases, the prosecution seeks to prove means, motive, and opportunity if direct eyewitnesses to the crime are not forthcoming. Then there is also the charge of *criminal negligence*—perhaps one did not *intend* to do damage, but one *should have known* (given one's background) that damage would or could result. This would seem to fit Morris' case.

In 1989, shortly after the Internet Worm was let loose, Pamela Samuelson, a law professor with a deep interest in the law relating to computers, wrote a short piece for the *Communications of the ACM* titled, "Can Hackers Be Sued for Damages Caused by Computer Viruses?" In it she observes that the "law can be a rather blunt instrument" in dealing with hackers. Legal theory and precedent has not yet clearly caught up with the new phenomena related to computers: hacking, piracy, and the like. Thus there are a number of reasons that a person who has suffered damage and/or loss from the activity of a computer hacker might not want to rush to take the case to a law court.

First, there is the matter of current law not applying clearly and unambiguously to cases involving computers. Samuelson writes:

> The law generally recognizes only established categories of legal claims, and each of the categories of legal claims has its own particular pattern to it, which must be matched in order to win a lawsuit based on it. While judges are sometimes willing to stretch the legal category a little to reach a fair result, they are rarely willing to create entirely new categories of law or stretch an existing category to the breaking point. Because of this, much of what lawyers do is pattern-matching or arguing by analogy. (Samuelson, 1989, p. 666)

Thus the law may evolve to fit new situations, but it does so *very* slowly. In the meantime, the injured parties in a hacking incident may find that the law simply does not have a "pattern" to fit their particular case. In the absence of a specific law dealing with damages caused by computer viruses, the lawyer for the plaintiff will have to look among the categories of suits that seek financial settlements in compensation for harm caused by "wrongful conduct." These suits are called *torts*.

Computer users need protection from bad programs, from each other, from people who want to steal their data (and often their money), and from systems that are too easily penetrated. The National Institute of Standards and Technology (NIST) could provide leadership in setting *standards* for system security, but they have not done much so far, and claim that their first responsibility is to federal agencies. Part of what is needed is more education regarding potential security problems and how they may be avoided. NIST says they have issued security guidelines, but the guidelines are generally ignored.[2]

An interesting question regarding liability arises if we ask whether companies (or colleges) are liable for what their employees (or students and faculty) say on the Internet. A 1989 article in the *Chronicle of Higher Education* suggested that colleges and universities are particularly vulnerable to lawsuits arising from damage created by viruses. However, David R. Johnson, coauthor of a report on college liability for viruses, said, "It's clearly not reasonable to attribute to the institution liability for the irresponsible actions of an individual student" (Moore, 1989, pp. A1, A20). However, if the college provides the *means* by which the crime (of setting loose a destructive virus) is carried out, by analogy with other criminal cases, might it be considered an *accessory to the crime*?

This again seems to be a case of something with the potential for good use—worldwide sharing of information—being misused for bad purposes by a few. It is their human *choice* that has caused the evil. To blame the university, which is merely trying to broaden the horizons of its students, would be analogous to holding a flashlight manufacturer responsible for the uses of its product in burglaries.

 ## COMPUTERS AND THE LAW

Just as the emergence of computer technology has raised many new (or at least *different*) problems for ethics, it clearly has raised new (or different) legal questions as well. (This was described in Chapter 4, when we discussed how to protect rights in software.) Some of the problems seem to be compounded because those in the computer world may not clearly understand the intricacies of the law, and those in the law (including judges, lawyers, legislators, and even juries) may not clearly understand the new technology. The best we can do, in hopes for the future, is to try to meet somewhere in between, each side making an effort to understand the other (as with the scientists and the humanists we discussed early in the book).

We look for some enlightenment on this from two respected legal scholars. Larry Lessig suggests that we should not expect the law to be the sole regulator of behavior. In the "real" physical world, there are four constraints on behavior: law, social norms, the market (I try to live within my means), and the architecture of nature (physical constraints on what I can do; for example, I cannot drive my car through that mountain, even though it would be the shortest route to my destination). These four constraints operate together to *regulate* behavior. Lessig goes on to deny the claims that cyberspace is "unregulable." Initially, cyberspace may seem to represent a previously unexperienced level of freedom, but there are four constraints at work there as well.

There are existing laws (against sexual harassment, or libel, or stealing) that apply in cyberspace as well as physical space. There are also social norms in cyberspace (one could be "kicked out of"—denied access to—a chat room for unseemly behavior, for example). The market also determines which and how many cyber-sites we may access, if they impose a charge. Finally, the analog to the architecture of physical space is the *code* of cyberspace—"the set of protocols, the set of rules, implemented or codified, in the software of cyberspace itself, which determine how people interact, or exist, in this space" (Lessig, 2001, p. 126). These four constraints operate together to regulate behavior, and it is important to look carefully at *how* they interact.

The analogies suggested by Lessig are very rich. Notice that, in our real-world example, we do not rely on a law against driving through mountains; the architecture of physical reality takes care of this for us. In cyberspace, the code can be written so as to prevent, say, pornography from being distributed to children by implementing various tests and conditions. Social norms generally prevent much undesirable behavior, both in the world and in cyberspace, because it is generally recognized with what disapproval it will be met. Similarly, we do not want *over*-regulation by the government, with laws restricting much of our behavior—either in the political physical world or in cyberspace. Thus we must be careful what we ask for in laws for cyberspace, lest they take away some of the freedoms we cherish. Fortunately, there are several groups that are on the alert to defend our civil liberties, among them the ACLU, CSPR, and EPIC. But they need our support.

Constitutional scholar Laurence Tribe takes on the question of how the Constitution is to be "mapped" onto cyberspace, and concludes that its framers "were very wise indeed," since the mapping can be understood clearly in terms of five basic axioms (or assumptions) of constitutional law that provide for us "a framework for all seasons."

1. The Constitution (with one exception) "regulates action by the *govern-ment* rather than the conduct of *private* individuals and groups" (Tribe, 1990, p. 211). New technology does not change this. The government does not regulate what books bookstore owners may put on their shelves; by analogy, the operator of a bulletin board merely organizes what is posted there but is not responsible for its content.
2. "A person's mind, body, and property belong *to that person* and not to the public as a whole" (Tribe, 1990, p. 211). Just because information can be transmitted and duplicated with perfect accuracy as 1's and 0's does not negate this basic right of an individual to his or her property.
3. "Information and ideas are *too important* to entrust to any government censor or overseer" (Tribe, 1990, p. 212). Free speech, however, does not extend to harmful speech; so, just as I could be prosecuted for the consequences of my falsely yelling "Fire!" in a crowded theater, the creator and unleasher of a virus or worm that does damage should be prosecuted.
4. "The human spirit is something beyond a physical information processor" (Tribe, 1990, p. 215). The Constitution protects what is uniquely human; one should never be forced to be a witness against oneself. If the content of information (on a computer or a printing press) triggers a governmental interest in seizing it, this is still a violation of First Amendment rights.
5. "The Constitution's norms, at their deepest level, must be invariant under merely *technological* transformations" (Tribe, 1990, p. 216). To claim that wiretapping, or other electronic surveillance, involves no improper search and seizure is surely a perversion of the intent of the law. Tribe writes: "Ironically, *fidelity* to original values requires *flexibility* of textual interpretation" (Tribe, 1990, p. 218). To say that we assume certain risks by using modern technology (such as the telephone) is tantamount to saying that our constitutional rights to free speech, privacy, and equality apply only if we remain in a simple, largely ignorant state.

Tribe thus lays a clear groundwork for attempts to map the Constitution onto cyberspace. How hard can it be? If our fundamental rights get compromised in the translation, then something is wrong with the translator. At the end of his article, Tribe proposes a Twenty-seventh Amendment that just might help clarify matters:

> The Constitution's protections for the freedoms of speech, press, petition, and assembly, and its protections against unreasonable searches and seizures, and the deprivation of life, liberty, or property without due process of law, shall be construed as fully applicable without regard to the technological method or

medium through which information is generated, stored, altered, transmitted, or controlled. (Tribe, 1990, p. 220)

It would seem as though such an amendment should not be necessary; it is just common sense. But given some of the actions of the courts and the legislature regarding issues involving computers, one has to wonder.

PROFESSIONAL ETHICS

J. R. Lucas says, "Professional people give themselves airs. They regard themselves as more responsible than other men, and like others to think so too" (Lucas, 1993, p. 193). This may well be the case with some professionals, who consider themselves very important, people who others should look up to. They generally have earned advanced degrees and often their positions have required the approval of a formal group of their peers, so they may just feel that all of their effort has earned some recognition. Occasionally, though, they may consider that their expertise in a particular area makes them experts in other areas as well (such as politics, ethics, art, and the like), even though they have no comparable training there.

A professional generally is one who does not necessarily think the customer is always right. A professional ought to be guided by the interests "of the people, of God, or the ideals" served, not by personal interest (Lucas, 1993, p. 193).

> The assumed ignorance of the patient, the client, or the pupil is the correlative of the esoteric knowledge and values of the profession. Long training has given the professional an expertise and dedication which enable and entitle him to make up somebody else's mind for him and decide what is in his best interests. (Lucas, 1993, p. 194)

The professions are considered to include medicine, law, dentistry, nursing, teaching, accounting, and often engineering. They seem to have several things in common: they generally are "white-collar jobs," they require a high level of training (attested to by specialized degrees) and skill, and they must, in most cases, pass some test (such as the bar exam for lawyers) and/or get approval from a group of their peers. In several of the professions mentioned, a person may *lose* the professional status by violating a commonly agreed upon code of professional behavior; for example, a lawyer can be disbarred.

The computing field involves white-collar jobs, but it does not fit the other characteristics of professions very well. The exceptions are those in the field who are college professors, and who are thus professionals by virtue of their advanced academic degrees and having been screened by the usual Ph.D. processes (qualifying exams and an approved original dissertation in their field of expertise), but *not* simply by virtue of their being in the computing field. There are no certification examinations *required* to work in computing, and many who have been very successful in the field had no formal training in it. Youngsters who become enamored of computers early in their lives become quite expert, and get jobs that will pay them to do what they love to do. They do not necessarily have college degrees, and yet they may get rich from an innovative hardware design or software package. For example, Bill Gates, the founder of Microsoft, dropped out of Harvard after two years of undergraduate work, and went on to become the richest man in America.[3]

There are similarities between computing and other professions, however. Those who are "in the know" are generally held in awe by those who do not understand the inner workings of the "mystical machine" (Savage et al., 1986) which can accomplish such wonders. This is similar to the awe in which some doctors are held by the patients seeking their help; they are believed to have mysterious and wonderful secrets that will cure illness and prolong life. In the 1950s and 1960s, when computing first was coming into its own, the experts of the old computer community were considered "high priests" who held the secrets to the inner workings of the powerful machine.

However, the truth of the matter is that there is no established standard of competence or of behavior for those working in the computing field, in the way that there is for the other professions mentioned. A few computer experts working now for high pay were "computer criminals" only a short time ago. As we discussed earlier, banks fearing computer break-ins, for example, have been known to hire those who have demonstrated that they know how it is done. There has been talk, as we discussed, of the Computing Sciences Accreditation Board requiring ethics to be taught as part of the college computing curriculum, but it is not clear whether that has been enforced, or how many college curricula are accredited.

The Association of Computing Machinery is the most well-established group for the field (many of whom also belong to the Institute of Electrical and Electronics Engineers (IEEE)), but it does not officially sanction the competence of any of its members, and its code of ethics is only a suggested set of principles; the ACM has no viable enforcement powers for the code. If an ACM member were to be found in violation of the code, "membership in ACM may be terminated." However, this does not pose a serious threat to anyone whose employer might not even take notice of their ACM membership or lack thereof. One has to wonder, if someone lists ACM membership on a resume or in material for a promotion, whether anyone ever checks to see whether the claim of membership is true.

Michael D. Bayles, in his book *Professional Ethics*, indicates that there are generally at least six types of sanctions socially imposed for professional misconduct (eight for lawyers):

1. Others *blame* the professional.
2. The person may experience social and professional *ostracism* and *boycott* (other professionals will not refer clients, organizations may refuse to hire the person).
3. Professional societies or licensing boards can give public or private *reprimands*.
4. The person may be *excluded from membership* in a professional society.
5. The professional *may be sued for malpractice*.
6. The professional may have his or her *license to practice suspended or revoked* (Bayles, 1989, pp. 189–90).

The sorts of strong control over who may *practice* in the profession that exist in the traditional areas do not exist in computing.

The ACM is a praiseworthy group, seeking to give stature to the field of computing. The point is, though, that it really has no power to deny anyone the right to continue working in the field (in the way that the American Bar Association, for example, can disbar a lawyer, who then can no longer practice law). There is, in fact, no comparable group in the computing field with this power. Given the influence on human life that computers and those who manipulate them have, it would be most desirable if there *were* some group that in fact could set and enforce standards for those working in the computing field. Then it could be properly called one of the professions. As it stands now, people who call themselves software *engineers* are violating the law in forty-eight states, since the title of engineer connotes a professional status achieved by meeting specified standards, which "software engineers" are not measured by.[4] The suggestion is that they should call themselves software (or hardware) *specialists* instead.

PROFESSIONAL CODES OF ETHICS

Professionals are considered to enter into a complex network of obligations and duties when they become active members of a profession. These obligations include serving "clients" on a fair and *equal access* basis; obligations to clients to act in a competent and trustworthy manner and maintain discretion (client privacy); obligations to third parties (not to inflict harm on others in carrying out duties to the client); obligations to employers (to the law firm, hospital, accounting firm, corporation, or the like that provides the realm in which to practice for any professional who is not self-employed), to be competent, honest, discrete, and loyal; and obligations to the profession itself (by maintaining its standards and furthering its goals through research and other contributions). This list of obligations was suggested by Bayles (1989, chs. 3–7).

There are various codes of ethics drawn up by different groups in the computing area. It is informative to compare them and their disciplinary procedures with those of the professions we have mentioned—for example, with the Hippocratic Oath for doctors. The codes for computing include the British Computer Society Code of Practice and Code of Conduct; the Data Processing Management Association (DPMA) Code of Ethics, Standards of Conduct and Enforcement Procedures; the IEEE Code of Ethics; and the ACM Code of Ethics and Professional Conduct (the first version in 1973, the second version approved in 1992). The 1992 ACM Code appears in Appendix B of the text, and the IEEE Code of Ethics in Appendix C.

The ACM Code has many noble sentiments. It encourages its members to "contribute to society and human well-being," "avoid harm to others," "be honest and trustworthy," to be fair and not discriminate, to respect property rights, to "give proper credit for intellectual property," to respect privacy, and to honor confidentiality. (*ACM Code* #1) Members are further encouraged to "strive to achieve the highest quality" in their work, know the laws relating to their work, honor contracts and agreements, "improve public understanding of computing and its consequences," and access computing resources only when such access is authorized; this is a clear reaction to the rise in hacking activity. (*ACM Code* #2) There is also a set of imperatives for organizational leadership.

Each professional imperative is discussed in the *ACM Code* at greater length to make its intent clear. Members are "expected to" abide by the code and could be punished by loss of membership in the ACM if they do not do so. Professional ethics in the computing area, as in other areas, is basically a set of ethical guidelines that should apply to *any human being* who has dealings with other human beings—fairness, honesty, honoring of contracts, not causing harm, and respect for life, property, and privacy of others—plus a few specifics that arise from the role of the professional in society. In computing, those who design systems, especially safety-critical systems, have an added obligation to the public to make those systems as safe and reliable as possible, with built-in human controls if the automatic system should fail. Rules of nontrespass also need to be particularly emphasized, because access to the computer systems of others is so easy and so relatively invisible. So professional ethics here would seem to reduce to good common sense plus a few directives specific to the computer specialist's role in society.

What About Microsoft?

In 2001, U.S. courts ruled that Microsoft had repeatedly violated the Sherman Antitrust Act to maintain its monopoly with Windows. However, the company appealed the decision, won't be broken up any time soon, and it won't have to face the first tough judge it ran up against again in court. That said, though the court can now tell Microsoft what it may and may not do in its software and documentation.[5]

Some of the claims made against Microsoft were price fixing, preannouncing products that never materialized, and deliberately making its product incompatible with the products of rival companies. These charges are echoes of the antitrust charges brought against another computer giant, IBM, in 1969. It is perhaps ironic that the scrutiny IBM was under after the antitrust suit allowed a small company like Microsoft to grow. However, both computer companies (at different points in time) seem to have used illegal and unethical practices to control the areas in which they operated.[6]

One may wonder what drives companies like Microsoft and IBM to employ such extreme measures, but the answer seems pretty clear—greed and a thirst for power. The lack of any professional sanctions brought against either company or their employees illustrates rather clearly the lack of any kind of oversight in the computer profession. It took the United States government itself to bring any control to bear on these two giants in the computer world.

 ## ARE SCIENCE AND TECHNOLOGY MORALLY NEUTRAL?

The claim is often made that technology is *morally neutral*, that it has no ethical component or consequences, and so scientists should be left alone by moralists to do their work. If this is so, then those working in areas of science and technology have no moral obligations connected with their work, with the possible exception of obligations to the profession, such as maintaining standards of excellence and competence, and contributing to the field through research. If this is the case, then scientists cannot be held morally responsible for the consequences of their innovations.

Science and technology have a very significant impact on the world in which we live, and so on the quality (and the possibility) of human life. Advances in science have brought countless benefits, such as increasingly rapid travel, the wide dissemination of information and entertainment, improvements in health care, and new sources of energy. But scientific advancements have also greatly enhanced the ways in which human beings can kill each other through the use of more efficient and devastating weaponry, developments that have made possible the destruction of the entire planet. Scientific advances have created new moral problems for us to solve—in genetics, in reproduction, in human conflict, and in the proper use of information—and have exacerbated other problems. The impact on the environment by technology is reaching disastrous proportions.

Advances in medical care have reduced infant mortality rates and increased life spans, but they have also contributed significantly to a world-wide problem of overpopulation, which is at the base of most of the environmental problems today. Sigmund Freud noted this effect as early as 1930, in *Civilization and Its Discontents*. He says that in this we have "probably worked against the beneficial effects of natural selection" (Freud, 1961, ch. III, p. 35). Freud finds, as the title indicates, civilization as the source of our "discontents"—our unhappiness, our problems. He attributes this primarily to the restrictions that "civilization" places on our natural impulses, but also to the effects wrought by many "scientific improvements."

In 1930, fifteen years before Hiroshima and Nagasaki, Freud was deeply concerned about whether the human species would wipe itself out and the rest of life on Earth with it:

> The fateful question for the human species seems to me to be whether and to what extent their cultural development will succeed in mastering the disturbance of their communal life by the human instinct of aggression and self-destruction. . . . Men have gained control over the forces of nature to such an extent that with their help they would have no difficulty in exterminating each other to the last man. (Freud, p. 92)

We thus come back to the question of whether science and technology are morally neutral. How *could* they be, when it is advances in science and technology that *create* moral problems for our time? Can a scientist working on an atomic bomb be legitimately indifferent to the uses to which it will be put? One might try the line, "Bombs don't kill people; *people* kill people." But can those who are in the business of creating more powerful and effective tools of destruction claim to have *no* connection with their *use* for destruction? Many responsible scientists have refused to work on such projects, or to take money for research from the U.S. Department of Defense. Groups have been established, such as Computer Professionals for Social Responsibility and the Union of Concerned Scientists, which take stands against certain scientific research and practices.

When I was an undergraduate engineering major, the physics professor teaching the principles of mechanics course I was taking had been involved in the Manhattan Project. Clearly, when he realized the actual effect of the work he had been involved in, he was devastated, and felt an overwhelming moral responsibility for it. Since Hiroshima, he had not taught atomic physics, and had moved into more neutral areas such as mechanics. Recently, he has been involved with writing books and productions for PBS that acquaint nonscientists with science's attempts to answer questions about nature, of "How do we know?" I greatly respect this man and his principles, and only hope that more scientists will reflect on their responsibilities to humanity when they engage in their work. It would be preferable for these scientists to anticipate the potential bad consequences of their investigations *before* they embark on them.

Abbe Mowshowitz points out that "By refusing to make judgments on the propriety of his professional activities, the scientist gives tacit approval to the goals of the institution which employs him" (Mowshowitz, 1976, p. 270). It would be hypocritical for a scientist to protest against the evils of war, while at the same time work for the military establishment.

Geoffrey Brown, in *The Information Game* (1990), discusses further the issue of the supposed moral neutrality of technology. He points out that some take the position that science, like any other form of knowledge, is morally neutral or, if anything, good, since knowledge is good. One must then step back and critically assess this claim. Is *all* knowledge good? Is it good to know how to torture people more effectively, or how to efficiently wipe out a whole race of people? Is it good to know how to create a technology that may get out of hand (like "The Sorcerer's Apprentice," or the DNA cloning of dinosaurs in *Jurassic Park*), and put that knowledge into creating a reality?

Kant provides the clearest analysis of the claim that knowledge is unqualifiedly good, pointing to examples like those we just cited, and then pointing out that a God who is omniscient (all-*know*ing) but not also omnibenevolent (all-*good*) would be a nightmare—a being with complete knowledge and total power as well, who did *not* have a good will—a Satan with no restraints. From this analysis, Kant concludes that the only thing that is good *without qualification* is a good will.

Brown analyzes the claim that an activity is morally neutral into two possible meanings: "(a) that it is neither good or bad in itself, so that, other things being equal, no one should be praised or blamed for doing it, or (b) that there is no morally right or wrong way of doing it, and therefore that what goes on within this activity is not, as such, open to moral approbation or condemnation" (Brown, 1990, p. 23). As Brown points out, (a) might be applied to something like playing chess. It is not good or bad to play chess; it is a morally neutral activity, since it does not matter—morally—whether you play or not. Chess might also be described under (b), in that there is no morally right or wrong way to do it, as long as you don't cheat. But other activities fall under (b) that do not fall under (a), like science (or parenting, or cooking). It *does* matter whether one engages in these activities, but it also makes a huge difference *how* one does it. There are many instances of parenting done badly (among the worst of which are parents who molest their defenseless children), and there are instances of bad cooking (from the merely unpalatable to that done deliberately to poison). Similarly, science can be done well, for good purposes, or badly—ineptly or, more importantly, for bad ends, or having damaging effects or side effects.

It is useful to analyze scientific research, or causation of change, in terms of Aristotle's Four Causes: (1) the *material* which is changed, (2) the *efficient* cause of the change (presumably the scientist, or some natural force the scientist sets in motion), (3) the *formal* cause of the change (what was the plan, or blueprint), and (4) the *final* cause of the change (its purpose, or goal). Of these, scientists generally spend most of their time with the first two, and then in formulating the third (the design specifications, or the new law of nature discovered), but do not bother with the fourth, which is the most important. The question should not be just "*How* can we do this?", but more importantly, "*Why* should we do this?"

We saw in our discussions in Part One that to claim that one morally *ought* to do something implies the precondition that one *can* do it; otherwise the *ought* is empty of content and does not relate to a possible action. What we should derive from our discussion in this section is that, with respect to many *can*s, one should first ask whether one *ought* to do them. This does not imply a circle that one cannot get out of. Just because I *can* buy a gun and kill the president does not mean that I *should* do so. There is a whole realm of possibilities ("cans") that our moral intuition and ethical principles rule out. Each *can*, each choice, should be accompanied by the question, "*ought* I to do this?" If the answer to that question is "no," then the possibility represented by the "can" should not be actualized. The other side of the formula, "*ought* implies *can*," merely applies to cases in which we can rightly attribute responsibility. I cannot fairly say that I *ought* to have done X, if it is not a possibility that I *can* do X.

The issue with regard to science and technology then becomes one where science *can* lead in many new directions (including more effective means of killing, torture, genocide, and so on), but the scientists have a moral responsibility to humanity to stop and ask themselves whether they *should* pursue that direction.

The computer has opened up many new avenues of development in science and technology, and has made some existing areas of research more viable. Computer experts must often work with a range of more traditional professionals—from doctors and lawyers to engineers—on projects that for them carry explicit responsibilities. The computer professional who is involved, for example, in work on an expert system that will complement or replace some of the functions performed by a doctor, will work closely with the doctor on the features the system should have, and the safety precautions that should be taken. The doctor has a professional responsibility to try to heal patients, not to harm them; computer professionals working on such projects should thus recognize that their work entails similar responsibilities and moral decisions, because their programs will be functioning in the same role as the doctor.

■ ENDNOTES

1. However, Hume would question whether there *is* such a meaningful notion as causality. All we ever observe is the *contiguity* ("touching" in space and/or connected in time) of "cause" C and "effect" E and *succession* (E follows C), and the fact that this pattern has repeated. But Hume argues that there is no *necessary connection* that we observe between C and E, which would be requisite to causality. One can always imagine "cause" C having some "effect" *other than* E; thus the connection cannot be *necessary.*

2. Gary M. Anthes, "Government Security Efforts Neglect Corporate Needs," *Computerworld* 28, 19 (May 9, 1994), 30.

3. "Interview," *Playboy* (July 1994), 56.

4. Julia King, "Engineers to IS: Drop That Title!" *Computerworld* (May 30, 1994), 1, 19. See also Fran Allen, Paula Hawthorn, Barbara Simons, "Not Now, Not Like This," *Communications of the ACM* 43, 2 (February 2000), 29–30.

5. Frank Hayes, "Pyrrhic Victory," *Computerworld* (July 2, 2001), 62.

6. Marc L. Songini, "Is History Repeating Itself with Antitrust Battle?", *Computerworld* (March 5, 2001), 30.

■ SHORT ESSAY QUESTIONS

1. Discuss briefly how current law is inadequate to deal with computer hackers. If you can, make suggestions as to how it should be changed.

2. Read Peter G. Neumann's article, "Certifying Professionals," in *Communications of the ACM* (February 1991), p. 130. Summarize clearly the article and the issues involved, and make a case for one side of the argument: Do you think that computer professionals should have to be formally certified by taking a test or obtaining the approval of a professional group, or do you think that this is not appropriate to the computing field? Compare Neumann's position with that of John Shore in "Why I Never Met a Programmer I Could Trust," in *Communications of the ACM* 31, 4 (April 1988), pp. 372–75. (It also appears in Dejoie et al., 1991, pp. 97–102.) Argue your considered view clearly.

3. Compare the 1973 ACM Code with the 1992 Code. What differences are there, and how do you account for them? Is anything left out from the earlier Code that you think should have been retained? How would you further improve the 1992 Code?

4. The IEEE Code of Ethics is included in Appendix C of the book. In what ways does it differ from the ACM Code? Discuss the difference between an area in which a person is formally certified as a member of the profession and one where this procedure is not in effect.

5. Geoffrey Brown, in *The Information Game* (pp. 24–29), takes some time to examine the distinction often drawn between science and technology. Explicate what he has to say about this distinction, and what relevance it might have to the question of the moral neutrality (or nonneutrality) of either.

■ LONG ESSAY QUESTIONS

1. Pick an instance of a computer "error" that had serious effects (there are many to choose from in this book) and discuss the difficulties of assigning *responsibility* in the case. Explain why it is more difficult to accurately and fairly assign blame in cases where computers are involved.

2. Read Book III of Aristotle's *Nicomachean Ethics* on responsibility, and discuss critically how it relates to and provides guidance for current questions regarding responsibility in the computing field.

3. Examine the terms of the "shrink-wrap" license on a piece of expensive software and discuss whether these terms are enforceable, responsible, or moral, and the issues of liability on the side of the seller and the side of the purchaser.

4. Discuss the issue of the legal liability of someone who runs an electronic bulletin board. Refer to the readings by Cangialosi (1989), Charles (1987), DiCato (1990), and Jensen (1987). See if you can find any more recent relevant references (for example, Friedman and Buono (2000)). Note also the case of David LaMacchia.

5. Refer to the excellent discussion of whether technology is morally neutral in Brown (1990, ch. 2), and the discussion in Ladd (1989). Outline the issues clearly for someone who is not familiar with them, and then critically assess both sides of the argument—that science and technology *are* morally neutral and should be left alone, versus there *is* a moral component to technology and its effects, and those working in the area of science and technology should be fully aware of the moral implications of their work. Determine which position you think is correct and defend your assessment, using examples if possible.

6. Can a computer be considered to make choices (decisions) and, if so, should it be held responsible for those decisions? This is a complex question that gets into issues in artificial intelligence (which we discuss in Chapter 12), but you can get a start by considering a pair of articles by Bechtel (1985) and Snapper (1985). Summarize clearly the arguments raised in these two articles, and then come to a considered conclusion, supported by your own arguments, regarding an answer to the question posed.

7. Read critically the article by Ladd (1989), "Computers and Moral Responsibility." Summarize the main points and assess their validity. What do you conclude about the responsibility for computer errors (failures, malfunctions, and programming errors)? What does the concept of diffused or collective responsibility do to the fundamental concept of responsibility?

8. In some legal contexts, corporations can be considered as persons, because it is *persons* who make and break contracts and who can be held responsible for damage caused by their actions. Examine this concept of corporations as persons more closely, and then consider whether it can be extended to considering computers and computer systems (or robots) as persons in certain legal contexts. This is an open question with no "pat" answer.

■ REFERENCES AND RECOMMENDED READINGS

"ACM Code of Ethics and Professional Conduct." *Communications of the ACM* 32, 2 (February 1993), 100–105.

Anderson, Ronald E., Deborah G. Johnson, Donald Gotterbarn, and Judith Perrolle. *Communications of the ACM* 36, 2 (February 1993), 98–106.

Anthes, Gary H. "Government Security Efforts Neglect Corporate Needs." *Computerworld* 28, 19 (May 9, 1994), 30.

Aristotle. *Nicomachean Ethics*, Book III.

Bayles, Michael D. *Professional Ethics*. Belmont, CA: Wadsworth, 1989.

Bechtel, William. "Attributing Responsibility to Computer Systems." *Metaphilosophy* 16, 4 (October 1985), 296–305.

Beusmans, Jack, and Karen Wieckert. "Computing, Research, and War: If Knowledge Is Power, Where Is Responsibility?" *Communications of the ACM* 32, 8 (August 1989), 939–56.

Boyle, James. *Shamans, Software, and Spleens: Law and the Construction of the Information Society*. Cambridge, MA: Harvard University Press, 1996.

Brown, Geoffrey. *The Information Game: Ethical Issues in a Microchip World*. Atlantic Highlands, NJ: Humanities Press, 1990, chs. 2, 9, 10.

Cangialosi, Charles. "The Electronic Underground: Computer Piracy and Electronic Bulletin Boards." *Rutgers Computer and Technology Law Journal* 15 (1989), 265–301.

Charles, Robert. "Computer Bulletin Boards and Defamation: Who Should Be Liable? Under What Standard?" *Journal of Law and Technology* 2 (1987), 121–50.

Collins, W. Robert, Keith W. Miller, Bethany J. Spielman, and Phillip Wherry. "How Good Is Good Enough?" *Communications of the ACM* 37, 1 (January 1994), 81–91.

Computer Crime and Computer Security: Hearing Before the Subcommittee on Crime, U.S. House of Representatives, May 23, 1985. Washington, DC: Government Printing Office, 1986.

Dejoie, Roy, George Fowler, and David Paradice, eds. *Ethical Issues in Information Systems*. Boston, MA: Boyd & Fraser, 1991, ch. 2.

DiCato, Edward M. "Operator Liability Associated with Maintaining a Computer Bulletin Board." *Software Law Journal* 4 (1990), 147–59.

Dunlop, Charles, and Rob Kling, eds. *Computerization and Controversy: Value Conflicts and Social Choices.* Boston, MA: Academic Press, 1991, Part VII.

Ermann, M. David, Claudio Gutierrez, and Mary B. Williams, eds. *Computers, Ethics, and Society.* New York: Oxford University Press, 1990, Part III.

Feinberg, Joel. "Sua Culpa." From *Doing and Deserving: Essays in the Theory of Responsibility.* Princeton, NJ: Princeton University Press, 1970. Also in Deborah G. Johnson and John W. Snapper, eds. *Ethical Issues in the Use of Computers* (Belmont, CA: Wadsworth, 1985), 102–120.

Forester, Tom, and Perry Morrison. *Computer Ethics: Cautionary Tales and Ethical Dilemmas in Computing.* 2nd ed. Cambridge, MA: MIT Press, 1994, chs. 5, 7.

Freud, Sigmund. *Civilization and Its Discontents.* New York: W.W. Norton, 1961.

Friedman, Jonathan A., and Francis M. Buono, "Limiting Tort Liability for Online Third-party Content Under Section 230 of the Communications Act." *Federal Communications Law Journal* 52, 3 (May 2000), 647–665.

Hart, H. L. A. "Punishment and Responsibility." From "Postscript: Responsibility and Retribution," in *Punishment and Responsibility: Essays in the Philosophy of Law* (New York: Oxford University Press, 1968). Also in Johnson and Snapper, 1985, 95–101.

Hayes, Arthur S. "Establishing Liability for Computer Viruses." *Wall Street Journal*, 26 October 1990, sec. B, p. 1.

Hollander, Patricia A. *Computers in Education: Legal Liabilities and Ethical Issues Concerning Their Use and Misuse.* Asheville, NC: College Administration Publications, 1986.

"IEEE Code of Ethics." Institute of Electrical and Electronics Engineers.

Jensen, Eric C. "An Electronic Soapbox: Computer Bulletin Boards and the First Amendment." *Federal Communications Law Journal* 39, 3 (1987), 217–58.

Johnson, Deborah G. *Computer Ethics.* 2nd ed. Englewood Cliffs, NJ: Prentice-Hall, 1994, chs. 3, 7.

Johnson, Deborah G., and John W. Snapper, eds. *Ethical Issues in the Use of Computers.* Belmont, CA: Wadsworth, 1985, Parts I & II.

Johnson, Jeff, and Evelyn Pine. "Towards a Guide to Social Action for Computer Professionals." *SIGCHI Bulletin* 25, 1 (January 1993), 23–26.

Kaufman, Arnold S. "Responsibility, Moral and Legal." *Encyclopedia of Philosophy*, vol. 7. New York: Macmillan, 1967, pp. 183–88.

Ladd, John. "Computers and Moral Responsibility: A Framework for an Ethical Analysis." In Carol C. Gould, ed., *The Information Web: Ethical and Social Implications of Computer Networking* (Boulder, CO: Westview Press, 1989), pp. 207–27. Also in Dunlop and Kling, 1991, 664–75.

Lessig, Larry. *Code: And Other Laws of Cyberspace.* New York: Basic Books, 1999.

Lessig, Larry. "The Law of the Horse." **www.harvard.edu/lessig.html**

Lessig, Larry. "The Laws of Cyberspace." In Spinello and Tavani, 2001, pp. 124–34.

Leveson, N., and C. Turner. "An Investigation of the Therac–25 Accidents." *Computer* 26, 7 (1993), 18–41.

Lucas, J. R. *Responsibility.* Oxford, England: Clarendon Press, 1993.

Luegenbiehl, Heinz C. "Codes of Ethics and the Moral Education of Engineers." *Business and Professional Ethics Journal* 2, 4 (1983), 41–61.

Martin, C. Dianne, and David H. Martin. "Professional Codes of Conduct and Computer Ethics Education." *Computers & Society* 20, 2 (June 1990), 18–29.

Mayo, Bernard. *The Philosophy of Right and Wrong: An Introduction to Ethical Theory.* London: Routledge and Kegan Paul, 1986.

Moor, James H. "Are There Decisions Computers Should Never Make?" *Nature and System* 1 (1979), 217–29. In Johnson and Snapper, 1985, 120–30.

Moore, Thomas H. "Colleges Seem Vulnerable to Legal Actions Arising from Computer Viruses." *Chronicle of Higher Education* 35, 42 (June 28, 1989), A1, A20.

Mowshowitz, Abbe. *Conquest of Will: Information Processing in Human Affairs.* Reading, MA: Addison-Wesley, 1976, chs. 11–13.

Nissenbaum, Helen. "Computing and Accountability." *Communications of the ACM* 37, 1 (January 1994), 73–80.

Nycum, Susan. "Liability for Malfunction of a Computer Program." *Rutgers Journal of Computers, Technology, and the Law* 7 (1979), 1–22. Also in Johnson and Snapper, 1985, 67–78.

Prince, Jim. "Negligence: Liability for Defective Software." *Oklahoma Law Review* 33 (1980), 848–55. Also in Johnson and Snapper, 1985, 89–94.

Samuelson, Pamela. "Can a Computer Be an Author?" In Ermann et al., eds. *Computers, Ethics & Society* (New York: Oxford University Press, 1990), pp. 299–307.

Samuelson, Pamela. "Can Hackers Be Sued for Damages Caused by Computer Viruses?" *Communications of the ACM* 32, 6 (June 1989), 666–69.

Samuelson, Pamela. "The Copyright Grab." *Wired* 4, 1 (1996). www.wired.com:80/wired/archive/4.01/white.paper_pr.html

Savage, John E., Susan Magidson, and Alex M. Stein. *The Mystical Machine: Issues and Ideas in Computing.* Reading, MA: Addison-Wesley, 1986.

Sawyer, Fay H. "What Should Professional Societies Do About Ethics?" *Journal of Professional Issues in Engineering* 110, 2 (April 1984), 88–99. Also in Johnson and Snapper, 1985, 43–50.

Smith, Brian Cantwell. *Limits of Correctness in Computers.* (Presented at a Symposium on Unintentional Nuclear War at the Fifth Congress of the International Physicians for the Prevention of Nuclear War, Budapest, Hungary, June 28–July 1, 1985.) Stanford, CA: Center for the Study of Language and Information, 1985. Reprinted in Dunlop and Kling, 1991, pp. 632–46.

Snapper, John W. "Responsibility for Computer-Based Errors." *Metaphilosophy* 16, 4 (October 1985), 289–95.

Spinello, Richard A. *Cyberethics: Morality and Law in Cyberspace.* Sudbury, MA: Jones and Bartlett, 2000.

Spinello, Richard A., and Herman T. Tavani, eds. *Readings in Cyberethics.* Sudbury, MA: Jones and Bartlett, 2001.

Tribe, Laurence H. "The Constitution in Cyberspace." In Ermann, 1990, pp. 208–20.

Waldrop, M. Mitchell. *Man-Made Minds: The Promise of Artificial Intelligence.* New York: Walker, 1987, ch. 11.

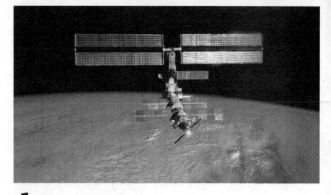

Chapter 11

Computers, the Government, and the Military

 INFORMATION AND POWER

It has been said that "knowledge is power"; it has also been said that "power corrupts." The logical inference is obvious, that "knowledge corrupts." But surely this does not refer to all kinds of knowledge: Some knowledge is good, such as the knowledge of how to heal the sick, or feed the hungry. Kant made the appropriate distinction when making his case that the only thing that is good without qualification is the *good will*. He pointed out that knowledge without a good will, such as the knowledge of an expert torturer, could be bad.

Knowledge can be power in the sense of a power to *understand*—the world, human nature, and the like. Again, such knowledge, like free choice, can be used for good or for evil. One person might use a knowledge of human nature to manipulate and dominate people; it is *this* kind of knowledge that would corrupt.

Knowledge is related to information in various ways (see Chapter 9). One may know *that* (some piece of information is true), or one may be said to know *how* (to do certain things, which may involve manipulating information about them). I may be said to *know that* today is Tuesday (a piece of information I checked against my calendar, a repository of information); I *know how* to play tennis—which means a number of things, including that I at one time or other exercised this knowledge by actually playing, since before that I had only theoretical knowledge about the game, but might not have been sure how to apply it.

Since information has become such a "hot" commodity (as we discussed in Chapter 7), those who have lots of information—about the stock market, or consumer preferences, or the presence of oil deposits—can get rich. The rich are also very powerful in our society, and can control people, companies, and even, at times, politicians.

It is also true that a government that has control of a great deal of information will have control over a great many people. In Orwell's *1984*, "Big Brother" maintained its power by having information on what everyone in the society was doing. It exercised that power by bombarding the population with Newspeak phrases ("war is peace," "freedom is slavery," "ignorance is strength") which kept them off-balance and easily manipulated. But of course the United States is not at all like Orwell's Oceania—or is it becoming more like it every day?

 ## BIG GOVERNMENT

Locke, whose writings served as a model for much of the design of the fledgling government of the United States, believed in minimalist government—a government governs best that governs least. Of course, he did not anticipate the sheer size of governments that would arise in the twentieth century; perhaps this is one reason that our current government does not meet Locke's criterion, but rather is a huge bureaucratic structure.

Record-Keeping and Surveillance

We have seen that computers create hitherto undreamed-of capabilities to collect, handle, analyze, and disseminate vast amounts of information. Some of the largest and fastest computers belong to the federal government, in its various agencies. We saw that there are over 2,000 federal databases, some of which do not even come under the coverage of the Privacy Act. Government investigative agencies (the FBI, the CIA, and the NSA) handle huge amounts of information, using extremely sophisticated computers and programs that generally are years ahead of the technology in the public or industrial domains. Some of that sophistication is hinted at in movies like *A Clear and Present Danger* and *Enemy of the State.*

The government has used extensive surveillance on suspected dissidents for many years. For example, the Kennedy administration kept close track of those who were active in the civil-rights movement, especially Dr. Martin Luther King Jr. In *The Rise of the Computer State,* David Burnham writes:

> This surveillance ultimately involved the placement of electronic bugs in the motels where King stayed as he moved about the country and the subsequent effort to peddle the secretly recorded material to newspaper columnists. During the Johnson administration, concern about race-riots, civil-rights demonstrations and antiwar protests prompted the president to order the army to greatly enlarge its surveillance of citizens, almost all of whom were only exercising the right to speak their minds. The surveillance led to the creation of intelligence files on about 100,000 persons (including Catholic priests and one U.S. senator) and on an equal number of domestic organizations (for example, the National Organization for Women, the John Birch Society and the NAACP). (Burnham, 1983, p. 13)

The CIA carried on similar surveillance under the Johnson administration, even though such activity was in violation of the law under which Congress approved the original establishment of that agency. Burnham writes that President Nixon "knowingly encouraged the White House staff to violate the law by obtaining the computerized tax files on individuals Mr. Nixon did not like. This action served as the basis for one of the proposed articles of impeachment drawn up against Mr. Nixon by the House Judiciary Committee shortly before he resigned" (Burnham, 1983, p. 13).

There have also been stories around for years that some government agencies might have tampered with the files (criminal, credit, and the like) of people believed to be subversives, thus undermining their chances for jobs, loans, and so forth. Whether or not this is actually true, the computerized files (some of which most people are not even aware exist) provide a natural playground for such activity. It was such suspicions, or the awareness of the potential for such activity, that gave rise to the creation of the Privacy Act in 1974.

If the government databases contain, on the average, 25 files on each adult American, there is a total of over 6 billion such files in existence. The sheer volume of this information increases the likelihood for errors in these files. The superbureaus like TRW (now Experian) operate on a somewhat smaller scale, but demonstrate the possibility of such errors. TRW was taken to court in 1976 by an Ohio resident who had been denied a mortgage due to incorrect data in his file, about which he informed TRW but they failed to correct. TRW argued that "it has no obligation to determine the accuracy of the information it receives from businessmen about the bill-paying habits of individual customers. 'Put another way,' said Avern Cohn, the federal district judge who handled the case, TRW contends 'it was an error to allow the jury to consider whether there is an obligation on the defendant [TRW] to test truthfulness and/or accuracy of the information it receives'" (Burnham, 1983, pp. 43–44).

Burnham reported that every year "about 350,000 individual subjects become sufficiently upset to register a formal complaint with the company's consumer relations department about the accuracy of TRW reports. And each year as many as 100,000 of these contacts result in TRW changing the information in the computers" (Burnham, 1983, p. 45). If there are that many errors that are noticed in a large system like this, it is probably only the tip of the iceberg, and many more are likely to go unnoticed. People are generally sensitive to things that affect their credit status, and so may be more likely to check with credit bureaus, Furthermore, there are other credit bureaus that collect credit data on you without your permission. How many more *unnoticed* errors are there in the government databases, and what effects could they have on people's lives?

Kent Greenwalt, a professor at Columbia University's Law School, suggested serious consequences of the government record-keeping in a report to the White House:

> If there is increased surveillance and disclosure and it is not offset by greater tolerance, the casualties of modern society are likely to increase as fewer misfits and past wrongdoers are able to find jobs and fruitful associations. The knowledge that one cannot discard one's past, that advancement in society depends heavily on a good record, will create considerable pressure for conformist actions. Many people will try harder than they do now to keep their records clean, avoid controversial or "deviant" actions, whatever their private views and inclinations. Diversity and social vitality is almost certain to suffer, and in the long run independent private thoughts will be reduced.[1]

One of the points illustrated here is that computers have incredibly long memories. They will retain a piece of data, right or wrong, forever, unless it is deliberately deleted. Some states, like Florida and Connecticut, require the erasure of all criminal and arrest records if the person is acquitted or not prosecuted (Freedman, 1987, p. 94). However, many other systems fail to delete or correct erroneous records, and the incorrect information may remain in the files for many years.

Government Applications of Computers

Large bureaucratic governments today could not run without computers. They have become so complex, and have such tremendous record-keeping requirements, that only computers can do the job. It is as if computers came into major use just in the nick of time to save governments that were about to sink into the chaos of paperwork they generate. Intelligence agencies today rely very heavily on computer analysis. The Defense Department uses computerized simulations ("war games") to assess the probable effects of various actions that might be taken, and also have computerized systems making military decisions.

In 1984, a mobile sentry robot called PROWLER (Programmable Robot Observer with Logical Enemy Response) was completed. It resembles a small tank and is programmed to patrol an area and identify intruders. Its obvious advantages are that it "obeys orders" unquestioningly and does not tire or need sleep. It can carry weapons, such as M60 machine guns and a grenade launcher, though the military said it had no plans to arm it, but just have it send a warning message to intruders.[2] Yet if it has been designed with the capacity to use weapons, why would this design feature not be used? One is reminded of the mobile police unit, ED–209 (Enforcement Droid 209), in the movie *Robocop*, which developed a "glitch" and blew away a civilian who had thrown down his weapon.

Data from weather satellites can be fed into government supercomputers to make much more accurate predictions of the weather, which can be used to track hurricanes and predict tornado warnings, and are particularly useful for aircraft and ships at sea. Such data, in addition to information on land under cultivation, can be used by the Agriculture Department to make crop predictions and thus help make agricultural policy.[3]

The Library of Congress has computer access to files containing the Congressional Record, and congressional committees make use of an on-line system to develop budgets. A Correspondence Management System contains a record of the stands taken on recent issues by various senators, and members of Congress can query a computer system called LEGIS for up-to-date information on the status of various bills and a system called SOPAD contains a summary record of recent debates in Congress.[4]

The National Security Agency

The average American may know little or nothing about the National Security Agency (NSA). We all hear a lot about the FBI and the CIA, but little about NSA. This may well have something to do with the fact that it is not directly responsible to Congress and is not covered by any laws passed by Congress. It was created in 1952 by a secret order from President Truman, and it has operated under White House directives since then. "So intense was the secrecy, in fact, that during the first few years of the NSA's life its mere existence as an arm of the Defense Department was not acknowledged in an official manual of the U.S. government" (Burnham, 1983, p. 122).

NSA deals primarily in surveillance, on a budget many times greater than that of the CIA. So much paperwork is generated in their work that they needed a $2 million incinerator capable of destroying 72,000 pounds of classified papers each day. Since we have been talking earlier about Orwell and his *1984*, one cannot help being reminded of the following passage from *Animal Farm*:

> There was, as Squealer was never tired of explaining, endless work in the supervision and organisation of the farm. Much of this work was of a kind that the other animals were too ignorant to understand. For example, Squealer told them that the pigs had to expend enormous labours every day upon mysterious things called "files," "reports," "minutes," and "memoranda." These were large sheets of paper which had to be closely covered with writing, and as soon as they were so covered, they were burnt in the furnace. This was of the highest importance for the welfare of the farm. But still, neither pigs nor dogs produced any food by their own labour; and there were very many of them, and their appetites were always good. (Orwell [1946], 1956, p. 119)

As Burnham points out, the lack of a legal charter means that the NSA is not bound by the principle that all government agencies must be subject to checks and balances. This means that NSA employees operate outside of the law, because the law does not cover them, and they are accountable not to the Congress or the people, but presumably only to the president.

> The National Security Agency has two broad goals, one offensive, one defensive. First, the NSA attacks the communication links of the world searching for the foreign intelligence that can be gained by intercepting telephone messages and other electronic messages and intercepting the signals generated by such events as the launching of a missile or the operation of a radar set. Second, the NSA defends the communication links that carry information bearing on the national security of the United States from penetration by the spies of other nations. (Burnham, 1983, p. 123)

The NSA is supported by billions of dollars to maintain its array of computers, satellites, operatives, and surveillance equipment.

After Watergate, the Senate Select Committee on Intelligence investigated suspected abuses by the NSA and other federal intelligence agencies. "In speeches and statements made during the course of this investigation, the committee's chairman, Senator Frank Church, repeatedly emphasized his belief that the NSA's intelligence-gathering activities were essential to the security of the United States. But he also emphasized that the NSA was a serious threat to freedom" (Burnham, 1983, p. 125). This view presents the country with a serious dilemma: "NSA—can't live with 'em, can't live without 'em."

Church once observed that the NSA equipment used to monitor the Russians could just as readily "monitor the private communications of Americans" and creates "a tremendous potential for abuse." If NSA's surveillance power was ever directed against communication in the United States, "no American would have any privacy left. . . . There would be no place to hide" (reported in Burnham, 1983, p. 124). Burnham continues the thought:

> It was the NSA, after all, that picked up the electronic order from Tripoli authorizing the Libyan diplomats in the United States to give money to the president's brother. It was an NSA spy satellite called Ferret that some years ago reportedly reached down from the edge of space and recorded the voice of Nikita Khruschev giving orders on the mobile telephone in his speeding limousine. (Burnham, 1983, p. 126)

If they can "tap" Khruschev in his limousine, why not you on the phone in the "privacy" of your own home?

The NSA also has the power to issue security directives. Some of these have been rather interesting, in light of our previous discussion of privacy and autonomy. National Security Division Directive (NSDD) 84 required 120,000 federal employees to agree to lifetime reviews by the government of *anything* they wanted to publish.[5] Admiral Inman, as an NSA official, requested (in the interest of national security) that all scientists working in the area of cryptography submit their research to NSA for review before it could be published (Burnham, 1983, pp. 139–44).

NSDD 145, signed by President Reagan in 1984, arose out of a fear of an information "mosaic" that could be interpreted, by anyone who attended carefully, to reveal national secrets. Admiral Poindexter, then head of the NSA, drafted this directive to restrict unclassified information relating to national security and "other government interests," and to take a "comprehensive and coordinated approach" to restricting all foreign access to telecommunications and computer systems. This directive was withdrawn in 1987 under pressure from the Congress, fearing that it opened the door to government monitoring of all computer systems; however, the policy is still in effect. NSDD 189 reflects an effort by the Department of Defense and the

National Science Foundation to restrict foreign students' access to super-computers in U.S. universities.[6]

Other Agency Restrictions on Freedoms

We discussed the passage of the 1994 FBI Wiretap Bill, that exists in spite of widespread opposition from various concerned groups. The impact of this law is yet to be seen, but the opposition raised many serious doubts regarding its impact on privacy. Certainly, at the very least, it will make FBI wiretapping much easier than it has been in the past, at our expense.

In his book *Decent Interval*, a former CIA official named Frank Snepp described the last days of the U.S. presence in Vietnam and his criticisms of the U.S. efforts. The Supreme Court (by a six-member majority) held that Snepp had violated his contractual obligations to the government by giving Random House the manuscript before it had been approved by the CIA's publication review board. Snepp's royalties ($140,000) were denied to him; all royalties, past and future, were assigned to the U.S. government (Burnham, 1983, pp. 171–72). One is reminded of the movie *Hopscotch* in which Walter Matthau, as a former CIA agent, spills the beans on a number of covert operations in a book—but Matthau gets away with it, by faking his death! Snepp has published an account of the government attack on him called *Irreparable Harm: A Firsthand Account of How One Agent Took on the CIA in an Epic Battle Over Free Speech* (Random House, 1999).

Blame the Computer!

In 1969, when President Nixon decided to keep secret the bombing raids against Cambodia, a programmer for the Defense Department simply adjusted the Pentagon computer program to report these raids as raids on targets in Vietnam. These reports were then submitted to the Senate Armed Forces Committee. This followed a memorandum from Defense Secretary Melvin Laird and General Earle Wheeler, Chairman of the Joint Chiefs of Staff, which said: "All sorties against targets in Cambodia will be programmed against preplanned targets in the Republic of Vietnam and strike messages will so indicate."

Admiral Thomas H. Morer, then Chairman of the Joint Chiefs of Staff, was called to testify four years later to the same Senate committee that had received the doctored reports. He argued that the errors were the fault of the computer system:

The raids against the Cambodian targets, he said, carried such a high classification that information about them could not be recorded in the Pentagon's computer, which was authorized to store only lesser categories of military secrets. But it was absolutely essential that the flying time consumed by these most secret raids somehow be noted in the central computer so that the fuel, bombs and other supplies actually used in sending the B–52s over Cambodia were accounted for and therefore replaced in the supply line. This was the only reason, he explained, why the program in the Pentagon computer had been adjusted so that the geographic coordinates of the actual targets in Cambodia appeared in the printouts as the coordinates of targets in Vietnam.

"It's unfortunate that we have become slaves to these damned things," Admiral Morer told the committee. (Burnham, 1983, p. 146)

What has become of government accountability if, whenever something goes wrong, it is blamed on the computer?

It is also disturbing that there is a tendency to take whatever comes out of a computer as gospel, when anyone familiar with software problems knows the probability of error. It is also possible for a programmer to get a computer to print out whatever the programmer wants it to, and make it look like the result of a long and arduous analysis and calculation. All the programmer has to do is set up the program to run a respectable amount of time, and then insert a statement that will output whatever result the programmer desires. For example, imagine a program that was supposed to determine, "scientifically," who the next president of the United States should be. The programmer could manipulate the result as desired. This is similar to a book about statistics that was called *How to Lie with Statistics*; someone could write a book called *How to Lie with Computers*.

Big Business Influences Big Government

The other groups that have the big computers and thus control large amounts of information are the large corporations in the United States. They control powerful lobbies in the Congress, and often influence political debate. A wealthy businessman (Ross Perot) ran for president in 1992, suggesting that the country should be run just like a business. The problem with that, of course, is that an employee is somewhat less than autonomous, determined greatly by what the "boss" wants; that is not a model for a free society.

The European community adopted a Declaration of Mass Communication Media and Human Rights in 1970, which affirmed the following:

> The right to privacy consists essentially in the right to live one's own life with a minimum of interference. It concerns private, family, and home life, physical and moral integrity, honor and reputation, avoidance of being placed in a false light, nonrevelation of irrelevant and embarrassing facts, unauthorized publication of private photographs, protection from disclosure of information given or received by the individual confidentially.[7]

The European Union (EU, formerly called the European Community) considered "the adoption of sweeping rules for computerized information like personal medical and insurance records and airline reservation records that would restrict their use by businesses and government agencies" (Markoff, 1991, p. A1), and this gave rise to the EU Privacy Directive, that went into effect October 25, 1998. The proposals would prohibit publishers from selling lists of subscribers without their agreement, banks would have to notify customers before selling their names to mail-order companies, and restrictions would be placed on the use that employers could make of their employees' records. Companies would also not be permitted to transfer personal data to another country unless that country offered similar records protection. See www.sans.org/infosecFAQ/infowar/shelter.htm for the regulatory principles of the Data Protection Directive.

The American business community is quite concerned about the impact this may have on the way they do business. The use of "smart cards" that contain financial information about customers has been under consideration but might be unacceptable in Europe given these new guidelines. Extensive lobbying was going on at the time of Markoff's article (1991), by corporations such as Reader's Digest and American Express, against the European proposal. Questions have arisen whether the Directive is illegal under World Trade Organization (WTO) rules such as the General Agreement on Tariffs and Trade (GATT). It will be interesting to see how much influence big-business interest has when weighed against private interest by the politicians in Congress (Markoff, 1991, pp. A1, D1). For a thorough discussion of the "Safe Harbor" agreement that tries to reconcile the EU Directive and United States business practices, see:

www.freetrade.org/pubs/pas/tpa–016.pdf

It is also interesting in this context to note that it took the United States until March 1, 1989, to enter the Berne agreement for the protection of literary and artistic works, which was originally signed by many countries on December 9, 1886. The United States became the eightieth member to sign the agreement, 103 years after its initiation. This seems to show U.S. reluctance to join with the international community in agreements to protect artistic rights or the rights of privacy. From the current case regarding privacy, one can only infer that it is because of the influence of big business interests.

Environmental Impact of Computers

We discussed earlier the question of whether computer technology was morally neutral. Another question that should be considered is whether it is *environmentally* neutral. Jerry Mander, in his book *In the Absence of the Sacred*, raises concerns about the threats of *megatechnology* in surveillance invasions of privacy, centralization of power, health hazards at work, and hair-trigger computerized responses to nuclear threats. He also has the following environmental concern:

> Computer manufacturing employs millions of gallons of acids and solvents that are eventually disposed of at toxic dumps. In communities where computers are manufactured, serious problems have arisen. In Silicon Valley, California, for example, high concentrations of trichloroethylene (a solvent that the EPA has called carcinogenic) have seeped into the drinking water. At one point, computer manufacturers, while not admitting guilt, passed out truckloads of bottled water in the affected communities. The Environmental Protection Agency has identified eighty similar chemical spill sites associated with computer manufacturing, and expects the problem to escalate.
>
> Suburban communities affected by toxic wastes have been able to organize to mitigate the problems. But workers who manufacture computers and who have suffered health problems have been less effective. This is because most computer factory workers are nonunion and many are non–English-speaking and undocumented. So they have a hard time telling their story to management and/or the press.[8]

If computer manufacture has serious environmental side effects, this should be examined carefully since the preservation of our environment is an important moral issue. If human beings have value (and we have been proceeding on that assumption as self-evident), then whatever is conducive to their flourishing in a healthful, nonthreatening environment has derivative value.

The industry fosters built-in obsolescence, at a very rapid rate. Not only software, but hardware, is quickly rendered useless, as new bells and whistles are added, and new versions are made incompatible with older systems. This is irresponsible, but unless the government steps in to change the ground rules, greed will prevail. It would seem at least that an industry that creates so much "garbage" in the form of outmoded systems that will choke our landfills should take some responsibility for recycling as much as possible. Japan and some European nations have made positive moves in this direction. So far in the United States, it is only voluntary (see Perry, 1983, and Biddle and Mann, 1993).

CENTRALIZATION VERSUS DECENTRALIZATION OF GOVERNMENT

In 1979, the computer scientist, psychologist, and 1978 Nobel Prize–winning economist Herbert A. Simon wrote a paper entitled "The Consequences of Computers for Centralization and Decentralization," which is still relevant to our concerns today. The serious question, which was addressed by the founding fathers of the United States government in the Federalist and Anti-Federalist papers, is that of just how much power should reside in a centralized government, and how much should be disseminated to state and local authority, and to the people themselves. The concern, expressed eloquently by Patrick Henry, was that if the emerging nation allowed too much centralization of power, they would be exchanging one form of tyranny (that of George III of England) for another.

Simon points out at the beginning of the article that the terms 'centralization' and 'decentralization' are heavily value-laden. "Decentralization is commonly equated with autonomy, self-determination, or even self-actualization. Centralization is equated with bureaucracy (in the pejorative sense of that term) or with authoritarianism and is often named as the prime force in the dehumanization of organizations and the alienation of their members" (Simon, 1980, p. 212).

In his article, Simon concludes that computers have not *caused* greater centralization, but that they can be used to facilitate it. He points out several advantages to centralization (in business and in government): (1) "economy of scale," which means that experts do not have to be distributed widely through the organization, but can operate effectively from a central location (thus requiring fewer experts); (2) the coordination of interdependent activities (presumably so that the "right hand" will know what the "left hand" is doing); (3) a guarantee that the activities of the parts are for the good of the whole. He says: "The cause of centralization, if there has been any, is not the computer but the need to address the whole problem rather than isolated fragments of it. The computer enhances our ability to do this; it does not create the necessity for it" (Simon, 1980, p. 218). Again, it is matters of efficiency that drive us toward centralization; the crucial question remains whether that motion will deprive us of freedom and privacy in its wake.

The computer can be a means of increasing either centralization or decentralization; the choice is ours. The tremendous record-keeping and analysis capabilities of computers could be used by a strong centralized government to monitor and control its citizens; we examined some of the disturbing trends in this direction in Chapter 7, on privacy. On the other hand, the computer can greatly increase individual autonomy (assuming that all have fair access to computing power, a question to be addressed in our discussion of the National Information Infrastructure), and perhaps contribute to making the United States more truly a *participatory* democracy.

 THE INFORMATION SUPERHIGHWAY

The Internet and its problems are a preview of difficulties that we may have with the "Information Superhighway"—officially known as the National Information Infrastructure (NII)—that is high on many agendas at the moment. One problem is *abuse* (from theft of data or funds, to tampering, to invasions of privacy, to imposters,[9] to flaming), and another is *access* (that is, whether everyone will have a fair chance to take advantage of the superhighway, or whether there will be on- and off-ramps restricted to a privileged few).

Goals

Thomas DeLoughry writes of a group of seventy-one organizations planning a campaign to ensure that the information superhighway serves the public interest. Seven principles are suggested to achieve this end:

1. Free access to any information that relates to full participation in society.
2. Guaranteed freedom of speech for users of the superhighway, as well as copyright protection of material accessed.
3. An "electronic commons" for discussion and debate.
4. A "healthy marketplace of ideas" that is open to everyone, and not controlled by the telecommunications carriers.
5. Opportunities to improve work and the workplace (equity).
6. Policies that protect users' privacy.
7. Public involvement in making policy for the network. (DeLoughry, 1993, A23)

To these seven, the Computer Professionals for Social Responsibility (CPSR) adds, based on their "experiences as both designers and users of networking systems," an eighth:

8. Functional integrity. "The functions provided by the NII must be powerful, versatile, well-documented, stable, reliable, and extensible." [10]

Some of these principles have ethical content, and others—such as "functional integrity" and an "electronic commons"—deal with means. The concern with freedom (of access, of speech) is a moral concern, since it is one of the fundamental goods. Privacy may be a fundamental good, a means to fundamental goods, or a natural right, as we discussed in Chapter 7. It is clear that advantages should be equally available to all (equity); this promotes a stable society, and a sense of community, in which friendship can thrive and knowledge can grow.

Some of the major concerns raised by CSPR that must be addressed if the NII is to be successful are whether it will unfairly discriminate regarding access, whether the government and a few powerful corporations will control the system, whether commerce will be emphasized at the expense of communication, whether privacy and security of data and financial assets will be threatened, and whether information will be controlled and even censored.

A Comparison of Concrete and Electronic Highways

An essay entitled "The Ghost in the Modem" by Richard Sclove and Jeffrey Scheuer contains some very insightful observations on the obvious (and not-so-obvious) parallels between the information superhighway and the U.S. interstate highway system. [11] It seems that then Vice President Al Gore, in vigorously supporting the information superhighway, is following in the footsteps of his father, U.S. Senator Al Gore, who championed the Interstate Highway Act in 1956. The authors of the essay point to the fact that the new interstate highway system was not at the time a public mandate, that many people did not even have private automobiles and used public transportation, and that the bill was largely the result of "aggressive lobbying by auto makers and road builders."

The results of the new system of interstate highways, though valuable to many, made things worse for others. In many cities, the new roads simply wiped out "once viable poor and minority neighborhoods"; in other cases, such neighborhoods were encircled by the new roads, thus effectively cutting them off and making them into ghettos. The point is that we must be alert and cautious that analogous things do not happen with the information superhighway—that it does not turn out to be primarily designed by and used by small but powerful special-interest groups, and that it does not make the segregation of poor and minority groups even worse. The goals are exciting and worthwhile, if they are designed for the benefit of all.

Another aspect of NII, one that has not been publicly discussed very much so far, is who will foot the bill for the tremendous costs that will be involved? If the analogy with the interstate highway system is continued, it will be the taxpayers (whether they want it or not, or benefit from it or not). If it is largely private industry that will fund it, will that give them too much control of the system—where it goes, what it will contain? The NII will soon become the GII (Global Information Infrastructure). Who will dominate and who will benefit then? Will the United States try to control the whole system? Will it become a platform for ideological conflict or for agreement?

One should realize that the information superhighway is not something entirely new. Such an information infrastructure has existed in the United States in many forms including the telephone system, radio and television networks, automated banking, credit card systems, airline reservation networks, and families of computer networks like the Internet. Any "superhighway" will be constructed on the roadbed that is already in place.

The Vision of the Government for NII

In 1994, the Clinton administration produced two documents outlining the plans and goals for the National Information Infrastructure. The first was called "Putting the Information Infrastructure to Work" (we will refer to it as *NII-1*); the second was called "The Information Infrastructure: Realizing Society's Goals" (*NII-2*).[12] In a letter introducing the second report, the Clinton Secretary of Commerce Ronald H. Brown says that the "administration is developing a broad vision of an advanced information infrastructure. As an interconnection of computer networks, telecommunication services, and applications, the National Information Infrastructure (NII) can make a difference not just in how people work but in how well they live." [13]

The first report began with a characterization of the "national vision" for the NII: It can "enhance the competetiveness of our **manufacturing** base; increase the speed and efficiency of **electronic commerce**; improve **health** care delivery and control costs; promote the development and accessibility of quality educational and lifelong learning for all Americans; improve environmental monitoring and assessment of our impact on the earth; sustain the role of libraries as agents of democratic and equal access to information; provide government services to the public faster, more responsibly, and more efficiently" (*NII–1*, 1994, p. 1). The premise of this vision should always be kept in view by the public and Congress as the Internet and legislation concerning it continue to develop.

Manufacturing and Commerce   Examples of how business can benefit are provided by both Wal-Mart and General Motors. Wal-Mart became number one in retailing in the United States by investing in "'quick-response' equipment linking each point-of-sale terminal to distribution centers and headquarters," enabling "the company to maintain high service levels and increase sales while preserving one-fourth the inventory investment." Inventory could be restocked quickly and sales could be tracked so that the store was able to stock popular items. In a different arena, "General Motors developed an infrastructure to enable Saturn and its numerous suppliers to operate as one company" (*NII–1*, 1994, p. 11). This contributed to the great success of the Saturn operation. In light of such examples of success stories for big business, we should ask if what one of the characters in Al Capp's *Li'l Abner* once said: "What's good for General Bullmoose is good for the U. S. A.!" is *really* true.

Health Care   In the area of health care, the report claims that the NII will make information about health care providers more readily available, scientific research will lead to more effective and economical medical care, all providers would be able to access the most recent information about medical technologies and treatments, and administrative processes could be simplified and speeded up. Many scenarios of the future are suggested: a sick child is diagnosed at a distance through information obtained via telecommunication connections; a state public health official is able to recognize a tendency toward whooping cough in the children of a community and arrange to send extra vaccine; a doctor is able to practice a new surgical technique on a virtual reality patient (*NII–1*, 1994, pp. 41–42).

Education   In the area of education, it is envisioned that people of all ages will have access to multimedia information sources and instructional software. The NII will allow students to collaborate with others at great distance on projects and give instruction in basic skills and job training. It is admitted that this will require "significant capital investment" (*NII-1*, 1994, pp. 57–68). Here some serious questions need to be asked. Will connection to the NII supplement or largely replace "live" teaching? Granted that multimedia tools can provide an integration of material, do they really surpass the much less expensive combination of textbook, atlas, movie clips, and slides? Or do they just repackage them and make them available to a student isolated at a single terminal instead of in a classroom interacting with other students experiencing the same material?

There has been a long discussion of computer-aided instruction (CAI) programs, and it has been feared that they encourage rote learning and undermine social skills; this undermining of social skills (and responsibility to community) is reflected in many of today's hackers, as discussed earlier. It is not clear that if CAI is repackaged in fancy multimedia guise, it will be any more fundamentally effective. These are serious questions that need to be asked now, before a tremendous investment has been poured down one path that could have been much more effectively used elsewhere in education.[14]

A related issue to that of all this record keeping in and transmittal of education made possible by NII is that of privacy. A disturbing alert from CSPR-announce titled "Privacy at Risk: Educational Records" was received in July 1994. It describes the development of a national network of electronic student records that will be linked to various social service agencies, employers (through WORKLINK), the military, and the justice system. CPSR warns that there is no guarantee that this information will be shared only with the knowledge of students and their parents. A national proposal is asking that children entering kindergarten have Social Security numbers, so that they can be tracked through the system.

Publication 93–03 of the National Education Goals Panel, "empowered by the Goals 2000 bill to oversee education restructuring nationally," recommends that information of each student should include birthweight, prenatal care, number of years in preschool, poverty status, physical and emotional development at ages five and six, data on medical and dental checkups, attitude and personality test results, number and names of people living in household, type of dwelling, and family income. A recent example of record-sharing is cited:

> In Kennewick, WA, over 4,000 kindergarten through fourth graders were rated by their teachers on how often they lie, cheat, sneak, steal, exhibit a negative attitude, act aggressively, and whether they are rejected by their peers. The scores, with names attached, were sent to a private psychiatric center under contract to screen for "at-risk" students who might benefit from its programs. All of this was done without the knowledge and consent of the children or their parents. (CPSR-announce, July 19, 1995)

It seems that the information in an "electronic portfolio" of this kind would follow students through life, and erroneous information—for example, a childhood fight that was recorded as extremely aggressive—could have deleterious effect on a child's future, much as bad credit data or arrest records (even though exonerated) can affect lives, as discussed in Chapter 7.

Environment The *NII-1* report stresses how much a national network will improve environmental monitoring, prediction, and analysis. This is certainly true; a shared, up-to-date information base will help enormously in assessing damage, sending emergency warnings (see also *NII-2*, pp. 89–90, on disaster management), and predicting the results of various remedial actions. We should not, however, let this increased information-handling capacity blind us to the fundamental questions of how to change human activities and attitudes so that the human damage to the environment is greatly slowed.

Libraries The section of *NII-1* on "Libraries and the NII" paints a glowing picture of ubiquitous information for all, of librarians as "managers of both information and knowledge." We have already discussed the importance of distinguishing between knowledge (understanding) and information; an initiative that would tend to conflate them, reducing them to the lowest common denominator of information, would be most unfortunate. The vision of the totally digitized library seems unrealistic. Clifford Stoll (1995) points out that the actual process of digitizing books and magazines is very slow, error-prone, and very expensive. Would the result be that only the most recent material would get digitized (say, from 1975 forward)? Just the prospect of keeping up with what is published new every year would seem overwhelming.

If electronic searches were to become the *modus operandi*, what would happen to earlier books that weren't deemed "cost-effective" to transform? Would they just get ignored? Would libraries even continue to stock them, once they have "gone digital"? Is it really going to be more cost-effective for every scholar at a university to download, or order through Interlibrary Loan, copies of articles of interest, when a single copy of the article in a physical journal would have served many scholars? And what of digitized books? Will you carry them around with you, read them in cars and buses, or late at night in bed? Stoll discusses how uncomfortable it was to take his lap-top to bed to read a novel. The evolution of e-books raises a whole new set of questions.

Even *NII-1* admits that copyrights present somewhat of a problem to the digitized libraries they envision. We discussed at some length in Chapter 4 the concerns for protecting intellectual property rights in a computer environment. Our discussion there concentrated primarily on computer software, but here we are concerned with the "software" of books and magazines. Protection of intellectual property is supposed to encourage the writers to do excellent work, not only to spread their ideas, but stimulated by the attendant rewards. How are such rewards to be preserved in a system where all intellectual property is digital and can be easily transmitted anywhere and perfectly copied?

Pamela Samuelson hypothesizes a future picture in which the Library of Congress buys one copy of a book (or actually just demands the copy in compliance with the copyright law, which states that a copy must be deposited with them). After this first sale (or no sale), the Library of Congress, free to all, then makes the book available to all comers through Interlibrary Loan. The libraries involved may even have facilities that allow the users to make (download) personal copies of the book. Samuelson then says, "If the economic assumptions underlying copyright law are valid . . . one could expect fewer authors to write fewer works and/or share less of their work with others" under this scenario.[15]

A possible solution to the problem of the first sale being the last sale might be to have a pay-per-use arrangement, where each user who accesses the work must pay to do so. How would this work, and how much should each user have to pay? I often just quickly skim a book to see if it is of interest to me; would I have to pay the same rate as a library user who accesses and downloads the entire book? If downloading facilities are not available, must users read the book in its entirety *at* the library, or must they own a home computer through which they can access the library copy? Samuelson suggests a sort of "celestial jukebox" where users connected to the network can order books or movies of their choice.[16] One advantage of this arrangement would be that the single copy of the digitized book could be accessed at the same time by many users, unlike current library copies.

Will access to the future digitized libraries be free and available to all? The costs will be greater than with conventional libraries, and computer systems must be purchased and maintained by both the libraries and the users. Is this really going to improve the way things are? Will computerized searches really be better than current searches which, granted, can be aided by computerized databases such as Periodical Abstracts, or will they fail to catch many of the related categories, and older references, an old-fashioned search finds?

As in the other areas we discussed, we should not be Luddites shaking our fists at the future. But we should look carefully and critically at the differences between promise and hype, between what realistically will bring real gains and what may, in the long run, create net losses (of privacy, information, understanding, and human closeness and sympathy).

Some Dissenting Voices

Discussion of the NII continues, and it certainly is lively. CPSR solemnly praises its possibilities for good, but expresses deep concerns about whether access will truly be equitable, and whether the Net will just be turned into a pervasive shopping network by profit-seekers. There are stronger voices of dissent as well.

Jacques-Yves Cousteau wrote an editorial in the August 1995 issue of *Calypso Log* that attributes "mental pollution" to the Information Highway:

> I took up the defense of the image, the beautiful image, that should reflect the real world and not the fads that pervert it. Today, I want to contribute to saving what we have left of good sense and intellect. Let us be serious: The toll imposed at the gateway to information superhighways is much too high. We already have great difficulty using the data available to us on the information byways. The mind is to be cultivated and irrigated, not flooded. (Cousteau, 1995, p. 3)

Jeffrey Johnson of CPSR, who characterized himself as the "designated curmudgeon" at the 1995 ACM Conference of Human-Computer Interaction (CHI '95), shared his comments while participating in a panel on the information superhighway.[17] The title of his remarks was, "Information Superhighway or Superhypeway?" The first flaw he sees in the hype is the vision of the NII as primarily a way to make money, order pizza, and get entertainment on demand. It should instead "provide access to government and government officials, better ways to deliver government services, ways to make democracy more participatory, and educational tools." It should connect people with each other.

The second flaw Johnson sees is that the discussion so far has been based too much on "best-case analyses." It is being "sold to the public primarily by companies that have a stake in its commercial success." One must be concerned with the cost and ease of access, and the fact that computer equipment quickly becomes obsolete and has to be replaced. We should be sensitive to the possibilities of an onslaught of junk mail, the posting on bulletin boards of offensive and even pornographic material, the possibilities of censorship and the potential for snooping.

There is disagreement about the value of the Net to the disabled. The *NII-2* report writes glowingly of how it will reduce barriers to full participation in society, to business and employment, and to communication and access. It will also reduce language and literacy barriers for the disadvantaged and the disabled. It also says it will reduce injuries to information workers (*NII-2*, 1994, pp. 10–12). Jeffrey Johnson, on the other hand, says that "handicapped people will find most of the network's services inaccessible." As with any serious ethical problem we face, we must begin by trying to assess the relevant facts. Only then can we proceed to evaluate the moral potential of this new technology.

Clifford Stoll, author of *The Cuckoo's Egg* and no stranger to computer networks, has serious reservations about the information highway, which he discusses at length in his book, *Silicon Snake Oil* (1995). He fears that today's computer networks isolate people, "cheapen the meaning of actual experience," act against literacy and creativity, and will undermine education and libraries (Stoll, p. 3). He writes, "for all this communication, little of the information is genuinely useful" (Stoll, 1995, p. 2).

If you look critically at what is written to most of the bulletin boards on the Net, you will find a lot of "kvetching" and uncritical personal reflections, but little of real worth. The idea of free access to publishing sounds great, until one reflects critically on what publishers and editors do for us. They screen out the chaff, they make authors write more clearly and to the point. If I read an article in a journal, I know that it has had to pass muster with some serious critics before getting published, so I am less likely to find it a waste of time.

Stoll warns against our becoming mystically lured by the Net, and becoming lotus-eaters (a reference to Homer's *Odyssey*, not *1-2-3*). He emphasizes that "life in the real world is far more interesting, far more important, far richer, than anything you'll ever find on a computer screen" (Stoll, 1995, p. 13). He refers to those who work in a "digital dungeon" (p. 96) tied to entering data into a voracious computer, and to the Net as a "trendy medium" (p. 104) for the rich, a "digital dumpster" (p. 193).

Stoll says that those who sell the silicon snake oil promise that "computers and networks will make a better society"; but, he argues, "there are no simple technological solutions to social problems. There's plenty of distrust and animosity between people who communicate perfectly well. Access to a universe of information cannot solve our problems; we will forever struggle to understand one another" (p. 50). We have discussed the difference between information and understanding: one is helpful—a means; the other is critical—an end in itself.

The important question with respect to the hype of NII is will it, and can it, deliver what it promises, and not just become a pawn of big business? Will it really be to the benefit of society as a whole, and will all be able to take advantage of it?

If so, how? Is giving the poor a tax break for buying a computer going to help those so poor that they pay no taxes? Is the promise of giving every citizen a computer more important than seeing that they have enough food, clothing, health care, and a decent place to live? We must be sure that we have our priorities straight, and to do this we must look to the hierarchy of goods. Knowledge (understanding) is one of the highest-level goods, but we must ask ourselves whether the Net will promote understanding or just convey information, much of which is of little value? How are we to sort through all the information to find what *is* of value? This requires real *education*, not just throwing more information/data at us. Furthermore, knowledge can only be sought by someone who is alive and healthy enough to carry out the quest.

Some time ago, Richard O. Mason articulated the four major issues of the information age as Privacy, Accuracy, Property, and Access (PAPA).[18] These four issues should be kept at the forefront of our vision when considering the information highway.

The information highway will be what we (and Congress, which is supposed to represent our interests) make of it. Messages coming from those who question the hype seem to say "consider the source" of the best-case scenarios, look carefully at the costs versus the benefits (how utilitarian!), and don't allow ourselves to be rushed into a huge commitment and expenditure at electronic speed without careful consideration. Winn Schwartau writes: "A national Information Policy shouldn't be thrown together piecemeal or be allowed to evolve from political, technical, or special-interest whims. It must be comprehensive and as all-inclusive as possible."[19]

Since these concerns were voiced, the Internet has enjoyed an amazing popularity, as a vehicle for commerce and for research (though one has to be careful about the quality of sources in doing research). However, some of the concerns voiced here at the inception of this phenomenon should be kept in mind as it continues to grow and mutate.

NUCLEAR THREATS

Norbert Wiener, the "father of cybernetics," wrote some very dire projections in *The Human Use of Human Beings* (1950) and expressed great concern over the future of humanity. He was writing in the aftermath of World War II, and the bombing of Hiroshima and Nagasaki. Humans have created weapons which can bring about their own extinction and the destruction of this planet. Wiener writes, "The effect of these weapons must be to increase the entropy of this planet, until all distinctions of hot and cold, good and bad, man and matter have vanished in the formation of the white furnace of a new star" (Wiener, 1950, p. 142).

Wiener bemoans the fact that those in political power often have too little perspective on the long-term good for the nation and humanity: "It is one of the paradoxes of the human race, and possibly its last paradox, that the people who control the fortunes of our community should at the same time be wildly radical in matters that concern our own change of our environment, and rigidly conservative in the social matters that determine our adaptation to it" (Wiener, 1950, p. 56). This can be seen in a government that spends billions on weapons and "defense" but is reluctant to spend much on social programs and education. Our scientific achievements have brought us to the brink of what could be a cataclysmic disaster. "The hour is very late, and the choice of good and evil knocks at our door" (Wiener, 1950, p. 213).

Wiener makes reference to the story "The Monkey's Paw," by W. W. Jacobs. In this story, a man comes into possession of a monkey's paw, which it turns out will give him three wishes. His first wish is for two hundred pounds. The next day, a man comes to tell him that his son has been crushed to death in the factory machinery, and the father will receive 200 pounds in liability compensation. About a week later, at his wife's urging, he uses the second wish to wish his son alive again. When something comes knocking at the door, he realizes that it is his son coming from the grave, a frightful thing. So, before his wife can open the door, he uses his third wish to wish the creature gone. The moral of the tale would seem to be, "Be very careful what you wish for." Wiener's reference to the story would seem to suggest that, in wishing for nuclear power, we have conjured up something we cannot control and which may come in the night to destroy us.

Computers and Nuclear Power

The role of computers in this area falls into two parts: the use of computers to monitor and control nuclear energy installations, and the use of computers to monitor and react to nuclear attack. We will discuss the "Star Wars" approach to the second category, that of protection against nuclear attack, in the next section.

The use of computers and computerized robots allows work with nuclear materials that would threaten human lives, so the use of these devices enhances our ability to handle nuclear materials. A "robot proxy" can go into contaminated areas and "see" for the human user through "magic glasses" and handle the material with "magic gloves" controlled by the human.[20] Computers can be used to monitor nuclear reactors, and to initiate emergency procedures should failures occur. This is all to the good, *except* that we have seen that there are difficulties with computer software and system reliability, and the last place we want a computer error to crop up is in controlling a nuclear facility. Thus, precautions and backup systems must make the system as close to foolproof as humanly and computer-ly possible.

 # COMPUTERS AND THE MILITARY

Computers are coming more and more into use in military planning and action, as was brought dramatically into the homes of Americans as they watched the Gulf War unfold on television. We saw in Chapter 8 that the Patriot missiles were not as successful in that war as we were initially led to believe, but it is clear that the idea of computer-controlled weapons is becoming more and more of the reality in warfare. Manuel De Landa, in *War in the Age of Intelligent Machines*, writes:

> For centuries, military commanders have dreamed of eliminating the human element from the battlefield. When Frederick the Great assembled his armies in the eighteenth century, he did not have the technology to eliminate human bodies from the space of combat, but he did manage to eliminate the human will. He put together his armies as a well-oiled clockwork mechanism whose components were robot-like warriors. No individual initiative was allowed to Frederick's soldiers. (DeLanda, 1991, p. 127)

When soldiers can make decisions, run for cover, surrender, or take the initiative on their own, they are out of the control of the generals, who would prefer to be *in control*. Thus an army of robot warriors that could fight well would be desirable to most generals. The generals could control their troops' every move, as Frederick controlled his armies through their fear of him. A robot soldier would never question the command of a superior, which is the way military training says things should be.

This scenario would put the generals in absolute control. The advantage would be that human lives would not be lost on the robot battlefield (of course, things could change if computers were to aim weapons at civilian populations). The battle would go to the side with the best technology, and the most robots. It would be a war decided by scientific and financial superiority. In past wars, it has been much cheaper to use human soldiers to die on the battlefield. That would still be true, and tomorrow's generals would have to weigh that in the balance.

In a *Strategic Computing* report from the Defense Advanced Research Projects Agency (DARPA), the following statement is found:

> Instead of fielding simple guided missiles or remotely piloted vehicles, we might launch completely autonomous land, sea, and air vehicles capable of complex, far-ranging reconnaissance and attack missions. . . . In contrast with previous computers, the new generation will exhibit human-like, "intelligent" capabilities of planning and reasoning. . . . Using the new technology, machines will perform complex tasks with little human intervention, or even with complete autonomy. . . . The possibilities are quite startling, and could fundamentally change the nature of human conflicts. . . .[21]

Could there be such a thing as an autonomous weapon? What would that *mean*? Where would *responsibility* then lie? Gary Chapman writes:

> Autonomous weapons subvert all international law concerning the just deployment of force because computers can never be punished. The basis of all law is responsibility and the prospect of retribution, which are meaningless to computers. . . . Autonomous weapons would turn what we call war into unreflective, organized, automatic, near-complete destruction. They would empty conflict of its human purpose, consequently making war more senseless than ever, even while it became more devastating.[22]

Could programmers adequately anticipate all of the circumstances that a soldier-robot would have to be ready for? If computerized systems have a very hard time with tasks like tying shoes, even though they can play a master-level game of chess, how will they be able to navigate and function in a complex battlefield situation? Adolf von Schell, a World War I German army captain, wrote in *Battle Leadership*: "Every soldier should know that war is kaleidoscopic, replete with constantly changing, unexpected, confusing situations. Its problems cannot be solved by mathematical formulae or set rules."[23]

Thus the technological problems facing battlefield robots are enormous, but computer-controlled weaponry is much more feasible. The question is, is it reliable? Who will be making the decisions to fire the weapons—a human or the computer? And where will the responsibility lie?

Simulations

Simulation, or modeling, is very important in much scientific and social science research. Models are used when the item modeled is too large (such as a galaxy) to get into the laboratory, or too small (a molecule, for example) to be observed as it exists. They are also used when predictions about the future are to be made; if we know the current state of a system and the laws that govern its behavior, we can look ahead and estimate what it will do in the future. This is what the Club of Rome investigators did in making predictions about when we will run out of various essential fuels and other resources, in their report, *The Limits to Growth*.

In many cases we are dealing with a process that is inherently random in nature, such as a dice game or a roulette wheel, or something we wish to force to be random, such as the old "draft lottery"; or else so little may be known about the laws governing a particular process (such as economic theories, or the structure of the brain) that an assumption of randomness is as good as any—better, perhaps, since it does not introduce any unwarranted bias in a particular direction.

In simulations, we perform "thought-experiments" (*Gedanken-experiments*) with our mathematical models, to see how the system will behave. We build into the model all we currently know about the system, to make it the best "likely story" we can construct. We can then look some time into the future with the model, and predict the system's behavior. We may even "tweak" the model slightly, to see how various changes might affect it. For example, in a global resource model, we might see what overall long-term effect governmental population controls, or restrictions on private transportation, might have. If we are building a model of the brain, we will incorporate all of the current physiological information available; we might then construct a model with as many *neuron* elements as possible, and see if we can simulate learning.[24]

For many of these models, random numbers are needed. We could go to the New York telephone directory, or consult the RAND Corporation's table of "A Million Random Digits," or we could use a computer program called a pseudo-random number generator. These programs are not *truly* random, since they do follow an algorithm, but they are constructed so that the numbers they generate have the *appearance* of being random—that is, they occur in random order, and they are uniformly distributed over the desired range of values. All basic generators create *uniform* distributions, but these can be manipulated to be Gaussian, chi-square, or other distributions.[25] The *New York Times* ran an article which expressed amazement at the lack of *true* randomness is these random-number generator programs ("Coin-Tossing Computers Found to Show Subtle Bias"[26]), but anyone familiar with computers and these programs knew that all along.

This is just the sort of example that illustrates that one should have a certain familiarity with computers and what they can and cannot do, in order to make rational decisions about whether to use computers in certain critical applications such as medicine, control of nuclear plants, strategic defense, or war.

"War Games"

The RAND Corporation and others have for years been writing programs that simulate various aspects of global activity, and prominent among these have been "war games." A war game simulation constructs a model, building in all of the currently known parameters of defensive strength, volatility of government, and so on, of various nations in the world, and then plays out various scenarios, in an attempt to predict reactions, estimated casualties, and the like for certain contemplated actions.

This kind of program had been around for years before 1983, but in that year the movie *War Games* catapulted this simulation into the national awareness. In the movie, a young computer whiz (played by Matthew Broderick) succeeds in breaking into a national defense computer and, thinking he is dealing with a company manufacturing new and challenging software games, chooses, from a list that includes "Fighter Combat," "Desert Warfare," "Guerrilla Engagement," "Air-to-Ground Actions," and the "Chemical and Biological Warfare," the option of "Global Thermonuclear War."

As he is innocently playing the "game" with the computer ("Joshua"), the computer's moves are setting in motion actual military responses to a perceived attack. The process seems unstoppable, and the country is on the verge of launching nuclear warheads against Russia, until the young man finally stimulates "Joshua" to play a series of games of Tic-Tac-Toe, first against him and then against itself, until it realizes that this is a game no one can win. The computer then (to no one's apparent surprise) makes the analogy between Tic-Tac-Toe and nuclear war: They are both games no one can win. "Joshua" calls off the launch, and the world is saved (at least temporarily).

False Alarms

With much of the nuclear response system in the United States (and in other countries) under computer control, one must wonder just how reliable and error-free these systems are. President John F. Kennedy gave a speech in September 1961, in which he said: "Today, every inhabitant of this planet must contemplate the day when this planet may no longer be habitable. Every man, woman, and child lives under a nuclear sword of Damocles, hanging by the slenderest of threads, capable of being cut at any moment by accident or miscalculation or by madness."[27] The question four decades later is whether a computer could be the cause of such an accident or miscalculation.

There have been some incidents reported regarding automatic computerized systems that should give us pause. One also wonders whether, as in the case of computer crimes, we have only heard about a small fraction of such incidents, since those in command do not want the bad press that would result.

The first incident reported occurred on October 5, 1960. The Ballistic Missile Early Warning System (BMEWS) had just been installed in Thule, Greenland, with a direct link to the Strategic Air Command (SAC) headquarters in the United States. BMEWS alerted SAC that it had picked up a signal that computer analysis indicated as missiles heading toward the United States from the area of the Soviet Union.

SAC went on full alert, to status level 5 (the highest), in response to the message. However, an alert person in control at SAC felt the need to double-check the information. At the time, Premier Krushchev was visiting the United States, and it seemed very unlikely that the Russians would choose that moment to attack. It turned out that the signal picked up by the BMEWS system had been the moon coming up over Greenland.[28] False alerts such as this remind us of the time (in the mid–1950s) that a radar station mistook a flock of geese for a Soviet bomber attack.[29] On another occasion, returning space junk was detected as incoming missiles.[30]

On November 9, 1979, the U.S. nuclear defenses sprang to the ready in response to a missile alert. Ten jet fighters "scrambled aloft" ready to retaliate, and it took six minutes to determine that this was a false alert. Apparently, a "mechanical error sent 'war game' information into the sensing system that provides early warning of nuclear attack, indicating that the United States was under attack from a few missiles launched by a Soviet submarine, probably located in the northern Pacific."

NORAD did discover the mistake, and "Defense officials said the system had a series of human and mechanical double checks to prevent computers from prompting orders to launch American missiles in a counterattack."[31] (That is good to know!) The same page of the *New York Times* included a news item from Moscow, indicating that the Soviet news agency Tass "warned that another such error could have 'irreparable consequences for the whole world.'" This incident shows, as did the *War Games* movie, the dangers of a simulation being mistaken for the real thing.

In 1980, there were two false alerts very close together on June 3 and June 6, less than six months after the "war games" simulation attack. Senators Gary Hart and Barry Goldwater undertook to report on these incidents to the Senate. They determined that the failure (which simply repeated on the second day) "was caused by a faulty integrated circuit in a communications multiplexer" (Hart and Goldwater, 1980, p. 7). Clearly, we must take all precautions to guarantee that a programming, human, or mechanical error cannot trigger a nuclear holocaust.

"Star Wars" by Any Other Name

On March 23, 1983, President Ronald Reagan made a speech in which he launched the Strategic Defense Initiative (SDI), which soon gained the nickname "Star Wars." Reagan was encouraged by two advisors in this initiative—physicist Edward Teller (one of the scientists responsible for the development of the atomic bomb) and ex-Pentagon defense leader Danny Graham, who became head of what he called the "High Frontier." Presumably the idea was that the last unclaimed frontier is space, and that we should claim it first. In Reagan's short speech, he called on the scientific community that had given us nuclear weapons to now work to make those weapons "obsolete and useless."

Danny Graham's High Frontier organization made a television commercial that showed a child's drawing of a house and family, and the rainbow "Peace Shield" that would protect them. The audio accompanying the cartoon, spoken by a child, said: "I asked my daddy what this Star Wars stuff is all about. He said that right now we can't protect ourselves from nuclear weapons, and that's why the President wants to build a Peace Shield. It would stop missiles in outer space so they couldn't hit our house. Then, nobody could win a war. And if nobody could win a war, there's no reason to start one. My Daddy's smart."

The "peace shield" was to involve technology that could hit a missile on its way toward the United States. There are many problems associated with such an endeavor, including timing, picking out the real missile from debris, and plotting a trajectory to intercept it. Some of the proposals involved using nuclear devices in space to carry out the defense; but the ABM treaties had prohibited the placing of nuclear weapons in space. Other strategies involved bouncing laser beams off of orbiting mirrors in space, but these mirrors are easily damaged.

Reagan's speech marked the beginning of a large-scale program of research and development to create a space-based *defensive* system against nuclear attack. Scientists were radically split on this program. Teller, of course, supported his idea strongly. Hans Bethe, Nobel Prize-winning physicist, called the program "nonsense," and said that it was "setting the country on a completely futile course" which "also might be a very dangerous course" (NOVA/Frontline, 1986). Many scientists ran to jump on the SDI bandwagon to take part in the stupendous funding that was available. Many of these scientists were looking primarily to how the funding would help their own areas of research interest, not to the SDI results.

Many other scientists very strongly opposed SDI from the outset. Computer Scientists for Social Responsibility (CPSR) came out against the project. Computer scientist Jim Horning said that no system of this complexity has performed as expected (or hoped) in its full-scale operational test; there is no good reason to expect that SDI will perform as hoped. It is a huge system that is intended to be used at most once, and which cannot be realistically tested in advance of its use.[32] Given the problems with large-scale programs, how could we possibly expect that it will work right, without testing, the first time it is used? We can't test it without actually using it, but to actually use it is to initiate an action that most likely would start a nuclear war, or else to wait and use it in the event of a nuclear attack, in which case it would be too late to find out that it does not work. We are caught in a Catch-22.

This was the view of many, including computer scientist David Lorge Parnas. Parnas was invited by the SDI Organization (SDIO) to serve on a $1,000-a-day advisory panel, the SDIO Panel on Computing in Support of Battle Management. Two months later, he resigned from the panel, and published a number of papers in strong opposition to SDI. He stressed the software reliability problems of large systems, and the inability to test the system.

When Danny Graham was presented with the views of those scientists who said that Star Wars would not work, he responded: "I just say, 'Fine, you say it won't work. We say it will. Why not give us a chance?'" (cited in Lilenthal, 1989). In this reply, Graham apparently was trying to appeal to the American sense of fair play. However, he did not address the issue of what the consequences would be if it did not work.

Filmmaker George Lucas brought suit against High Frontier, Inc., for the use of the term "Star Wars." He felt that he did not want his products associated with missile defense (Lilenthal, 1989), and that this would turn children off from his products. The District Court judge (Gerhard Gesell) ruled that, even though "Star Wars" was a Lucas trademark, the term could be used by the public to communicate their views on SDI.[33]

In a meeting of representatives of the Johnson administration with the Soviet premier Aleksey Kosygin in June 1967, Secretary of Defense Robert McNamara suggested that the United States, to maintain its deterrent, would have to expand their offensive forces. Kosygin replied, the blood rushing to his face: "Defense is moral, offense is immoral" (NOVA/Frontline, 1986). The real question with respect to Star Wars has been whether it is in fact moral. There are many moral issues that are connected with it. One can claim that the purpose of SDI is to save lives. But one can *claim* anything; the issue is whether it would in fact save lives, or make a nuclear confrontation more likely.

To do an ethical analysis on this issue, we should recall our outline for such analysis at the end of Chapter 3. The first step is to "get the facts." In this case, it is particularly crucial to get the relevant facts, and to sort out what the truth is. Proponents of Star Wars claim its great potential and accuracy; opponents, including major scientists like Hans Bethe and many computer scientists (Parnas, CPSR, etc.), argue that it is not feasible, that it cannot be tested, and moreover, that it is terribly dangerous. More recently (April 2000), the Union of Concerned Scientists said that National Missile Defense won't work, and that simple countermeasures would defeat it (see **www.ucsusa.org/security/**). The better your science and computer science background, the more qualified you will be to assess these conflicting claims. You might want to take into consideration our previous discussions of computer reliability.

The second step is to look to the ethical principles we have found to be well-grounded. The proponents of Star Wars technology are obviously appealing to utilitarian calculations regarding the consequences of having as opposed to not having such a system. The problem, as we have seen before, is that the future is notoriously difficult to predict. Can we judge the effects of such a system? We cannot afford Danny Graham's "try it and see" approach if the results could be disastrous. So we must try to make the best estimate of feasibility and possible side effects given the information we have. Perhaps a computer simulation might be helpful in this sort of "What if?" situation, but we must be sure that the simulation has accurate details, a realistic model for how things work, and a well-tested program.

Could we universalize our "build a shield" maxim here? It would seem that our government would not be happy if other countries were building similar shields, and putting space-based lasers into orbit. Certainly, other countries are alarmed at our proposals to do so. What should this tell us? To what virtues, or strengths of character, does this project contribute? Any? Will it even provide peace of mind, as the rainbow ad promises?

Obviously, SDI would be a means to an end—we should get clear in our minds just exactly what this end is supposed to be. World peace? A noble goal, but this does not seem to be a means that promotes that end; instead it makes our neighbors nervous. Is the goal protection? Here the analysis of facts comes in; just how effective would the protection be? What if it is 90 percent, but also the existence of the shield has escalated the possibility of an attack? Are 10 percent casualties acceptable? Is the goal retaliation, or revenge, against anyone presuming to attack us? Is this a noble goal, tied to a fundamental good?

We want to maximize fundamental goods. Life is a basic good, so it is moral to protect it. But we must critically examine the *means* used to protect life. It would not be acceptable to build a wall of innocent people around your home to protect it. If we have a "shield" and our NATO allies do not, have we in effect made them more vulnerable? Just life itself is a lower good; we need life to allow development, fulfillment—health, friendships, knowledge, and the other higher goods we have discussed. Another question we must ask here, then, is how much the cost of such a defense initiative undermines other human activities that the government could foster—health facilities, housing, education, environmental protection. After you have completed your analysis, see what your considered judgment is.

The previous approach that it was claimed would preclude nuclear war was called Mutually Assured Destruction (MAD); the deterrent was that neither side would initiate a nuclear war, since they would be inviting their own suicide. Would a defensive strike capability be more or less effective than MAD? If one side announced its plan to develop such a capability (as the United States announced to the world in 1983), would this prompt the enemy to try to get in a quick nuclear attack before the system was complete? All of these questions remained unanswered, but billions of dollars went into scientific research and development projects for SDI.

On May 13, 1993, Secretary of Defense Les Aspin proclaimed the end of the Star Wars era, and the Strategic Defense Initiative Organization was renamed the Ballistic Missile Defense Organization. The BMDO budget request for 1994 was $3.8 billion, the same as had been requested by SDIO. An article in *The Economist* says that BMDO "employs the same people to do the same things."[34] John Pike, a space technology expert for the Federation of American Scientists, observed: "They are still working on the same set of weapons the Bush administration worked on. They're basically telling SDI they need a new letterhead."[35] What is the point of this, claiming that SDI is over, when it just seems to have mutated into BMDO? Is this a "smoke and mirrors" operation to fool the public into thinking that Star Wars is over, when it is just operating under a new name, at the same level of funding? And, we might ask, is this an *ethical* thing for the government to do? Is deception justifiable? If some scientists who support the program do so because it provides them funding for the research they want to do, is that an adequate justification? Think about the arguments against relativism here.

A 1994 article said that $36 billion was spent on Star Wars since 1984, without a single working system to show for it. There is, however, evidence that some of the key experiments to show Star Wars technology would work were rigged.[36] Yet a Republican Congress was seeking to bring back funding for Star Wars projects.[37] Newt Gingrich is reported as saying, "One day mathematically something bad can happen and you ought to have a minimum screen on a continent-wide basis, and that's doable."[38] As happened before with the Soviet Union, talk of such a U.S. defense initiative deeply disturbs other countries. A senior Chinese foreign ministry official said that the development of a "theatre missile defense" to deploy around U. S. troops in Asia "will increase the danger of nuclear war" and "trigger an arms race in outer space."[39]

Here we have a technology that was strongly opposed by many major scientists, that had nothing tangible to show for a $36 billion investment,[40] that puts other major powers on edge, and that apparently resorted to deceptions to keep it alive. Yet many in Congress and President George W. Bush want to continue the program. Such a view has been referred to as the "faith-based missile defense."[41] We can only hope that the public and the Congress will become well informed on the details of any Star Wars–like proposals, and do not forget what almost two decades of Star Wars taught us.

Yet Star Wars refuses to go away. President George W. Bush is actively pursuing implementation of a National Ballistic Missile Defense and an overthrow of the ABM treaty. The tragedy of September 11, 2001, is being used as an impetus to pursue this ill-considered objective. Bush asks, what if Osama Bin Laden were to launch a nuclear missile at the United States? Wouldn't we want to be ready to shoot it down? On December 13, 2001, Bush told Russian president Vladimir Putin that the United States will leave the ABM Treaty in six months. Putin called this a "mistake," and the Russian prime minister said it was regrettable because it will undermine global strategic balance.

■ ENDNOTES

1. Reported in David Burnham, *The Rise of the Computer State* (New York: Random House, 1983), p. 47.

2. Donna S. Hussain and Khateeb M. Hussain, *The Computer Challenge: Technology, Applications, and Social Implications* (Santa Rosa, CA: Burgess Communications, 1986), p. 235.

3. Hussain and Hussain, p. 225.

4. Hussain and Hussain, p. 225.

5. John Shattuck and Muriel Morisey Spence, "The Dangers of Information Control," *Technology Review* (April 1988), 69.

6. Shattuck and Spence, p. 67.

7. Eur Consultative Assembly Res 428, p. 911; reported in Warren Freedman, *The Right of Privacy in the Computer Age* (New York: Quorum Books, 1987), pp. 126–27.

8. Jerry Mander, *In the Absence of the Sacred* (San Francisco, CA: Sierra Club Books, 1991), p. 55. Higher rates of illness are found in those working in Silicon Valley than in other areas of manufacturing (see Joseph LaDou, "The Not-So-Clean Business of Making Chips," *Technology Review* [May/June 1984], 23–36). The California Department of Health found miscarriages 2.4 times the normal rate and birth defects 2.5 times normal in Silicon Valley communities where water supplies were contaminated by the toxic byproducts of chip manufacture (see J. Burton, "Studies Relate Defects to High-tech Toxins in Water," *Computerworld* (January 28, 1985), 84).

9. See Dante's *Inferno*, Canto XXX, for their proper place in Hell.

10. *CPSR Newsletter* 11, no. 4 & 12, no. 1 (Winter 1994), 3.

11. Richard Sclove and Jeffrey Scheuer, "The Ghost in the Modem," *Washington Post*, 29 May 1994, *Outlook* section, p. C03.

12. The reports can be ordered from the Superintendent of Documents, U.S. Government Printing Office, Washington, DC 20402; tel. (202) 783-3238; the second report is also available as NIST Special Publication 868 from the National Technical Information Service, Springfield, VA 22161; tel. (703) 487-4650; NII-2 is available electronically (via Internet) iitf.doc.gov or nii.nist.gov/nii/niiinfo.html

13. "The Information Infrastructure: Realizing Society's Goals," Department of Commerce, Technology Administration (Washington, DC: Government Printing Office, September 1994). NIST Special Publication 868.

14. See Clifford Stoll's comments on this in *Silicon Snake Oil* (New York: Doubleday), chs. 2, 9.

15. Pamela Samuelson, "Copyright and Digital Libraries," *Communications of the ACM* 38, 3 (April 1995), 19.

16. Pamela Samuelson, "The NII Intellectual Property Report," *Communications of the ACM* 37, 12 (December 1994), 23.

17. Jeffrey Johnson, "Information Superhighway or Superhypeway." cpsr-nii (online), May 24, 1995.

18. Richard O. Mason, "Four Ethical Issues of the Information Age," in Roy Dejoie et al., *Ethical Issues in Information Systems* (Boston: Boyd & Fraser, 1991), pp. 46–47. Regarding *access*, Ben Schneiderman reports that the term "user interface" appears only once in the 96-page NII-2 ("The Information Superhighway for the People," *Communications of the ACM* 38, 11 (January 1995), 162).

19. Winn Schwartau, *Information Warfare: Chaos on the Electronic Superhighway* (New York: Thunder's Mouth Press, 1994), p. 352.

20. Hans Moravec, *Mind Children* (Cambridge, MA: Harvard University Press, 1988), pp. 85–88.

21. Quoted in Jonathan Jacky, "The Strategic Computing Program," in David Bellin and Gary Chapman, eds., *Computers in Battle—Will They Work?* (Boston: Harcourt Brace Jovanovich, 1987).

22. Gary Chapman, "The New Generation of High-Technology Weapons," in Bellin and Chapman, pp. 97–99.

23. Quoted in Gary Chapman, "The New Generation of High-Technology Weapons," in Bellin and Chapman, p. 91.

24. For example, see Erich M. Harth and Stacey L. Edgar, "Association by Synaptic Facilitation in Highly Damped Neural Nets," *Biophysical Journal* 7, 6 (1967), 689–717.

25. For a discussion of how to write a pseudo-random number generator, and how to turn uniform distributions into Gaussian and other distributions, see, for example, Stacey L. Edgar, *Fortran for the '90s* (New York: Computer Science Press, 1992), pp. 464–78.

26. Malcolm W. Browne, "Coin-Tossing Computers Found to Show Subtle Bias," *New York Times*, 12 January 1993, pp. C1, C9.

27. Quoted in Robert M. Baer, *The Digital Villain* (Reading, MA: Addison-Wesley, 1972).

28. E. Berkeley, "The Social Responsibility of Computer People," in Z. Pylyshn, ed., *Perspectives on the Computer Revolution* (Englewood Cliffs, NJ: Prentice-Hall, 1970), p. 461.

29. Richard Burt, "False Nuclear Alarms Spur Urgent Effort to Find Flaws," *New York Times*, 13 June 1980, p. A16.

30. Daniel F. Ford, *The Button: The Pentagon's Strategic Command and Control System* (New York: Simon & Schuster, 1985), p. 85.

31. A. O. Sulzberger, Jr., "Error Alerts U.S. Forces to a False Missile Attack," *New York Times*, 11 November 1979, p. 30.

32. See David Parnas, "SDI," *Abacus* 4, 2 (Winter 1987), 46–52. Tyler Folsom adds, "The Strategic Defense Initiative is a high-tech gravy train with little prospect of feasibility due to extremely demanding software requirements and the impossibility of adequately testing the system." ("The Search for an 'Electronic Brain'," in DeJoie et al., eds., *Ethical Issues in Information Systems* [1991], p. 302). See also Michael Nussbaumer, Judith DilOrio, and Robert Baller, "The Boycott of 'Star Wars' by Academic Scientists," *Social Science Journal* 31, 4 (1994), 375–88.

33. *New York Times*, 27 November 1985, p. B8.

34. "Strategic Defense–Second Coming," *The Economist* (May 22, 1993), pp. 31–32.

35. "Star Wars–Mainly the Name Has Changed," *U.S. News and World Report*, 24 May 1993, p. 11.

36. Heat-seeking missiles launched from Vandenberg AFB failed to hit their targets on the first three tries, so the nose of the "enemy" missile was heated before launch on the fourth try, and the target was approached from the side rather than head-on. This test was cited by the Pentagon as evidence that they could "hit a bullet with a bullet" (Vincent Kiernan, "'Successful' Star Wars Test Was Faked," *New Scientist* 143, 1937 (August 6, 1994), 8). See also William J. Broad, *Teller's War: The Top-Secret Story Behind the Star Wars Deception* (New York: Simon & Schuster, 1992).

37. Jonathan S. Landay, "GOP Plots 'Star Wars' Rescue as '96 Budget Battle Looms," *Christian Science Monitor*, 2 May 1995, p. 1. Herb Block, in a cartoon in the *Washington Post*, 27 November 1994, characterizes supply-side economics and Star Wars as Dracula and Frankenstein that came back with the new (1994) Congress.

38. Eric Schmitt, "Republicans Want to Try Again with 'Star Wars'," *New York Times*, 7 February 1995, p. A20.

39. Patrick E. Tyler, "China Warns Against 'Star Wars' Shield for U. S. Forces in Asia," *New York Times*, 18 February 1995, p. A4.

40. Of course, we probably should not discount the pizza warming tray that San Diego defense contractor Claude Hayes made out of a device built for Star Wars; Hayes has a contract with Pizza Hut for the tray. Rosie Mestel, "Cold War Technology on a Plate," *New Scientist* 141, 1908 (January 15, 1994), 10.

41. *Software Engineering Notes* (*SEN*) 26, 6 (November 2001), 6–7.

■ SHORT ESSAY QUESTIONS

1. In the quote from Kent Greenwalt (see footnote 1), he suggests that the keen surveillance and the lack of forgiveness of computerized record-keeping systems will tend to increase conformity in society. He suggests that this would be a bad thing. Why? Do you agree with him or not? Give thoughtful reasons. (You might want to check out Alexis de Tocqueville's *Democracy in America* for a critique of an overemphasis on *equality*.)

2. See what you can track down that is more recent on the impact of the European proposals to guarantee privacy rights of personal records (Markoff, 1991), and the American response to it.

3. Watch the movie *Colossus: The Forbin Project*. (Notice that the installation for the Colossus computer, imbedded in a mountain, looks a lot like the U.S. national control center in Cheyenne Mountain, Colorado.) Discuss the purposes for which Colossus was created, and the point at which things begin to get out of the hands of its creator, Dr. Forbin (when he says, "It's built even better than we thought!"). The society that Colossus controls at the end of the movie is one in which there is no threat of nuclear war. Discuss why it still might not be a society in which human beings want to live.

4. *Computers in Battle—Will They Work?* (edited by David Bellin and Gary Chapman), discusses how human beings are being taken more and more "out of the loop" in computerized military systems (as they are in airplanes as well). Discuss whether this is a good thing. Could someone *surrender* to a computer or a computerized robot?

5. If computers are controlling most of the battle decisions, would it be possible to take humans dying "out of the loop"? That is, could we just pit *our* computer against *their* computer, both supplied with all of the data on weapons, troops, strategies, and the like, and let them play out the scenario strictly as a "war game" with no casualties? In times past, sometimes the leaders of two armies would fight it out to decide a war, so that no others had to die on either side; could this be done with computers instead? (There was an old *Star Trek* episode in which Kirk and crew visited a civilization in which wars were fought this way; it did not work out for them.) Discuss the feasibility of this plan, and any disadvantages.

6. The Clinton administration increased support for the effort to construct a space station. See what you can find out from recent newspapers, journals, and government publications about the International Space Station Alpha, and try to determine whether its intent is just for peaceful, beneficial purposes, or whether it could be connected with aggressive (or defensive) actions by the military. Check out the "Space Station User's Guide" on **www.spaceref.com/iss/**

7. Read and discuss "Four Unsound Arguments for Strategic Defense" in Douglas P. Lackey, *Ethics and Strategic Defense* (Belmont, CA: Wadsworth, 1989).

■ LONG ESSAY QUESTIONS

1. Read Chapter 4 in Fred Dretske's book, *Knowledge and the Flow of Information*. The chapter is about the connection between knowledge and information. Write a critical exposition of Dretske's ideas in this chapter, and try to assess whether he is right in the views he puts forward. Imbedded in the chapter is a discussion of Edmund Gettier's argument that purports to show that knowledge is not (or not only) justified true belief. Analyze Gettier's argument as part of your discussion.

2. Look into Jerry Mander's charges concerning the environmental dangers presented by computer manufacture. Consult EPA reports and other sources. Evaluate whether his concern is well grounded.

3. Read up on the latest information available on the information superhighway. Sort out how much of it is "hype," and try to find any factual data that indicate what its *real* advantages (to humans in general) will be, as opposed to more sports channels and more at-home shopping channels. How many of your more recent sources concern themselves with the question of *fair access*, and what do they have to say about it?

4. Consider carefully the effects of the information superhighway on public libraries. Will books cease to be published on paper, and will they become available only (or primarily) electronically? What effect

will that have? Will this have a further negative effect on widening the gap between rich and poor? (Check out www.digitaldivide.gov). What disadvantages can you see to electronic libraries? What advantages? Check out the article by Pamela Samuelson under Recommended Readings to see what concern librarians and scholars had in 1995 over the possible limitations on availability of government documents, and a legal perspective on the copyright issues.

5. Analyze the position put forward by Walter E. Morrow, Jr., in his article "SDI Research is Critical."

6. See what information you can find in recent newspapers and journals regarding the activities of the Ballistic Missile Defense Organization (BMDO), or the operations designated as National Missile Defense. Does it really still seem to be the SDI (Star Wars) program under a new name, or is it significantly different? Do the concerns over Star Wars apply to the operation of this organization as well?

7. James H. Moor wrote a thought-provoking article entitled "Are There Decisions Computers Should Never Make?" (*Nature and System* 1 [1979], 217–29), in which he makes the case that it does make sense to say that computers make decisions. The serious question then becomes whether their decision-making is (or will become) at least as good as that of human beings and, if and when it does, whether there should be any restrictions on the decisions computers are *allowed* to make. Read the article, present a critical account of its contents, and discuss what limitations (if any) *you* would suggest.

8. Examine critically the concept of a "just war." The "classic formulation" of the idea is attributed to Augustine, in *The City of God*. Check out this source, read Robert P. Churchill's article on "Nuclear Arms as a Philosophical and Moral Issue," and compare Paul Ramsey's *The Just War* (New York: Scribner's, 1968) and Michael Walzer, *Just and Unjust Wars* (New York: Basic Books, 1977). Keep in mind the role of computers in war.

9. Paul Ramsey writes that "whatever is wrong to do is wrong to threaten" ("A Political Ethics Context for Strategic Thinking," in *Strategic Thinking and Its Moral Implications*, ed. Morton A. Kaplan [Chicago: University of Chicago Center for Policy Studies, 1973], pp. 134–35). Examine this notion and the light it sheds on nuclear deterrence strategies such as MAD and SDI.

■ REFERENCES AND RECOMMENDED READINGS

Arendt, Hannah. *The Origins of Totalitarianism.* New York: Harvest/HBJ, 1973.

Asker, James R. "Allies Show New Interest in SDI, Theater Missile Defense Research." *Aviation Week & Space Technology* (June 17, 1991), 105–108.

Asker, James R. "Research, Development for SDI Major Source of New Technology." *Aviation Week & Space Technology* (April 8, 1991), 57.

Baer, Robert M. *The Digital Villain.* Reading, MA: Addison-Wesley, 1972.

Bellin, David, and Gary Chapman, eds. *Computers in Battle—Will They Work?* Boston, MA: Harcourt Brace Jovanovich, 1987.

Beusmans, Jack, and Karen Wieckert. "Computing, Research, and War: If Knowledge Is Power, Where Is Responsibility?" *Communications of the ACM* 32, 8 (August 1989), 939–51.

Biddle, Michael B., and Ray Mann. "Recipe for Recycling." *IEEE Spectrum* 31, 8 (February 1993), 22–24.

Borning, Alan. "Computer System Reliability and Nuclear War." *Communications of the ACM* 30, 2 (February 1987), 112–31. Also in Dunlop and Kling, 1991, pp. 560–92.

Broad, William J. *Teller's War: The Top-Secret Story Behind the Star Wars Deception.* New York: Simon & Schuster, 1992.

Brodeur, Paul. "The Annals of Radiation." *New Yorker* (June 12, 19, 26, and July 19, 1989); or see his book, *Currents of Death* (New York: Simon & Schuster, 1991).

Brown, Harold, ed. *The Strategic Defense Initiative: Shield or Snare?* Boulder, CO: Westview Press, 1987.

Browne, Malcolm W. "Coin-Tossing Computers Found to Show Subtle Bias." *New York Times,* 12 January 1993, pp. C1, C9.

Buffey, Philip M., and W. J. Broad. *Claiming the Heavens.* New York: Times Books, 1988.

Burnham, David. *The Rise of the Computer State: The Threat to Our Freedoms, Our Ethics, and Our Democratic Process.* New York: Random House, 1983.

Churchill, Robert P. "Nuclear Arms as a Philosophical and Moral Issue." In A. Pablo Iannone, ed., *Contemporary Moral Controversies in Technology* (New York: Oxford University Press, 1987), pp. 215–24. Originally published in

Annals of the American Academy of Political and Social Science 469 (September 1983), 46–57.

Codevilla, Angelo. *While Others Build: A Commonsense Approach to the Strategic Defense Initiative.* New York: Free Press, 1988.

Cooper, Henry F. "Cooperation on Building Global Defenses." *San Diego Union-Tribune* (May 13, 2001). Also can be found at:

www.highfrontier. org/SDUnionTribCooper.htm

Cousteau, Jacques-Yves. "Editorial: Information Highway: Mental Pollution." *Calypso Log* 22 (August 1995), 3.

Dalai Lama. *Ethics for the New Millennium.* New York: Riverbank Books, 1999.

DeLanda, Manuel. *War in the Age of Intelligent Machines.* New York: Zone Books, 1991.

DeLoughry, Thomas J. "Guaranteeing Access to the Data Highway." *Chronicle of Higher Education* 40, 11 (November 3, 1993), A23.

Dretske, Fred I. *Knowledge and the Flow of Information.* Cambridge, MA: MIT Press, 1982.

Dunlop, Charles, and Rob Kling, eds. *Computerization and Controversy: Value Conflicts and Social Choices.* Boston, MA: Academic Press, 1991, parts I & IV.

Einstein, Albert, and Sigmund Freud. *Why War?* International Institute of Intellectual Cooperation. League of Nations, 1933.

Ermann, M. David, Claudio Gutierrez, and Mary B. Williams, eds. *Computers, Ethics, and Society.* New York: Oxford University Press, 1990.

Florman, Samuel C. "Odysseus in Cyberspace." *Technology Review* 97, 3 (April 1994), 65.

Ford, Daniel F. *The Button: The Pentagon's Strategic Command and Control System.* New York: Simon & Schuster, 1985.

Forester, Tom, and Perry Morrison. *Computer Ethics: Cautionary Tales and Ethical Dilemmas in Computing.* 2nd ed. Cambridge, MA: MIT Press, 1994, chs. 5, 7. In the First Edition (1990), see Appendix.

Freedman, Warren. *The Right of Privacy in the Computer Age.* New York: Quorum Books, 1987.

Gavrilov, V. M., and M. Iu. Sitnina. "The Militarization of Space: A New Global Danger." *Soviet Studies in Philosophy* 25 (Winter 1986–1987), 27–45.

Gibson, William. *Neuromancer.* New York: Ace Books, 1984.

Gilmartin, Patricia. "Plan to Deploy Limited SDI System Faces Tough Fight in Senate." *Aviation Week & Space Technology* (July 29, 1991), 29.

Gray, Colin. "Strategic Defense, Deterrence, and the Prospects for Peace." *Ethics* 95 (1985), 659–72.

Graybosch, Anthony J. "The Ethics of Space-Based Missile Defense." *The Monist* (January 1988), 45–58.

Hart, Senator Gary, and Senator Barry Goldwater. "Recent False Alerts from the Nation's Missile Attack Warning System: Report to the Committee on Armed Services, United States Senate." U.S. Government Publication No. 81-2992. Washington, DC: Government Printing Office, 1980.

Horgan, John. "Star Wars of the Seas: Do Lessons of the Iranian Airbus Tragedy Apply to SDI?" *Scientific American* (September 1988), 14–18.

Hussain, Donna S., and Khateeb M. Hussain. *The Computer Challenge: Technology, Applications, and Social Implications.* Santa Rosa, CA: Burgess Communications, 1986.

Jacobs, W. W. "The Monkey's Paw." From *The Lady of the Barge.* New York: Dodd, Meade, [1902] 1930. Reprinted in Van H. Cartmell and Charles Grayson, eds., *The Golden Argosy.* New York: Dial Press, 1955.

Johnson, Deborah. *Computer Ethics.* 2nd ed. Englewood Cliffs, NJ: Prentice-Hall, 1994.

Johnson, Deborah G., and John W. Snapper, eds. *Ethical Issues in the Use of Computers.* Belmont, CA: Wadsworth, 1985.

Kizza, Joseph M. *Ethics in the Computer Age: ACM Conference Proceedings (November 11–13, 1994).* New York: ACM, 1994.

Krauthammer, Charles. "Killing Star Wars—To Save It." *Washington Post,* 21 May 1993, sec. A, p. 25.

Lackey, Douglas P. *Ethics and Strategic Defense.* Belmont, CA: Wadsworth, 1989.

Lilenthal, Edward Taylor. *Symbolic Defense: The Cultural Significance of the Strategic Defense Initiative.* Urbana, IL: University of Illinois Press, 1989.

Mander, Jerry. *In the Absence of the Sacred: The Failure of Technology and the Survival of the Indian Nation.* San Francisco, CA: Sierra Club Books, 1991.

Manno, Jack. *Arming the Heavens.* New York: Dodd, Mead, 1984.

Markoff, John. "Europe's Plans to Protect Privacy Worry Business." *New York Times,* 11 April 1991, pp. A1, D6.

Moor, James H. "Are There Decisions Computers Should Never Make?" *Nature and System*, vol. 1 (1979), 217–29.

Moravec, Hans. *Mind Children: The Future of Robot and Human Intelligence.* Cambridge, MA: Harvard University Press, 1988.

Morrow, Walter E., Jr. "SDI Research Is Critical." *Technology Review* (July 1987), 24–25, 77; also in Ermann et al., 1990.

Mowshowitz, Abbe. *Conquest of Will: Information Processing in Human Affairs.* Reading, MA: Addison-Wesley, 1976.

NOVA/Frontline. "Visions of Star Wars." PBS production, 1986.

Nusbaumer, Michael R., Judith A. DilOrio, and Robert D. Baller, "The Boycott of 'Star Wars' by Academic Scientists: The Relative Roles of Political and Technical Judgment," *Social Science Journal* 31, 4 (1994), 375–88.

Orwell, George. *Animal Farm.* New York: Signet/NAL, [1946] 1956.

Orwell, George. *1984.* New York: Signet/NAL, [1949] 1973.

Orwell, George. "Politics and the English Language." In *The Orwell Reader.* New York: Harvest/HBJ, [1933] 1956.

Parnas, David Lorge. "SDI: A Violation of Professional Responsibility." *Abacus* 4, 2 (Winter 1987), 46–52; also in Ermann et al., 1990, 359–72.

Parnas, David Lorge. "Software Aspects of Strategic Defense Systems." *Communications of the ACM* 28, 12 (December 1985), 1326–35.

Payne, Kenneth B. *Strategic Defense: "Star Wars" in Perspective.* Lanham, MD: Hamilton Press, 1986.

Perry, Tekla S. "Cleaning Up." *IEEE Spectrum* 30, 2 (February 1993), 20–26.

Raloff, Janet. "Building the Ultimate Weapons: Lasers and Particle Beams Are Being Assessed for Military Deployment." *Science News* 126 (July 21, 1984), 42–45.

Roberts, Eric. "Programming and the Pentagon." *Abacus* 4, 4 (Summer 1987), 54–57.

Rothfeder, Jeffrey. *Privacy for Sale: How Computerization Has Made Everyone's Private Life an Open Secret.* New York: Simon & Schuster, 1992.

Russell, Bertrand. *Unarmed Victory.* New York: Penguin, 1963. On the Cuban missile crisis.

Samuelson, Pamela. "Copyright and Digital Libraries." *Communications of the ACM* 38, 3 (April 1995), 15–21, 110.

Samuelson, Pamela. "The NII Intellectual Property Report." *Communications of the ACM* 37, 12 (December 1994), 21–27.

Shattuck, John, and Muriel Morisey Spence. "The Dangers of Information Control," *Technology Review* (April 1988), 62–73.

Simon, Herbert A. "The Consequences of Computers for Centralization and Decentralization." In Michael L. Dertouzos and Joel Moses, eds., *The Computer Age: A Twenty-Year View* (Cambridge, MA: MIT Press, 1980), pp. 212–27.

Simons, Barbara. "Questions About the NII." (Inside Risks column) *Communications of the ACM* 37, 7 (July 1994), 170.

Simons, Geoff. *Bugs and Star Wars: The Hazards of Unsafe Computing.* Manchester, England: NCC Blackwell, 1989.

Smith, Brian Cantwell. *Limits of Correctness in Computers.* (Presented at a Symposium on Unintentional Nuclear War at the Fifth Congress of the International Physicians for the Prevention of Nuclear War, Budapest, Hungary, June 28–July 1, 1985.) Stanford, CA: Center for the Study of Language and Information, 1985.

Stallman, Richard. "Can Freedom Withstand E-Books?" *Communications of the ACM* 44, 3 (March 2001), 111.

Stoll, Clifford. *Silicon Snake Oil: Second Thoughts on the Information Highway.* New York: Doubleday, 1995.

Strategic Defense Initiative Organization. *The 1989 Report to the Congress on the Strategic Defense Initiative.* Washington, DC: Government Printing Office, 1989.

Tirman, John, ed. *The Fallacy of Star Wars: Based on Studies Conducted by the Union of Concerned Scientists.* New York: Vintage Books, 1984.

U.S. Department of Commerce, Technology Administration. *Putting the Information Infrastructure to Work.* Washington, DC: Government Printing Office, May 1994. NIST Special Publication 857. (*NII–1*)

U.S. Department of Commerce, Technology Administration. *The Information Infrastructure: Reaching Society's Goals.* Washington, DC: Government Printing Office, September 1994. NIST Special Publication 868. (*NII–2*)

Weinberg, Steve. "Former CIA Agent Blows the Whistle on a Government Out to Silence Him." *St. Louis Post-Dispatch,* 22 August 1999, p. C12.

Wiener, Norbert. *The Human Use of Human Beings.* Boston, MA: Houghton Mifflin, 1950.

Zuckerman, Lord. "The New Nuclear Menace." *New York Review of Books,* 24 June 1993, pp. 14–19.

Chapter 12

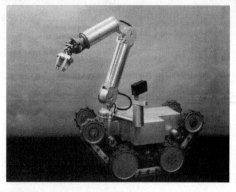

The Artificial Intelligensia and Virtual Worlds

ARTIFICIAL INTELLIGENCE—SOME GENERAL BACKGROUND

There are many definitions of artificial intelligence. Eugene Charniak and Drew McDermott say that "Artificial Intelligence is the study of mental faculties through the use of computational models" (1985, p. 6). Most of the definitions boil down to something like, "Artificial intelligence (A.I.) is getting machines (computers) to exhibit behavior that, if it were performed by a human, we would call intelligent." The term itself was coined in 1956 by John McCarthy, a participant at the Summer Research Project at Dartmouth College in Hanover, New Hampshire. Among the other ten people present at the project were Marvin Minsky and Claude Shannon. A year later, McCarthy went to MIT to set up the A.I. Lab there, and in 1962 he went to Stanford to organize the second main A.I. laboratory in the country. The third is at Carnegie-Mellon, where two people—Allen Newell and Herbert Simon—devised a program known as Logic Theorist, for proving theorems in mathematical logic.

That same year George Miller came up with his "magical number seven"—the claim that human beings can deal consciously with only about seven ("plus or minus two") items of information at a time—thus moving from the popular behaviorist input-output view to looking at the mind as an *active* entity that could *do* things with information, a beginning to cognitive science. It was also in the mid–1950s that Noam Chomsky, a professor at MIT, came up with the notion of a "formal grammar," providing linguistics with a formal rigorous mathematical framework for analyzing the structure of language.

Some earlier work was relevant to these developments, such as Alan Turing's articles on the universal (Turing) computing machine (Turing, 1937), and the "Can A Machine Think?" article in 1950 (Turing, 1950). In the 1930s, Claude Shannon showed that switching circuits could be used to represent logical operations like "and," "or," and "not." In 1943, Walter Pitts and Warren McCulloch showed how hypothetical networks of nerve cells could perform the operations of formal logic. In 1948, Norbert Weiner coined the term *cybernetics* as the "science of communication and control in man and machine"; it included the theory of feedback systems, information theory (first defined by Shannon in 1948), and the electronic computer.

Computers (even earlier, more primitive ones) were quite good at **algorithmic** reasoning—following a finite sequence of instructions until a solution or stopping place is reached. But the move to thinking in terms of artificial intelligence came when programs (like Logic Theorist) began to be written to do **heuristic problem solving**—a "discovery" approach, sometimes using trial-and-error methods, in which words like *hunch* and *intuition* began to be part of the problem-solving vocabulary. The "brute-force method" simply would not do for certain sorts of problems where the "combinatorial explosion" is at work—for instance, when Shannon calculated that there were on the order of 10^{120} possible moves in a game of chess.

Newell and Simon created another program called the "General Problem Solver" (GPS), which was supposed to model human thought processes. They wrote a book in 1992 called *Human Problem Solving.* GPS used an approach called *means-end reasoning,* where the present state of the system is constantly being compared to the "goal state" (like winning the game, or dominating the center of the board in chess), and the program is attempting to reduce the "distance" between the two states. It makes use of a table that associates the system's goals with various operators to achieve them.

GPS often took the "long way" in solving problems, and occasionally got trapped in dead ends, so it was eventually abandoned as an approach by most workers in the field who wanted fast solutions, whether or not they mimicked the ways in which humans solve problems. However, one interesting development of GPS was SHAKEY, a robot at Stanford University that was developed in 1971 to move in a world of doors, rooms, and boxes. In the 1960s, Marvin Minsky's students at MIT were writing programs to do visual analogies and to solve high-school algebra problems (Daniel Bobrow and the STUDENT program). In 1962, John McCarthy designed LISP (for LISt-Processing language), still the major language of A.I.

Expert Systems

In 1971, Edward Feigenbaum created a program called DENDRAL, which could figure out, from mass spectrometry data, which organic compound was being analyzed, and its success rate was comparable to that of expert human chemists. Considered the first **expert system**, DENDRAL was able to apply rules about which organic groups can bond combined with general knowledge and chemists' "tricks" for interpreting data. All of this was gleaned from interviews with chemistry *experts* and then built into the program, thus making use of a *knowledge base* and *heuristic rules*. Many other expert systems have been designed since, and are still being created to solve different problems.

Two early expert systems in the medical area were MYCIN and INTERNIST. MYCIN was developed in 1972–76 to advise doctors in the diagnosis of blood and meningitis infections and on selecting drugs for treatment. In one formal test, MYCIN prescribed correctly in 65 percent of the cases, while human specialists on the same cases were correct only 42.5 percent to 62.5 percent of the time. The program has been used at the Stanford Medical Center. INTERNIST was designed at the University of Pittsburgh in the early 1970s, to make diagnoses in internal medicine. Now called CADUCEUS, it is the most complex knowledge-based system ever built, containing over 100,000 pieces of medical information by 1982.

Two other well-known expert systems are **Prospector**, developed in the late 1970s to aid geologists in finding ore deposits, and **Xcon** (originally known as **R1**, because, so the lore goes, if asked about expert systems, it could reply "I are one")—used by Digital Equipment Corporation to design configurations of its minicomputers. (Using computers to design and configure other computers! It is beginning to sound like they can replace humans soon. One should note that, with regard to the reproduction challenge, John von Neumann *proved* in the 1940s that a computer could "reproduce"—that is, build a copy of itself if given access to a supply of materials, and provided with an internal "blueprint" of itself. Isn't that what humans do, except not so "self-consciously"? We certainly make use of external materials.)

Terry Winograd's SHRDLU, a "language-understanding" program, was developed in 1970 at Stanford University to operate in a very restricted world of colored blocks and pyramids and a tabletop, and to respond to commands like *stack, put, remove,* and *move.*

Walter Maner raises serious ethical issues with respect to medical expert systems. Should doctors be considered negligent if they fail to consult a computer diagnostic program? Who will be considered responsible if a "computer error" results in a patient's injury or death? Should a computer be allowed to make decisions such as whether to take a patient off a life-support system, thus relieving the doctor of having to make that decision? Would we find such a shifting of responsibility acceptable? It certainly would take a great deal of pressure off the doctor; but *is* this a decision a computer should make?

There is some reassurance in having recourse to charging a human doctor (or a lawyer) with malpractice, in which case the offending professional, if guilty, undergoes punishment overseen by the professional organization. There would be no similar recourse for "malpractice" by a computer program. One would be inclined to lay blame with the programmer, but there is no professional body with teeth to punish the programmer, and no malpractice insurance for programmers. Should there be?

Doctors are supposed to preserve life and health (both fundamental goods) whenever possible. A doctor swears a professional oath to uphold this duty, and that commitment should give the patient confidence in the doctor. There is no similar professional obligation formally committed to on the part of the computer or the programmer. An ethical programmer should realize that dealing with something as precious as life and health involves an implicit obligation to preserve it, and not to do harm; one should not need the threat of professional sanction to be especially careful in such circumstances. The programmer should create the most effective and well-tested program possible.

Patients who spend most of their time interacting with computers will lose the benefit of the "human touch" and the bond that can develop between doctor and patient. What will become of trust and morale? Or should a computer be the physician of choice because it is more reliable and objective? Is there any legal problem in having a computer (albeit an expert system) engaging in the practice of medicine, when it has not qualified in the same way that human physicians must (Maner, 1979)?

Implementation of voice-activated expert systems for doctors and nurses is made more complex by issues of training, speed, patient confidentiality, and various other human factors. The doctors in particular are finding it difficult to work into their routines; the nurses are having more success since they had a hand in the design of their system (Betts, 1994, p. 73).

Game-Playing

As early as 1948, Arthur Samuel, at Stanford, began writing a checkers-playing program. He gave the program techniques so that it would "learn" from its mistakes and, after a time (so the story goes), the program could beat Samuel! The best that an algorithmic program incorporating the principles that Samuel used in playing checkers should have been able to do playing against him should have been a draw. Claude Shannon thought it would be more interesting to have the computers play chess, and people have been writing programs to play chess ever since—programs that kept getting better and better, until Deep Blue (IBM) defeated chess grandmaster Gary Kasparov in May 1997; since then, interest in chess-playing computers has waned, the "problem" seemingly solved.

Theorem-Proving

Computer programs have been used to prove mathematical theorems. In one case, a computer proof was said by expert mathematicians to be more *elegant* than the corresponding proof in *Euclid's Elements*.

For years, the "Four-Color Hypothesis"—a hypothesis that refers to the minimum number of colors that are needed to color in a planar map such that no two adjacent areas are the same color—remained unproved and unfalsified. It had been proved that it could be done with five colors, but many mathematicians believed that it could be done with four. However, none of them could prove this. Then, in 1976, the Four-Color Theorem was "proved" with the aid of a computer—using 1,200 hours of computer time.[1] This raises interesting new questions regarding the nature of mathematical proof. In the past, one mathematician could always check the steps in a proof proposed by another mathematician. In the case of the Four-Color Theorem proof, no human could follow all of the steps that the computer made in confirming the proof.

THE TURING TEST

Alan Turing, a brilliant mathematician and early computer enthusiast whose help in cracking German codes during World War II saved Britain from considerable additional bombing, wrote a (now famous) paper for the journal *Mind* in 1950, in which he carefully examined the question, "Can Machines

Think?" Turing suggested that the issue might be approached by first defining the words 'machine' and 'think' in the question. However, dictionary definitions would be of no help to us here, as (besides being circular) they are merely reports of common usage. They only tell us what people currently believe thinking is, and what they call machines nowadays; they do not delve into the true nature of thinking, nor do they carefully examine what constitutes a machine. Furthermore, such definitions would reflect current biases, and probably answer the question quickly and vehemently in the negative, without really pondering it.

To seriously consider whether machines can think, we have to get past the normal reaction of looking at a blender or washing machine and saying "of course they can't think." The machines being referred to in Turing's question are different—they are sophisticated, with *memory* and *decision-making* capabilities. Their processes are much closer to being like what we normally call *mental* (at least when a human performs them) than to the *physical* processes carried out by your dryer and washing machine.

Furthermore, to raise a philosophical issue, it is very difficult (if not impossible) for you to determine with certainty whether anyone other than yourself thinks. You cannot get inside the heads of others and think their thoughts. So how do you know that they are thinking? One attempt to answer this is by **analogy**. Other people look like me, act like me, and use language the way I do; because *I* think, by analogy, they must think also. This is not a strong argument, and it can certainly be seen to go wrong in a number of cases.

One can easily be fooled about *what* someone else is thinking. Some people are just good actors and can, for example, feign deep grief when they feel none. One can at least imagine an androidlike machine that appears human and seems to be thinking, but is "just" a machine. Science fiction abounds with them, from the *Alien* and *Terminator* series to the android officer "Data" in *Star Trek: The Next Generation* and the replicants in *Blade Runner*. If one can imagine being fooled, then it is at least possible.

It is also quite possible that beings other than humans might think; then the "they look like me" part of the argument from analogy does not cover this case and so does not take care of testing for thinking in general. For example, dolphins may think. They seem to have a very complex language (one of the signs of thought), and they enjoy play (often thought to be unique to humans). Two standard measures used for intelligence are density of interconnections in the brain and the ratio of brain weight to body weight. Dolphins have a density of neural interconnections close to or greater than that of humans, and their brain weight to body weight ratio is higher than that of humans; the higher ratio is supposed to indicate greater intelligence.

Given all of the galaxies, there is a relatively high probability of intelligent life elsewhere in the universe. Paul Churchland, in *Matter and Consciousness*, does a nice job of performing a reasonable calculation regarding this possibility. His calculation takes into account that there are on the order of 10^{11} stars with planetary systems in just our own galaxy, the placing of a planet, and the proper conditions (water, for one), and ends up with a "conservative estimate" that "the evolutionary process is chugging briskly away, at some stage or other, on at least 10,000,000 planets within this galaxy alone" (Churchland, 1984, p. 151).

Churchland began with the view that "intelligent life is just life, with a high thermodynamic intensity and an especially close coupling between internal order and external circumstance," taking into account the very low probability (1 in 10^7) that we were the *first* planet in our galaxy to develop intelligent life, and assuming an average duration for intelligent life (before it self-destructs; he refers to "internal instabilities") of from 1 billion to 5 billion years, he estimates at least 10^5 planets (in just *our* galaxy) currently on a level or ahead of us in evolutionary development (Churchland, 1984, pp. 150–57). If the possibility of intelligent ("thinking") life on other planets in this and other galaxies is reasonable, then they will most probably not all *look like* us or even *act like* us, and so we need a better test of thinking.

We will make a Kantian move here, and argue that to deal with the very real issues of what constitutes thinking, we will postulate the external world and at least the possibility of other thinking beings besides ourselves in it as a necessary presupposition to our inquiry, just as freedom is a necessary presupposition to considerations of moral law, and causality is a necessary presupposition to considerations of natural law.

Having put all of this preliminary discussion behind us, we come back to Turing's original question of whether machines can think. To avoid recourse to inadequate dictionary definitions, or conducting an opinion poll, Turing proposes an **objective test** as to whether a machine (or your mother, or your lover) thinks. His test is based on the "Imitation Game."

The Imitation Game

In the usual version of the Imitation Game, there are three players—a man, a woman, and an interrogator. The interrogator must ask questions of the man and the woman, who are both claiming to be the woman, and on the basis of the answers to those questions, the interrogator is to try to determine which one really *is* the woman. To avoid unfair clues, there is no visual contact between the interrogator and the contestants, and (to avoid their voices giving them away) all responses to questions are typed and sent to the interrogator.

The man has studied up for the game, reading women's magazines and books about women, and he feels that he can answer much as a woman would answer. There is no use in the woman saying, "Don't listen to him! *I* am the woman!", because the man could say (that is, type) exactly the same thing. The man wins if he can fool the interrogator; the woman wins if the interrogator correctly picks her.

Turing then suggests modifying the game to help us answer our perplexing question. Let any randomly chosen human being take the place of the woman; the job of this contestant is to try to convince the interrogator to choose him or her as the human. In the place of the man in the game, Turing puts a computer, whose job it is to try to fool the interrogator into picking it as the human. Just as in the earlier game, the computer can "study up" on what humans say and do.

Turing maintains that if the computer can do better than "chance" in the game, we should admit that it thinks. The reason for this is that we have been unable to distinguish it from something that we *do* admit thinks—a human being. Note that Turing had great confidence, in 1950, when computers were still rather primitive, that the test would be passed by a computer.

Objections   Turing says that people will raise various objections to a positive answer to the question, "Can a machine think?" He, in good Aristotelian manner, attempts a "negative demonstration" where he takes on the objections one by one, and tries to show that they do not harm his position.

1. *The theological objection.* "Only humans have God-given souls and think. Therefore no machine can think." But where is the cutoff between humans and animals? If evolution is true, at what point in evolution did God confer souls on humans? If a computer reached a sufficient level of complexity, couldn't God give it a soul? We surely do not want to say that God could not give a soul to a computer, because that would imply a limitation on God, who is all-powerful. Are thinking things necessarily made out of protein? (Minsky calls them "meat machines.") Why not silicon-based as well as carbon-based matter? (Of course, this reply to the objection does not even get into the matter of the difficulty of proving the existence of God or a soul.)

2. *The "heads in the sand" objection.* An ostrich buries its head in the sand so as not to see what is going on around it. Those who bring this objec-

tion simply say, "It would be too awful if computers could think!" But this is not an argument, and it carries no weight. Someone could have said, before World War II, "It would be too awful if there were another world war; therefore there will not be another world war." This feeling would not have affected the coming of the war.

3. *The mathematical objection.* This is based on research in the foundations of mathematics. Gödel's proof shows that no system complex enough to represent arithmetic can be both consistent and complete; there are *true* statements expressible in the system that cannot be proved true or false in the system. But humans can somehow "see" the truth of Gödel's proof, and the truth of the expressible-but-not-provable statement (G). Thus it is claimed that, since the computer could only know the truth of G if it could prove it true, and this is impossible, humans can know something the machine does not.[2]

This is a complex objection, and perhaps one of the most serious that can be raised. However, it is not clear just how we humans come to "see" the truth of G, or that it would be impossible for the computer to do something similar to what we do. It relies on the assumption that we can deal with meaning (semantics) whereas the computer is restricted to manipulating syntax. However, this may not be the case, especially if we think in terms of a "learning" computer, perhaps one equipped with a battery of sensors.

4. *The argument from consciousness.* It is said that a machine cannot *feel*, cannot have emotions. One problem we have here is that I cannot ever *know* that another human feels as I do; all I have to go on is that person's behavior. If a computer *behaves* as if it has emotions, how can I be sure it does not? Furthermore, is it emotion on which we want to stake our humanity, our thinking ability—or is it our reason? And reason is exhibited in activities like doing mathematics, playing chess, making considered decisions—but a computer can do all of these things. Lastly, we could always build a Scriven machine (described later in this chapter in the section on Consciousness) and see!

5. *Arguments from various disabilities.* Someone may claim, "A computer will never be able to do X," where X may be a variety of things (suggests Turing): be kind, have a sense of humor, tell right from wrong, enjoy strawberries and cream, learn from experience, and so on. This is the path taken by Hubert Dreyfus in his two books, *What Computers Can't Do* and *What Computers Still Can't Do*. These objections can be taken one by one. Why couldn't a computer be kind, or have a sense of humor, or tell right from wrong? Perhaps it just needs a good education. And strawberries and cream? Some humans are *allergic* to strawberries, and cream has a high fat content, which is unhealthy. This is not a serious objection.

6. *Lady Lovelace's objection.* Ada, Lady Lovelace, said that "the Analytical Engine has no pretensions to *originate* anything. It can do *whatever we know how to order it to perform.*" But much of what humans do is conditioned (by nature and nurture); some (materialists) argue that we are just machines, deterministic—so if we can "think," another machine could do so too. On the other side, there are machines that can modify their own programs (like some chess-playing machines) and be said to "learn." In such cases, Lady Lovelace's objection does not apply.

7. *The argument from continuity in the nervous system.* Our nervous system is continuous, computers are discrete. Well, perhaps, but the functional units of our brains are discrete, *binary* neurons that either fire or don't fire, just like memory components in a computer.

8. *The argument from informality of behavior.* Humans are illogical and unpredictable, whereas computers are logical and predictable. But is it our irrationality on which we base our claims to think? If we are too unpredictable, someone will throw us into a home for the mentally unstable. On the other side, there are the computers that can modify their programs, and so their behavior is not always predictable.

9. *The argument from ESP.* The objection says that humans have extrasensory perception (ESP), computers do not. Aside from questions regarding the credibility of ESP experiments, whatever the mechanism for ESP (is it like an electromagnetic field?), why couldn't it also operate on a computer?

Turing threw out the challenge in 1950, attempted to meet the objections, and said we must wait and see.

ELIZA   In 1976, Joseph Weizenbaum created a computer program to imitate the dialogue of a psychiatrist with her patient. The program picks up on words in context, and constructs a question based on each response given by the person. This can be done very nicely at a computer terminal, with the person typing in responses, and the ELIZA communications also appearing on the screen. A dialogue ensues, and since it is expected that a psychiatrist would try to draw out the person more on the topics that are mentioned, it seems quite realistic.

Weizenbaum tells a number of stories about how ELIZA "passed" the Turing test. One involved a person working at Bolt, Beranek, and Newman, a firm Weizenbaum consulted for. Someone had left the ELIZA program running on a terminal and the man logged on, unaware of ELIZA. He thought he was contacting Weizenbaum at home. ELIZA asked: WHAT IS YOUR PROBLEM? The man responded: I would like to use the computer facility this weekend. ELIZA asked: WHY DO YOU WANT TO USE THE COMPUTER FACILITY THIS WEEKEND?, and to the next response, said ARE YOU SURE? The man quickly got frustrated, and called Weizenbaum up on the phone to chew him out for being such a wiseacre. Weizenbaum was quite amused when he realized that the man had been communicating with ELIZA, thinking he was communicating with a human.

Another story Weizenbaum tells is about his secretary, who knew all about the ELIZA program and what it did. One day she asked him if she could try it, and Weizenbaum showed her how. After a few questions and responses, she asked Weizenbaum if he would please leave the room. Apparently she felt as if she were really talking to a psychiatrist, and wanted some privacy!

Weizenbaum himself does not believe that ELIZA has passed the Turing test, and makes no such claims. In fact, he has rather strong opinions about the limitations that should be placed on the tasks assigned to computers (see his book *Computer Power and Human Reason*, ch. 8). Yet a *functionalist* would say that ELIZA and a human are functionally equivalent, since they behave the same; thus they are interchangeable. The question that arises is, isn't there something present in the human that is lacking in ELIZA?

If you would like to try out the ELIZA program, there are currently several interactive versions online. I recommend:

http://livingroom.org/eliza/

Of those I tried, this one seemed closest to the original. There is a famous interaction with ELIZA reported by Weizenbaum, which includes, as an early entry from the user, "MY BOYFRIEND MADE ME COME HERE." This online version gives the same good responses to the entries, and so seems closest to Weizenbaum's program.

The Chinese Room

John Searle—sometimes referred to as the "black knight" of Artificial Intelligence because he gainsays many of the high-flown claims of the A.I. community—presents the following very interesting example in his article, "Minds, Brains, and Programs" (in Rosenthal, 1991). He says that one should imagine Searle, who knows no Chinese, placed in a room that has two windows that open into it. Through one of these windows he receives pieces of paper with Chinese characters on them. He also has a set of instructions, in

English, that tell him how to match up the input Chinese characters to other Chinese characters, and to hand them out the other window (as "output").

From the outside, it appears that Searle is actually reading the input strings and creating the output as if answering questions. The functionalist would say this is what is going on, since the "outputs" are correct. However, Searle points out, he *understands* nothing of either the input or the output strings. As he says, "my answers to the questions are absolutely indistinguishable from those of native Chinese speakers. Nobody just looking at my answers can tell that I don't speak a word of Chinese" (Searle in Rosenthal, 1991, p. 510).

He contrasts this case with one in which he is given English sentences as input and he hands out English sentences as output. In the English case, he *understands* what information is being conveyed; in the Chinese case, he understands nothing. He uses this example to counter claims made by "strong AI" that the current natural-language-processing AI programs *understand* the stories they deal with, and that their operation can shed some light on human understanding. He says that the computer program is doing something analogous to what he did with the Chinese input characters— manipulating symbols according to preset rules—but that there is no understanding whatsoever.

There has been much discussion of Searle's example, but it does seem to make an important point. The functionalist approach says that if the behavior of two boxes (rooms) is the same, what is going on inside the rooms is the same. Searle manages to put his finger right on a significant difference, that of *understanding*, which goes on in one case but not the other.

Another analogy might be to a blind person who has learned to use other cues to get around well, and who knows how to use the language of colors and patterns that sighted people use, in all the right contexts. The blind person would then behave the same as a sighted person in similar settings, and the functionalist would claim that they are equivalent. Yet there is definitely something in the sighted person's inner experience that is missing from that of the blind person—the *seeing* of a patch of red, the sweeping grace of a tree. What is missing is referred to as *qualia*.

 # ARTIFICIAL INTELLIGENCE AND ETHICS

So what is the relevance of all this discussion of artificial intelligence to computer ethics? Well, part of it has to do with the proper use of computers in sensitive and/or critical areas. With the advent of expert systems, questions arise about what are ethical uses of, for example, medical expert systems, and what uses might be unethical? Should computers be allowed to make battlefield decisions in war? Should the retaliatory potential of a country be left in the control of computer-automated systems?

The other question that arises is that, *if* machines were to become intelligent, what moral obligations we would have toward them. Would we treat them as slaves or as equals? Should they have rights (to go along with the responsibilities we ask them to take on)? Could an artificial intelligence learn the difference between right and wrong? Could it be autonomous? Recall that Kant, in his ethics, talks about rational beings, and about the obligations of duty among such beings. Rationality is the basis of the categorical imperative. We build and program the robots and computers, but that is not all that different from having and educating children.

Our word 'robot' comes from Karel Capek's 1923 play, *R.U.R.*–which stands for "Rossum's Universal Robots." 'Rossum' is the Czech word for reason, and it was old Rossum who created the 'robota', or *workers*. The robots are made to look like human beings, and take over human tasks. The humans get lazy, and don't do anything but sit around and make trouble. So the robots decide to wipe out the humans, because they are violent, aggressive, and bad for the environment. They do this only to discover that they do not know Rossum's secret formula for making more robots. But at the end of the play, a male-type robot and a female-type robot seem to be discovering each other and perhaps a "natural" way to create more robots.

One of the questions that arose when others were designing the robots was whether they should give them pain nerves. It was argued that they must do so, for pain would protect the robot from harm (it would withdraw its arm from a machine that would crush the arm, for example). Of course, the purpose of giving the robots pain was for the benefit of the humans. It does raise a more interesting moral question, though: that of whether, if we were to develop sentient robots, we *should* give them pain.

Is pain a necessary correlate of pleasure? If we wanted to give the robots the experience of pleasure, would they also have to have pain? Is pain necessary for survival? It seems to work that way sometimes for animals, but there are also many cases where the pain serves no warning or teaching purpose, such as the excruciating pain of terminal cancer. Would it be possible just to have certain warning sensors that would send a signal to the robot's CPU that could be interpreted as, for example, a signal indicating the fire, which could then be avoided? Would it *have* to inflict pain, or would the information that there is danger be enough?

The rational robot would act on such information, but of course the programmer would have had to anticipate all possible danger situations, and to program in the appropriate signals in reaction. If our advanced robot is to learn from experience, from interacting with the world, one cannot rely on a human programmer to anticipate all new danger situations that might arise. There is just so much we can teach our children, and warn them about, and then they have to go out and cope with the world on their own. The same would be true of our new breed of intelligent robots. So perhaps it would be necessary to give them "pain," as diabolical as that might seem. What do you think?

 # CONSCIOUSNESS

The theme of **consciousness** seems to be coming to the fore in the most recent artificial intelligence discussions. Turing's question of whether machines can think now seems to have moved to the question whether machines can be conscious, and what it means in *any* being to be conscious. Some of the more recent books in this area include the following: Paul M. Churchland, *Matter and Consciousness* (MIT Press, 1984); Daniel C. Dennett, *Consciousness Explained* (Little, Brown, 1991); Colin McGinn, *The Problem of Consciousness* (Blackwell, 1991); Owen Flanagan, *Consciousness Reconsidered* (MIT Press/Bradford, 1992); John R. Searle, *The Rediscovery of the Mind* (MIT Press, 1992); Martin Davis and Glyn W. Humphreys, *Consciousness* (Blackwell, 1993); Austen Clark, *Sensory Qualities* (Clarendon Press, 1993); Roger Penrose, *Shadows of the Mind* (Oxford University Press, 1994); David J. Chalmers, *The Conscious Mind* (Oxford, 1996); Norton Nelkin, *Consciousness and the Origins of Thought* (Cambridge University Press, 1996); Michael Tye, *Ten Problems of Consciousness* (MIT Press, 1999); and Michael Tye, *Consciousness, Color, and Content* (MIT Press, 2000). These books seem to be going to a more fundamental question—can something be intelligent (think) if it is not conscious? If the answer is *no*, then we should be talking about consciousness *before* we can talk meaningfully about thinking and intelligence (and if the answer is yes, some illuminating examples and explication should be forthcoming).

The move to consider consciousness with respect to machines is not new in the 1990s. In 1953, Michael Scriven wrote an article in *Mind* called "The Mechanical Concept of Mind." In this article he suggests constructing a sophisticated computer, giving it access to all of human literature (especially to that which relates to consciousness), teaching it not to lie (which, he says, will make it unadaptable as an advertising executive or a politician), and then asking it if it is conscious. We will refer to such a computer as a "Scriven machine." If the Scriven machine says "yes," then we know that it is conscious, and the long-disputed question has been finally answered. If it answers "no," Scriven says we will just have to build another computer! ("We must get a winner one day!")

Kurzweil's "Age of Spiritual Machines"

Ray Kurzweil, inventor of reading machines for the blind as well as speech recognition and music synthesis machines, wrote a visionary book in 1999 entitled *The Age of Spiritual Machines: When Computers Exceed Human Intelligence.* He begins by predicting that computers will achieve "the memory capacity and computing speed of the human brain by around the year 2020" (Kurzweil, 1999, p. 3). He goes on to make a number of fascinating predictions for the future (in 2029, a $1,000 computing unit will have the computing capacity of 1,000 human brains, and so on).

Hawking's Perspective

Physicist Stephen Hawking recently made the following observation:

> With genetic engineering, we will be able to increase the complexity of our DNA, and improve the human race. But it will be a slow process, because one will have to wait about 18 years to see the effect of changes to the genetic code. By contrast, computers double their speed and memories every 18 months. There is a real danger that computers will develop intelligence and take over. We urgently need to develop direct connections to the brain, so that computers can add to human intelligence, rather than be in opposition. (e-mail communication through his graduate assistant, Neel Shearer, October 2, 2001)

Hawking's ideas are at least as provocative as Kurzweil's. He seems to feel an urgency that we not get outstripped by machine intelligence, but rather co-opt it to enhance our own.

THE ECO-COMPUTER

In 1987, Geoff Simons wrote a book called *Eco-Computer: The Impact of Global Intelligence,* which focuses on the interaction of two current technologies—computers and communications networks (which actually are not clearly distinguishable these days). The eco-computer will be provided with artificial sensors that link it to the world, as well as an artificial intelligence to process the information gathered and initiate actions. Simons suggests that it will be able to have touch, vision, heat detectors, and auditory recognition:

> [It] will be equally interested in geological data and information about demographic change; it will interpret weather patterns and agricultural cycles; it will carry out market research, investigate theoretical social models—and embark upon optimized programmes of production and distribution. At the same time, mistakes will be made: there will be scheduling problems and human casualties. . . .
>
> The elements of the eco-computer are countless: through linkages and interfaces (through "connectivity") all the world of electronics will become part of its anatomy. It will permeate the biosphere and go beyond it: its nerves and muscles and probes will penetrate outer space and the depths of earthly oceans; its senses will see in the dark, hear molecules vibrate and smell the smallest chemical change. The planet will become a person: Gaia—cybernetic, independent, one.

Simons goes on to say that one can get a sense for what an eco-computer will be like from the Strategic Defense Initiative, or from an "intelligent building" that automatically controls its own air-conditioning, heat, fire detection, and the like. His vision here (which is not a utopian one) sounds a great deal like the Colossus computer in *Colossus: The Forbin Project.*

 ## CYBERSEX

People are constantly communicating over the Internet. When they do, they can write anything they want, as long as someone will read it (and no censors interfere). Thus, some people interchange scientific advances, others critique movies, some complain about the weather and the government, and some . . . write about sex. This can be suggestive, a kind of foreplay, or it can be quite explicit—when they write like this, and when someone reads it and responds, they are said to be engaging in **cybersex**. The correspondence can be strictly one-on-one, or it may be played out in a shared domain, a MUD (Multi-User-Domain). These are referred to as "chat rooms," places in cyberspace where a number of players can interact, constitute a sort of on-line singles bar.

One writer has characterized this as a kind of "X-rated Dungeons and Dragons";[3] in these domains, users often take on other identities—either not to be recognized, or just to heighten the fantasy. The "chat" can get very *hot* in such a MUD; people drop many inhibitions when they can hide behind another identity and a computer screen. These are primarily verbal sexual exchanges, though some "multimedia" connections might provide additional stimuli, such as pictures and sounds. However, the majority of such compu-sex encounters are primarily verbal. Branwyn writes: "In compu-sex, being able to type fast and write well is equivalent to having great legs or a tight butt in the real world" (at least among compu-sex enthusiasts).[4]

Some group "encounters" may involve one player giving sexual directions to another, or another pair. Many fantasies can be played out, especially if there are other "consenting" players. These fantasies are not much different than those played out when someone reads an erotic text, or watches an X-rated film, except that there are other "living" contributors to the story, so it does not come out the same way every time. No real harm is done; "a good time was had by all."

However, some of these encounters can have a serious downside. It is so easy, on the Net, to masquerade as someone you are not, that false hopes and expectations may be generated in the other party to the erotic exchange. There have been a number of cases of men masquerading as women, to entice other women to "let down their guard" and engage in sharing explicit sexual fantasies. When the deception is discovered, these women feel betrayed. In other cases, one party leads the other on for a time, only to cut off communication abruptly (this is not too unlike many real-life relationships). The most frightening aspect of such "chats" is when young children enter the picture and can be lured into face-to-face encounters with online perverts.

Langdon Winner writes that these Net connections provide "techno-erotic alternatives for bored, middle-class Americans."[5] The "data gloves" designed to help humans direct robot explorers are now extended to accoutrements for other extremities and organs. A pair of writers for *Liberation* in France describe the virtual sexuality system from "Cyber SM," in which participants put on their "sensation suits" and then can "stimulate" each other with computer-controlled voltages to the suits.[6] This sounds a bit beyond the current technology, and it also sounds dangerous! Would you want to trust your most valued bodily parts to shocks controlled by a new, and who-knows-how-well-tested, computer program? Recall our discussions of errors and reliability.

There are also various bulletin boards that cater to sexual fantasies. Users could log onto Amateur Action (in spite of charges against the owners pending in court) and select sexually explicit fiction and/or pictures from "Oral Sex," "Bestiality," "Nude Celebrities," or "Lolita Schoolgirls." Recent sites include Cybersex Matrix ("redhead in pigtails"), Oriental Cybersex, Cybersex Teens, Cybersex Lesbians, and many more. Since the police bust of this BBS that claims to be "the nastiest place on earth!", they begin their program with a message: "Amateur Action BBS is for the private use of the citizens of the United States! Use by law enforcement agents, postal inspectors, and informants is prohibited!"[7] This raises an interesting point: Is such a disclaimer sufficient to undermine any police involvement?

In 1995, EPIC lawyer David Banisar said that if "Net Police" wanted to try to filter out any "obscene, lewd, lascivious" material from all the traffic on the Net, it would be "like shooting an ICBM at a gnat. . . . it can't be done without the most Draconian methods being used" (see http://venus/soci.niu. edu/~cuidigest/CUDS7/cud724).

So, we might ask, is any of this immoral? The answer should come down to an assessment of whether any *harm* is done, and in what respect. Clearly, enticing minors into secret rendezvous for the purposes of sexually exploiting them is *harmful*—no question. But interactions among "consenting adults" would seem to be covered by privacy considerations. The *real* problem is, is this a productive way to spend a human life? Are at-a-distance, hidden-behind-the-computer relationships *real* relationships? Compu-sex may be "safe," with no serious entanglements, but is it satisfying? Does it take the place of *real* relationships with *real people* (not false personae)? Or does it contribute to a tendency to avoid society and commitments to others? It is on this basis that an ethical assessment of cybersex should be made.

VIRTUAL WORLDS

Multi-user domains are used for many encounters other than cybersex. People play out fantasies in medieval knights-and-dragons roles, or in outer space futuristic star treks. Generally the player takes on a persona (or several) in one or many MUDs. Is this deception? Only if the other player(s) take it seriously, as we indicated in several of the cybersex cases. But generally it is a fantasy, and no matter how engrossing it is, everyone really knows it is a fantasy. (Or do they?) Fantasies are fine; they stretch our imaginations, give us temporary escape from a humdrum world. But some players get addicted to these fantasies, spending up to seven hours a day in different MUDs. This obviously is not productive, and it may skew their perspective on the real world when they *do* return to it. This would have moral consequences if they did not meet their obligations to others, or carried the violence of some of the fantasies over into the real world, inflicting harm on others.

John Fodor raises the question whether the *deceptions* of taking on other identities in a MUD (or just in e-mail) are violations of Kantian ethics.[8]

Deceiving someone is analogous to making a promise and then breaking it; this would be treating others as a means rather than as ends in themselves. On the other hand, as we have said, those engaging in the fantasy *should* realize that it *is* a fantasy, and understand the game-playing rules that go along with that. When you create a persona (or several) in your medieval MUD, would you really be surprised to learn that the character you are inter-acting with right now is *not* Lancelot?

Fodor also points out that this kind of interaction is beneficial to persons with disabilities; they can "enjoy the full benefits of interacting with other per-sons without prejudice to their disabilities."[9] This is certainly true, and it is one of the good things about computer networking: It provides a "space" in which rational individuals can interact on an equal basis, independent of their physical endowments. Fodor suggests that this may force us to critically reexamine the universalizability of our ethical theories.[10] This may be so, but we have already recognized that there are very few actions that are truly universalizable without exception. This is why David Ross came up with the *prima facie* duties, and why a number of moral theorists returned to *virtue ethics* due to weaknesses in both Kantian and utilitarian ethics. This does not mean that a Kantian "golden rule" test is not a good one in many cases. And perhaps the real question here, as we already asked, is whether these are serious deceptions—that is, is anyone *really* deceived in a MUD? If not, then it is no more harmful that getting deeply engrossed in reading *Sir Gawain and the Green Knight* or watching *Star Wars*.

Perhaps the most serious problem that such game-playing presents, especially when it becomes an obsession that dominates someone's life, is the kind of "moral distance" it seems to place between the player and the real world. Richard Rubin identifies "Seven Temptations" in computer tech-nology that contribute to this moral distancing, change our perspectives, and "divert our attention from ethical concerns."[11] They are as follows:

1. *Speed.* One can commit an action at the speed of light in a MUD, or steal a computer file or divert electronic funds so quickly that there is little likelihood of being caught.
2. *Privacy and anonymity.* An act can be committed, such as destroying a database, with no trace left of who committed it; one can engage anonymously in the exciting, normally forbidden act of eavesdropping on someone else's private data and communications.
3. *Nature of the medium.* The fact that information can be stolen (copied) without being removed lends to the view that no damage has been done.
4. *Aesthetic attraction.* Writing a clever program, or hacking into a "secure" installation, represents a creative challenge.

5. *Increased availability of potential victims.* One can access billions of records at the touch of a button, and a damaging message posted on a public BBS can reach thousands or more in the blink of an eye.

6. *International scope.* Robin observes that "acting unethically around the world is quite possible." [12]

7. *The power to destroy.* Not only can all sorts of information be accessed, but it can be destroyed, for example, by unleashing a virus. Many of the games played in MUDs are ones in which the goal is to *destroy* the enemy.

As rational and moral agents, we must resist the temptations created by this new medium; we must not be seduced by the appearance of a "moral distance" between us and our "victims," a distance that in fact does not exist. Killing became easier with the invention of the gun; it could be performed at a much greater distance, and one's physical characteristics (such as strength and speed) were no longer relevant. This ease of killing may have increased its frequency, but it was made no less hateful.

The world of computers is drawing us farther and farther away from the real physical world in which bodies move more slowly and with greater difficulty, and real people with real feelings and concerns interact with each other. Cybersex takes the place of real sex (will children come from laboratories?), playing in the MUD takes the place of playing a sport or playing with real children. Children play Nintendo or electronically gamble at casinos instead of playing outdoors with each other.[13] They are not developing their bodies, their health deteriorates, and they are only developing a small part of their brains. In a video game or a MUD, someone can be killed and come back to life; what if children come to believe that is the way things really are?

When the baseball strike of 1994 went on interminably, the newspapers started publishing results of computer-simulated "games" to satisfy the fans; it would seem that the layoff and substitute satisfaction took the edge off the real thing, as attendance at ballparks since the settlement of the strike appeared to be down considerably. There was a notice on the TV broadcast of a live tennis match that one could hook up for "Fantasy Football" on the Internet! Will this soon take the place of high school, college, and professional football?

Virtual Reality

"It's a jungle out there. It's a Martian colony, too, or an underwater cavern. Or even a distant galaxy." [14] This is the hype imagined for tomorrow's virtual reality theme parks. Step up and take your choice; you can explore the steaming jungles of the Amazon, ride on a pterodactyl, or visit a Martian colony. Shades of the movie *Total Recall*!

Virtual reality began with "magic glasses" and a "data glove" that would allow a human observer to control a robot inside a dangerous environment (for example, one high in radiation). The observer could "see" through visual sensors and "feel" what was being touched through the data glove. This has expanded to virtual reality helmets that create a visual and auditory world for the wearer; this can be supplemented by a treadmill on which the person can move, and these movements are reflected in the virtual environment. Unlike a movie, what the wearer of the helmet does is *interact* with the environment and alter it by bodily motions. What is the point of this? It can be for entertainment (which is where most of today's hype comes from) and escape, or it can have some very productive applications.

Today's virtual reality systems are very expensive; the computers that run them can cost hundreds of thousands of dollars,[15] plus the cost of the VR equipment, so a good system is not likely to be available for use in the home or mall any time soon. When it is, it will have the same negative aspects of escaping into a MUD that we discussed. However, it also has great potential for exploration of places you could never normally go, for experiencing worlds of the past (or future), and for learning about the structure of objects.

The Cave Automatic Virtual Environment (CAVE) at the University of Illinois is used by scientists to simulate actually climbing *inside* physical objects; it allows them to rearrange molecules to create a stronger alloy, to "watch" gravitational waves move through space, and to point to where radiation must be aimed to dissolve a tumor without damaging surrounding tissue.[16] The CAVE project was jointly funded by the NSF, ARPA, the Department of Energy, NASA, Caterpillar Inc., and General Motors.

Other exciting applications of virtual reality are in flight simulators (that are more sophisticated than those that have been around for years) in which pilots can train, virtual surgery for fledgling doctors to practice,[17] virtual chemical experiments for scientists[18] (without laboratory explosions!), and a virtual museum with animated hieroglyphics and a feature that lets you actually "pass into paintings" and walk around.[19] A company called Virtual Vision, of Redmond, Washington, developed glasses that help Parkinson's disease sufferers correct their halting walks.[20] Scientists are using virtual elevators to overcome people's fear of heights,[21] and virtual reality environments are being used to overcome other phobias by exposing patients to the source of their fears.[22] UCLA is working on an elaborate "Rome Reborn" project.

All of these virtual reality experiments are valuable because they help us deal with various real-world situations, and allow us to learn more about the structure of reality. They *simulate* what *is real*, or *was real*, in order for us to learn more about, or cope better with, what is real. The applications of virtual reality to create fantasy worlds is much more suspect; it can have the effect of distancing its users from reality and from society. The wearer of a virtual reality helmet is alone in a world, and needs no other real people there; any company or challenge can be provided by the fake environment. Becoming addicted to such worlds makes users unfit to live in *this* world. An article we looked at in Chapter 6 suggested creating MUDs (that could also have virtual reality environments) where people act out crimes: "We need new scripts to keep virtual crime more entertaining than real crime. Wouldn't want perps to leave their terminals and start whacking real people on the real streets."[23] Is *this* the way to reduce crime, by making it into a game? What we need is moral education, not VR crime sprees "to let them get it out of their systems."

The name of the University of Illinois VR system—CAVE—immediately brings Plato's Cave to mind.[24] But Plato's motive for the metaphor was to encourage people to get out of the cave of appearances and into reality. MUDs and non–scientific-research VR just create new, more spectacular caves for people to hide in.

■ ENDNOTES

1. Kenneth Appel and Wolfgang Haken, "The Solution of the Four-Color-Map Problem," *Scientific American,* October 1977, pp. 108–121. Wolfgang Haken, "An Attempt to Understand the Four-Color Problem," *Journal of Graph Theory* 1 (1977), 193–206.

2. J. R. Lucas also uses this as a basis for claiming free will for humans, in *The Freedom of the Will* (Oxford, England: Clarendon Press, 1970).

3. Matthew Childs, "Lust Online," *Playboy,* April 1994, p. 156.

4. Gareth Branwyn, "Compu-Sex: Erotica for Cybernauts," *South-Atlantic Quarterly* 92, 4 (Fall 1993), 784.

5. Langdon Winner, "Cyberpornography," *Technology Review* 97, 2 (February 1994), 70.

6. Christian Simenc and Paul Loubiere, "Love in the Age of Cybersex," *World Press Review* 41, 4 (April 1994), 40.

7. Peter H. Lewis, "Despite a New Plan for Cooling It, Cybersex Stays Hot," *New York Times,* 26 March 1995, sec. 1, p. 1.

8. John L. Fodor, "CyberEthics," in Joseph Kizza, ed., *Ethics in the Computer Age: ACM Conference Proceedings (November 11–13, 1994)*. New York: ACM, 1994, p. 185.

9. Fodor, p. 185.

10. Fodor, p. 186.

11. Richard Rubin, "Moral Distancing and the Use of Information Technologies: The Seven Temptations," in Kizza, p. 152.

12. Rubin, p. 153.

13. Mitch Betts and Gary Anthes, "On-line Boundaries Unclear; Internet Tramples Legal Jurisdictions," *Computerworld* (June 5, 1995).

14. Murray Slovick, "Virtual Thrills & Chills," *Popular Mechanics*, April 1995, p. 86.

15. David L. Wilson, "A Key for Entering Virtual Worlds," *Chronicle of Higher Education* 41, 12 (November 16, 1994), A18.

16. Wilson, p. A19. This is like the movie *Fantastic Voyage*, in which scientists and their vehicle are shrunk so that they can go inside a person's body to repair damage.

17. Kevin T. McGovern, "Applications of Virtual Reality to Surgery," *British Medical Journal* 308, 6936 (April 1994), 1054–55. Cf. Gary Taubes, "Surgery in Cyberspace," *Discover* 15, 12 (December 1994), 84–94, which describes surgery at a distance.

18. Ted Nield, "Albert's Adventures in Hyperspace," *New Scientist* 144, 1947 (October 15, 1994), 62–64.

19. Stephen Burd, "Carnegie Mellon Researcher Invites You On a Trip to 'Virtual Reality'," *Chronicle of Higher Education* 41, 3 (September 14, 1994), A48.

20. Gail Dutton, "Perpetual Pathway," *Popular Science* 245, 1 (July 1994), 34.

21. Constance Holden, "Virtual Therapy for Phobias," *Science* 268, 5208 (April 14, 1995), 209.

22. Mark Hodges, "Facing Real Fears in Virtual Worlds," *Technology Review* 98, 4 (May 1995), 16–17.

23. Tom Dworetzky, "Crime and Punishment: Raskolnikov Does MUD Time," *Omni* 16, 11 (August 1994), 16.

24. The Cave image begins Book VII of Plato's *Republic*. Socrates introduces it to explain the effect of education (or the lack of it) on human nature. In the cave, prisoners are tied so that they can see only the wall of the cave, on which shadows play. The shadows are created by a fire burning behind them that shines on people (probably poets and statesmen) carrying statues of natural objects; these people walk along an elevated road, and their shadows are the only reality the prisoners know. One day a prisoner gets loose from the shackles, turns, and is blinded temporarily by the fire. He then sees an opening out of the cave and is dragged up the rough, steep path to the outside.

There he is initially blinded by the Sun, and cannot see what is around him. Finally, his eyes adjust and he sees, first, images reflected in water, then the things themselves, and finally the Sun itself. However, the Sun is blinding, and so he can only look for any extended time at its image reflected in water. For Plato, education is a *turning* of the soul in the right direction, to see (comprehend) reality. The prisoner who left the Cave must go back (it is his duty, but he must be forced), to bring the truth to those still there. However, just telling them will not put the truth into their souls; they must experience the journey and the revelation themselves.

The best rulers for the *polis* must be forced to rule, because they have no natural inclination to do so. Those who *want* to rule want to do so for the wrong reasons (power, money, glory). The true ruler can only be compelled to rule by the fear of being ruled by someone inferior who will botch things up and harm the state and those in it.

The good (moral) individual must also make the journey up the Divided Line (or out of the Cave), from ignorance to knowledge, as the lover of beauty and the true politician did.

■ SHORT ESSAY QUESTIONS

1. Marvin Minsky wrote a book entitled *The Society of Mind*. Check out the beginning of this book to find out what he means by this title.

2. Discuss the questions raised by Walter Maner about medical expert systems.

3. Discuss whether the Turing test is a good test of intelligence/thinking.

4. In the movie *Blade Runner*, the Tyrell Corporation creates robot "replicants" that are almost impossible to distinguish from humans. They have superior strength and agility, and equal or greater intelligence than the genetic engineers who created them. Replicants are used for slave labor on other planets and space stations. The replicants have mutinied and are not allowed to return to Earth. Special police squads—blade runners—have orders to shoot to kill any replicant found on Earth; this is not called execution, it is called "retirement." Comment on the morality of creating and using such entities in this way.

5. When Colossus takes control at the end of the movie *Colossus: The Forbin Project*, the all-powerful computer, a paragon of reason, issues the following message to the people of Earth: "This is the voice of World Control. I bring you the peace of plenty and content or the peace of unburied death. I will not permit war; it is wasteful. I will restrain man. You will come to defend me. Under my absolute authority, problems insoluble to man will be solved." Discuss Colossus as a rational, autonomous being. Is Colossus moral? Make comparisons to Hobbes' *Leviathan*. What constitutes justice in this state?

6. One problem with programming computers is that they have no "common sense," so you have to tell them everything and think of everything that might go wrong. They also take everything literally. They are much like the children's book character Amelia Bedelia, who worked around the house and took everything strictly literally. Thus, if Amelia was told to "Draw the curtains," an illustration of the curtains would result. Comment on this in regard to making computers "understand" and operate on their own in the real world, as AI predicts they will.

7. In the book *Being Digital* (1995), Nicholas Negroponte writes that virtual reality "can make the artificial as realistic as, and even more realistic than, the real" (p. 116). Comment on this observation and its implications.

8. It was reported in *Time* (March 20, 1995, pp. 63–64) that the CIA is using virtual reality devices to train its operatives. Speculate on how these VR devices might be used in this context.

■ LONG ESSAY QUESTIONS

1. Ned Block has a nice little argument that I like to refer to as the "Chinese nation argument." In it he constructs a system which could be *said* to have mental states even though it does not in fact have mental states. This occurs in a section of an article called "Troubles with Functionalism," which can be found in Lycan (1990, pp. 450–53) or in

Rosenthal (1991, pp. 215–17). Describe Block's example, making clear what functionalism is and what he means by a homunculus. (This may take a little more digging on your part.) Apply this example to the question of whether a computer, if it had the same "table" of relations between inputs and outputs as a human being, could be considered (functionally) equivalent to the human being.

2. Daniel Dennett wrote a fascinating article called "Where Am I?" in his book *Brainstorms* (1978, pp. 310–23). Read it, write a critical exposition of what point(s) Dennett is making in the article, and then connect it to our discussions of computers and computer ethics. What implications does Dennett's "split personality" (if it can be so characterized) have for his status as a person, for his moral responsibility?

3. At the end of his book *Eco-computer*, Geoff Simons suggests that the idea of a *person* may be extended to a complex computer system, and that the eco-computer might evolve "multiple personalities" because of inherent contradictions in its goals (such as trying to reduce pollution but also aid industrial productivity, which contributes to pollution). Discuss this notion of a schizophrenic eco-computer, which Simons says will be an amoral system running beyond our control.

4. Do you think consciousness could be an "emergent" property, that occurs at a certain level of complexity of an entity? This question was raised in a segment of *Star Trek: The Next Generation* called "The Quality of Life," where devices called ex-o-comps are introduced aboard the Enterprise. These tool-makers and problem-solvers are designed to "reconfigure their pathways" and "learn" so that they can make better tools. They apparently develop (the android officer Data is the first to notice) a sense of self-preservation, of protecting "life." They have a survival instinct, and Data takes a stand against allowing them to be destroyed to save a human life, since they also represent a life form. At the end, one of the ex-o-comps sacrifices itself to save two others. See if you can get a copy of this segment to watch. Comment critically on the idea of an emergent consciousness and self-awareness, and the development of survival instincts and those of sacrifice of oneself for others.

5. In another *Star Trek: Next Generation* episode, Commander Maddox is going to dismantle Data to learn more about how he works. There is no guarantee that Maddox will be able to put Data back together without loss of his experiences, the "ineffable quality to memory." So Data decides to resign from Star Fleet to avoid this. "When Dr. Sung created me, he added to the substance of the universe. If by your experiments I

am destroyed, something unique, something wonderful, will be lost. I cannot permit that." Maddox claims that Data cannot resign, since he is the *property* of Star Fleet. Captain Picard defends Data in the ensuing hearing. Just when things are looking bleak, Picard puts forward the following defense: "It has been said that Data is a machine; we too are machines, just of a different sort. A man created Data, but humans create children; are *they* property?" Maddox claims that Data is not sentient. When questioned by Picard about what is involved in sentience, Maddox responds intelligence, self-awareness, and consciousness. Picard goes on to demonstrate Data's intelligence, and that he is self-aware. When asked what is at stake in the hearing, Data responds: "My right to choose; perhaps my very life." It is left open whether Data has the third characteristic—consciousness. Picard argues that a race of Datas would be enslaved by Maddox's view, and slavery is wrong. The court grants Data's right to choose not to submit to Maddox's experiment. Discuss this episode from the point of view of our discussions of artificial intelligence. Discuss whether we have ethical obligations to any Datas we might create.

6. The *Los Angeles Times* reported (25 June 1994, p. B7) that in a computer game recreating World War II, Japanese players change the Pacific phase of the war to a Japanese victory. Discuss.

■ REFERENCES AND RECOMMENDED READINGS

Adam, Alison. *Artificial Knowing: Gender and the Thinking Machine.* London: Routledge, 1998.

Albus, James S. *Brains, Behavior, and Robotics.* Peterborough, NH: Byte Books, 1981.

Albus, James S. "The Robot Revolution: An Interview with James Albus." *Communications of the ACM* (March 1983), 179–80.

Anderson, Alan R., ed. *Minds and Machines.* Englewood Cliffs, NJ: Prentice-Hall, 1964.

Arbib, Michael A. *Computers and the Cybernetic Society.* 2nd ed. Orlando, FL: Academic Press, 1984.

Benedikt, Michael, ed. *Cyberspace: First Steps.* Cambridge, MA: MIT Press, 1992.

Betts, M. "Designing Doctor-Friendly Systems a Chore." *Computerworld* 28, 26 (June 27, 1994), 73, 76.

Blakemore, Colin, and Susan Greenfield, ed. *Mindwaves: Thoughts on Intelligence, Identity and Consciousness*. Cambridge, MA: Blackwell, 1987.

Boden, Margaret. *Artificial Intelligence and Natural Man*. New York: Basic Books, 1977.

Boden, Margaret A. "Escaping from the Chinese Room." In Boden (1990), pp. 89–104.

Boden, Margaret A., ed. *The Philosophy of Artificial Intelligence*. New York: Oxford University Press, 1990.

Bolter, J. David. *Turing's Man: Western Culture in the Computer Age*. Chapel Hill, NC: University of North Carolina Press, 1984.

Branwyn, Gareth. "Compu-Sex: Erotica for Cybernauts." *South Atlantic Quarterly* 92, 4 (Fall 1993), 779–91.

Burd, Stephen. "Carnegie Mellon Researcher Invites You on a Trip to 'Virtual Reality'." *Chronicle of Higher Education* 41, 3 (September 14, 1994), A48.

Cain, Philip. "Searle on Strong AI." *Australasian Journal of Philosophy* 68, 1 (March 1990), 103–8.

Capek, Karel. *R.U.R.* London: Samuel French, 1923.

Cartwright, Glenn F. "Virtual or Real? The Mind in Cyberspace." *Futurist* 28, 2 (March 1994), 22–26.

Cavazos, Edward A., and Gavino Morin. *Cyberspace and the Law: Your Rights and Duties in the On-Line World*. Cambridge, MA: MIT Press, 1994.

Charniak, Eugene, and Drew McDermott. *Introduction to Artificial Intelligence*. Reading, MA: Addison-Wesley, 1985.

Childs, Matthew. "Lust Online." *Playboy*, April 1994, pp. 94–96ff.

Churchland, Paul M. *Matter and Consciousness*. Cambridge, MA: MIT Press/Bradford, 1984.

Clark, Austen. *Sensory Qualities*. Oxford, England: Clarendon Press, 1993.

Codrington, Andrea. "High-tech Sex." *Self* 15, 11 (November 1993), 82–84.

Copeland, Jack. *Artificial Intelligence: A Philosophical Introduction*. Cambridge, MA: Blackwell, 1993.

Crevier, Daniel. *AI: The Tumultuous History of the Search for Artificial Intelligence*. New York: Basic Books, 1993.

Davies, Martin, and Glyn W. Humphreys, eds. *Consciousness: Psychological and Philosophical Essays*. Oxford, England: Blackwell, 1993.

Dejoie, Roy, George Fowler, and David Paradice, eds. *Ethical Issues in Information Systems*. Boston, MA: Boyd & Fraser, 1991.

Dennett, Daniel C. *Brainstorms: Philosophical Essays on Mind and Psychology*. Montgomery, VT: Bradford Books, 1978.

Dennett, Daniel C. *Consciousness Explained*. Boston, MA: Little, Brown, 1991.

Dennett, Daniel C. *The Intentional Stance*. Cambridge, MA: MIT Press/Bradford, 1987.

Dretske, Fred I. *Knowledge and the Flow of Information*. Cambridge, MA: MIT Press, 1982.

Dreyfus, Hubert L., and Stuart E. Dreyfus. *Mind Over Machine*. New York: Free Press, 1986.

Dreyfus, Hubert L. *What Computers Still Can't Do*. Cambridge, MA: MIT Press, 1993.

Dutton, Gail. "Perpetual Pathway." *Popular Science* 245, 1 (July 1994), 34.

Dworetzky, Tom. "Crime and Punishment: Raskolnikov Does MUD Time." *Omni* 16, 11 (August 1994), 16.

Firebaugh, Morris W. *Artificial Intelligence: A Knowledge-Based Approach*. Boston, MA: Boyd & Fraser, 1990.

Flanagan, Owen. *Consciousness Reconsidered*. Cambridge, MA: MIT Press/Bradford, 1992.

Florman, Samuel C. "Odysseus in Cyberspace." *Technology Review* 97, 3 (April 1994), 65.

Fodor, John L. "CyberEthics." In Kizza, 1994, pp. 180–87.

Forester, Tom, and Perry Morrison. *Computer Ethics: Cautionary Tales and Ethical Dilemmas in Computing*. 2nd ed. Cambridge, MA: MIT Press, 1994, ch. 7.

Freedman, David H. *Brainmakers: How Scientists Are Moving Beyond Computers to Create a Rival to the Human Brain*. New York: Simon & Schuster, 1994.

Gershenfeld, Neil. *When Things Start to Think*. New York: Holt, 1999.

Graubard, Stephen R. *The Artificial Intelligence Debate: False Starts, Real Foundations*. Cambridge, MA: MIT Press, 1989.

Hamilton, Robert A. "Using a Computer to Diagnose Illness." *New York Times*, 13 June 1993, p. CN4.

Haugeland, John. *Artificial Intelligence: The Very Idea*. Cambridge, MA: MIT Press, 1989.

Haugeland, John, ed. *Mind Design: Philosophy, Psychology, Artificial Intelligence.* Cambridge, MA: MIT Press, 1988.

Hirschorn, Michael. "The PC Porn Queen's Virtual Realities." *Esquire,* June 1993, pp. 57–60ff.

Hofstadter, Douglas R. *Godel, Escher, Bach: An Eternal Golden Braid.* New York: Vintage Books, 1980.

Johnson, Deborah G. *Computer Ethics.* 2nd ed. Englewood Cliffs, NJ: Prentice-Hall, 1994, ch. 8.

Kizza, Joseph M. *Ethics in the Computer Age: ACM Conference Proceedings (November 11–13, 1994).* New York: ACM, 1994.

Kurzweil, Raymond. *The Age of Intelligent Machines.* Cambridge, MA: MIT Press, 1990.

Kurzweil, Ray. *The Age of Spiritual Machines: When Computers Exceed Human Intelligence.* New York: Viking, 1999.

LaChat, Michael R. "Artificial Intelligence and Ethics: An Exercise in the Moral Imagination." *AI Magazine* 7, 2 (1986), 70–79. Also in Dejoie et al. (1991).

Levinson, Paul. "Picking Ripe: There Are Just Some Things You Can't Do in Cyberspace." *Omni* 16, 11 (August 1994), 4.

Lewis, Peter. "Despite a New Plan for Cooling It Off, Cybersex Stays Hot." *New York Times,* 26 March 1995, sec. 1, p. 1.

Lloyd, Dan. "Frankenstein's Children: Artificial Intelligence and Human Value." *Metaphilosophy* 16, 4 (October 1985), 307–17.

Lycan, William G. *Mind and Cognition: A Reader.* Cambridge, MA: Blackwell, 1990.

Maner, Walter. *Ethics in Computing: The Computer as Physician.* Final Report (March 12, 1979–November 30, 1979), prepared for the Virginia Foundation for the Humanities and Public Policy, University of Virginia, Charlottesville.

McCulloch, W. S., and W. Pitts. "A Logical Calculus of the Ideas Immanent in Nervous Activity." *Bulletin of Mathematical Biophysics* 5 (1943), 115–33.

McGinn, Colin. *The Problem of Consciousness: Essays Towards a Resolution.* Oxford, England: Blackwell, 1991.

Minsky, Marvin. *The Society of Mind.* New York: Simon & Schuster, 1986.

Minsky, Marvin. "Steps Toward Artificial Intelligence." In Feigenbaum and Feldman, *Computers and Thought* (New York: McGraw-Hill, 1963), 406–50.

Minsky, Marvin. "Why People Think Computers Can't." *AI Magazine* (Fall 1982), 3–15. Also in Ermann et al. (eds.), *Computers, Ethics, and Society* (New York: Oxford, 1990).

Moravec, Hans. *Mind Children: The Future of Robot and Human Intelligence.* Cambridge, MA: Harvard University Press, 1988.

Negroponte, Nicholas. *Being Digital.* New York: Knopf, 1995.

Nield, Ted. "Albert's Adventures in Hyperspace." *New Scientist* 144, 1947 (October 15, 1994), 62–64.

Offit, Avodah. "Are You Ready for Virtual Love? A Psychiatrist Looks at Cybersex." *Cosmopolitan*, January 1995, pp. 154–57.

Partridge, Derek, and Yorick Wilkes, eds. *The Foundations of Artificial Intelligence: A Sourcebook.* New York: Cambridge University Press, 1990.

Peat, F. David. *Artificial Intelligence: How Machines Think.* New York: Baen, 1988.

Penrose, Roger. *The Emperor's New Mind: Concerning Computers, Minds, and the Laws of Physics.* New York: Oxford University Press, 1989.

Penrose, Roger. *Shadows of the Mind.* Oxford, England: Oxford University Press, 1994.

Rapaport, William J. "Philosophy, Artificial Intelligence, and the Chinese-Room Argument." *Abacus* 3, 4 (Summer 1986), 7–17.

Rheingold, Howard. *The Virtual Community: Homesteading on the Electronic Frontier.* Reading, MA: Addison-Wesley, 1993.

Rheingold, Howard. *Virtual Reality.* New York, Summit, 1991.

Rich, Elaine. *Artificial Intelligence.* New York: McGraw-Hill, 1983.

Robinson, Phillip, and Nancy Tamosaitis. *The Joy of Cybersex.* New York: Brady Compu Books, 1993.

Rogers, Adam. "Through a Glass, Darkly." *Newsweek*, 23 January 1995, p. 52.

Rubin, Richard. "Moral Distancing and the Use of Information Technologies: The Seven Temptations." In Kizza, 1994, pp. 151–55.

Rosenthal, David M. *The Nature of Mind.* New York: Oxford University Press, 1991.

Samuel, A. L. "Some Studies in Machine Learning Using the Game of Checkers." In Feigenbaum and Feldman, *Computers and Thought* (New York: McGraw-Hill, 1963), 71–105.

Savage, John E., Susan Magidson, and Alex M. Stein. *The Mystical Machine: Issues and Ideas in Computing*. Reading, MA: Addison-Wesley, 1986, ch. 12.

Scott, A. Carlisle, and Philip Klahr, eds. *Innovative Applications of Artificial Intelligence 4*. Cambridge, MA: MIT Press, 1992; see also the first three volumes of this series, 1989–1991.

Scriven, Michael. "The Mechanical Concept of Mind." *Mind* LVII, no. 246 (1953). Reprinted in *Minds and Machines*, ed. Alan Ross Anderson (Englewood Cliffs, NJ: Prentice-Hall, 1964), pp. 31–42.

Searle, John R. "Minds, Brains, and Programs." *The Behavioral and Brain Sciences* 3, 3 (September 1980), 417–24.

Searle, John R. *Minds, Brains and Science*. Cambridge, MA: Harvard University Press, 1984.

Searle, John R. *The Rediscovery of the Mind*. Cambridge, MA: MIT Press, 1992.

Shields, Rob, ed. *Cultures of Internet: Virtual Spaces, Real Histories, Living Bodies*. London: Sage, 1996.

Simenc, Christian, and Paul Loubiere. "Love in the Age of Cybersex." *World Press Review* 41, 4 (April 1994), 40.

Simons, Geoff. *Eco-Computer: The Impact of Global Intelligence*. New York: Wiley, 1987.

Taubes, Gary. "Surgery in Cyberspace." *Discover* 15, 12 (December 1994), 84–94.

Torrance, Steve. "Breaking Out of the Chinese Room." In Yazdani, 1986, 294–314.

Turing, Alan. "Can A Machine Think?" *Mind* 59, 236 (October 1950), 433–60. Also found in James R. Newman, ed., *The World of Mathematics*, volume 4 (New York: Simon & Schuster, 1956), 2099–123; Feigenbaum and Feldman, eds., *Computers and Thought* (New York: McGraw-Hill, 1963), pp. 11–35; Alan Ross Anderson, ed., *Minds and Machines* (Englewood Cliffs, NJ: Prentice-Hall, 1964), pp. 4–30; Douglas R. Hofstadter and Daniel C. Dennett, eds., *The Mind's I* (New York: Basic Books, 1981), pp. 53–67.

Turing, Alan. "On Computable Numbers, with an Application to the Entscheidungs Problem." *Proceedings of the London Mathematical Society*, xlii (1937), 230–65.

Turkle, Sherry. "Artificial Intelligence and Psychoanalysis: A New Alliance." *Proceedings of the American Academy of Arts and Sciences* 117, 1 (Winter 1988), 241–67. Also in Ermann et al., *Computers, Ethics, and Society* (New York: Oxford, 1990).

Turkle, Sherry. *Life on the Screen: Identity in the Age of the Internet.* New York: Simon & Schuster, 1995.

Waldrop, M. Mitchell. *Man-Made Minds: The Promise of Artificial Intelligence.* New York: Walker, 1987.

Weizenbaum, Joseph. *Computer Power and Human Reason: From Judgment to Calculation.* San Francisco: W. H. Freeman, 1976.

Wertheim, Margaret. *The Pearly Gates of Cyberspace.* New York: Norton, 1999.

Wiener, Norbert. *Cybernetics: Or Control and Communication in the Animal and the Machine.* Cambridge, MA: MIT Press, 1961 [1948].

Wilson, David. "A Key for Entering Virtual Worlds." *Chronicle of Higher Education* 41, 12 (November 16, 1994), A18–19ff.

Winner, Langdon. "Cyberpornography." *Technology Review* 97, 2 (February 1994), 70.

Winston, Patrick Henry. *Artificial Intelligence.* 2nd ed. Reading, MA: Addison-Wesley, 1984.

Yazdani, M., and A. Narayanan, eds. *Artificial Intelligence: Human Effects.* West Sussex, England: Ellis Horwood, 1984.

Yazdani, Masoud, ed. *Artificial Intelligence: Principles and Applications.* New York: Chapman and Hall, 1986.

Appendix A

 PAPER 1—COMPUTER ETHICS

In *I, Robot*, Isaac Asimov suggested that there should be three Laws of Robotics :

1. A robot may not injure a human being, or, through inaction, allow a human being to come to harm.
2. A robot must obey the orders given to it by human beings, except where such orders would conflict with the First Law.
3. A robot must protect its own existence as long as such protection does not conflict with the First or Second Law.

—Handbook of Robotics
56th Edition, 2058 A.D.

There seem to be three (at least) positions from which to view robots and "intelligent" computers—as mere mechanisms (like some "Rube Goldberg" device, or even a car, that operates as it was built to do, given the proper impetus), as slaves, or as some "other" "intelligent" species. The first position really has no ethical import. However, given even the language Asimov uses ("may not," "allow," "obey," "protect," and the implication that decisions must be made as to whether a situation involves a test of one of the Laws, etc.), plus the language we use today with respect to computers (what Daniel Dennett has called the "intentional stance"—it is *useful* for us to regard computers, chess-playing machines, etc. from the point of view of something that has intentions—it *wants* to take my King, etc.), it seems that we are talking about something different than a car (though, admittedly, some people LOVE their cars!).

Assume the scenario (not far from the truth) that computers and computer-driven devices are playing an ever-increasing role in controlling things and making decisions that affect our lives, and that they are getting "smarter" by the moment. Should we then regard them as slaves? What are the ethical implications of this position, and how could we justify it? How should Asimov's Laws be rewritten for this situation (though they may be fairly close)? Now take it one step further, and imagine that the machines have gotten "smart" enough that they are doing many responsible jobs and making many decisions that had been done by humans. Does this change the picture at all? Are we going to give them responsibilities and duties, but no rights? On what grounds (if any) could that be justified? Discuss this based on some ethical principles (ones we have discussed, or others). How should the Laws of Robotics/Computers be modified? Should there be a complementary set of Laws for Humans Dealing with Computers?

Write a three-to four-page paper discussing these questions, and any other relevant issues they bring to mind. Do not just say "I feel", or "my friends/parents/teachers/politicians said"; find some principles on which to base what you say. Have some fun with this.

"My loyalties go to intelligent life, no matter in what medium it may arise."—Ross Quillian (distinguished computer scientist)

 # COMPUTER ETHICS TERM PAPER TOPICS

The following are suggestions for term paper topics in the course.

Directions for Students

The paper should be eight to ten pages long (double-spaced, typed or word-processed, with reasonable margins), or more if you get carried away, with appropriate footnotes/endnotes for references.

1. **Privacy in a Computer Age:** The *privacy* issue is one of the largest raised by the tremendous advances in computer technology. Briefly state the problem (as discussed in class and in your text and other references), assess whether the problem seems to be getting worse and why, and then discuss possible solutions or partial solutions. Take into account the complexity of

life on the planet today, so don't just give a simplistic solution like "unplug all of the computers"; if you want to look at a solution along such lines, then be sure to examine the vast consequences of such a move. Use at least three to four references besides your textbook for this.

2. **Privacy, from an ethical perspective:** As in topic 1, first briefly state the "privacy problem" as it faces us today. Then apply different ethical perspectives to the problem (and perhaps, if you feel so moved, add a new theory of your own to suit the situation). Clearly spell out where rights and responsibilities lie in this issue. How would Kant, Plato, Aristotle, Mill, Epicurus, a Stoic, a cultural relativist, etc. deal with this problem? This is a rich topic.

3. **"2084":** Read George Orwell's *1984* (written around 1948) and update it based on advances in computer technology. Make it clear how this can make the problems Orwell suggests even more critical, and what new problems he might not have anticipated will arise by the year 2084. Try to be as imaginative as he was. (Note that the *Seattle Times* ran a series called "2020world"—a futuristic look at what our world might be like in the year 2020, given the changes brought about by information technology. The series was authored by Kurt Dahl, vice president of information technology at the *Seattle Times*. This is no longer available, but interesting vignettes on technology can be accessed by sending a message saying **subscribe technology** to:

Majordomo@seatimes.com

(You may find this interesting.)

4. **The computer state:** David Burnham wrote a book called *The Rise of the Computer State* (1983). Assess and update his concerns. You might also want to look at the article "Would You Sell a Computer to Hitler?" by Laurie Nadel, and other sources on totalitarianism/power; Hannah Arendt's book, *The Origins of Totalitarianism* (1951), is an excellent, though difficult, book in this area.

5. **Star Wars:** Assess the Strategic Defense Initiative (changed to the Ballistic Missile Defense Organization, now referred to as National Missile Defense), looking at why many computer professionals take a strong stand against it, and evaluate the arguments for it. Remember you are doing this from the perspective of an *ethics* course. There are several articles listed in the recommended readings for Chapter 11. You should also do some research on this for even more recent material.

6. **Computer crime:** Do some research to come up with *recent* instances of computer crime that have not made it into the books we have looked at. This can include damaging hacking and viruses, but be sure you also look

for embezzlement, breaches of security, and the like. Assess whether current criminal law is adequate to deal with these problems and, if it is not, suggest changes.

7. **Professional ethics:** Develop a simple moral basis for so-called "professional ethics," and then assess how well the professional *codes of ethics* (IEEE, ACM, etc.) come up to meeting general moral standards. If they need improvement, suggest changes that would be beneficial.

8. **Who owns what is in your head?** Discuss the ethical basis of personal property, and how it could apply to *ideas* as well as *things*. Then discuss how this becomes more complicated when you are *employed* to create ideas, not things. What obligations do you have to your employer and to yourself? Compare this situation to the case of someone employed to make a physical product, such as a chair. What are the important similarities, and what are the crucial differences, if any?

9. **Ethical issues of artificial intelligence:** This is a rather open-ended question. What *are* the relevant ethical issues of AI? They seem to involve *responsibility*, and the extent to which machines should be relied upon to do jobs that were formerly done by humans. What sorts of guidelines are appropriate here? Michael LaChat says, "If AI is a real possibility, then so is *Frankenstein*." Discuss this remark, and perhaps look again at *Frankenstein*, *R.U.R.*, the movie *Colossus: The Forbin Project*, the movie *2001*, the movie *A.I.*, and the like.

10. **Software piracy:** Clearly this is only one of the major issues of computer ethics, though it seems to be the only one that many computer science departments address. State the issue, the arguments (if any), on both sides, and then develop a moral basis that would clarify the issue. Feel free to rely on Kant, or Utilitarianism, or whatever ethical framework you deem appropriate. Just deal clearly in good, sound moral *arguments*.

11. **Moral and social responsibilities of computer professionals:** What *are* the moral and social responsibilities of those working in the computer field? Are they insulated from all such responsibilities, saying they are just "doing their job"? Compare this position with the possible moral and social responsibility of nuclear scientists developing a bomb (as those who worked on the Manhattan Project). Can scientists really attend just to science without concern for its applications? This is a broad issue; discuss it critically.

12. **Weakness of will:** Socrates said in several places something to the effect that no one does wrong willingly. Kant says a similar thing in the *Foundations of the Metaphysics of Morals*. This is called *akrasia* in Greek. Look at Plato (*Symposium, Republic, Meno, Protagoras*) and Kant on this issue, and Aristotle (*Nicomachean Ethics* and *Eudemian Ethics*), Thomas Aquinas (*Summa Theologica*, especially I, 19, 48–49, 82–83; I–II, 18–20, 44, 77), and Hume, *Treatise* II, iii, 1–3, and III, i, 1). There are also some more

modern authors writing on this question, such as Donald Davidson and Harry Frankfurt, if you want to look at their ideas. Assess whether the position is correct, and what implications it has for ethics. This is a more philosophical topic, for those so inclined.

13. **Critical review:** Write a *critical* review of *one* of the following books (or articles), assessing its importance for the themes of this course.

Hubert and Stuart Dreyfus, *Mind over Machine*

Joseph Weizenbaum, *Computer Power and Human Reason*

Jerry Mander, *In the Absence of the Sacred*

Clifford Stoll, *Silicon Snake-Oil*

Marvin Minsky, "Why People Think Computers Can't," *AI Magazine* (Fall 1982), 3–14

William Bechtel, "Attributing Responsibility to Computer Systems," *Metaphilosophy* 16, no. 4 (October 1985), 296–305

Donna Haraway, "A Manifesto for Cyborgs: Science, Technology and Socialist Feminism in the 1980s," *Socialist Review* 15 (1985), 65–107.

14. **Computers and aesthetics:** Granted, this is a course in *ethics*, but the issues of computer ethics are not all that far removed from those of computer *aesthetics*. Pick an area—art, music, or literature—and ask pertinent questions about the viability of computer-generated "art" in that area; then attempt to answer your questions. What would we say about, say, a piece of music that is assessed by experts to likely be an undiscovered piece by Mozart, if it turns out to have been composed by a computer? What of computer-generated modern art? Should galleries be giving shows for the current best computer and its art? (Look at examples of computer art in various sources, including Raymond Kurzweil's *The Age of Intelligent Machines*, and do not restrict yourself to what computers are doing today—try to look to future possibilities). What about computer literary works? Look in Kurzweil at some computer-generated poetry ("A (Kind of) Turing Test"). Could a computer receive a Pulitzer Prize? See also the Pamela Samuelson article, "Can a Computer Be an Author?", in Ermann et al., 1990, pp. 299–307; and Margaret Gorove, "Computer Impact on Society: A Personal View from the World of Art," in Walter M. Mathews, ed., *Monster or Messiah? The Computer's Impact on Society* (Jackson, MS: University of Mississippi Press, 1980), pp. 125–141.

15. **Computer psychiatrists (or doctors):** Look at the ELIZA program, and consider the potential of more sophisticated programs of this nature. What is the future along these lines (or, for the alternate topic, of a computer

becoming a doctor, since there are already successful programs that do medical diagnoses)? Discuss thoroughly the pros and cons of a computer acting as a psychiatrist (or a doctor), given great advances in the technology. Try the ELIZA interactive version at: **http://livingroom.org/eliza/**

16. **The computer and the brain:** Look at parallels between the computer and the brain (including von Neumann's book of that title, Shannon's article "The Brain and the Computer" and Robert Jastrow's "Our Brain's Successor" in Van Tassel, ed., *The Compleat Computer*, Hans Moravec's *Mind Children*, and possibly some work on massively parallel computer systems. How much can we learn about the brain by computer simulation? How intelligent can we make computers by incorporating what is known about the structure of the human brain? Are there any ethical issues or limitations on such work?

17. **Computer president:** Sam Ervin, Jr., in an article, "Justice, the Constitution, and Privacy" in *The Compleat Computer*, suggests he had thought about writing a Constitutional amendment to allow a computer to become president. Discuss Ervin's thoughts on this, and then assess the proposal critically on your own.

18. **Hammurabi's computer code of laws:** The following was suggested as a modern update on Hammurabi's Code of Laws: "If a programmer builds a program for a man and does not make its construction firm, and the program he has built collapses and causes the death of the owner of the program, the programmer shall be put to death. If it causes the death of the son of the owner of the program, they shall put to death a son of that programmer." Discuss thoroughly this variation of "an eye for an eye."

19. **Technological utopia.** Philip Bereano writes "There are writers such as Cullenbach, LeGuin, and Bookchin who offer a political, utopian vision of a different kind of society and a different way to organize the "good life" socially. They would use technological systems very differently... [to] be much more conducive to the fulfillment of human values..." Research, give an exposition, and assess.

20. **Destroy the machines.** Samuel Butler wrote, in a letter to the editor of the *Press*, Christchurch, New Zealand, on June 13, 1863 (!):

> We refer to the question: What sort of creature man's next successor in the supremacy of the earth is likely to be... it appears to us that we are ourselves creating our own successors; we are daily adding to the beauty and delicacy of their physical organization; we are daily giving them greater power and supplying by all sorts of ingenious contrivances that self-regulating, self-acting power which will be to them what intellect has been to the human race. In the course of ages we shall find ourselves the inferior race. Inferior in power, inferior in that moral quality of self-control, we shall look up to them as the acme of all that the best and wisest man can ever dare to aim at. No evil passions, no jeal-

ousy, no avarice, no impure desires will disturb the serene might of those glorious creatures. Their minds will be in a state of perpetual calm, the contentment of a spirit that knows no wants, is disturbed by no regrets... [M]an will have become to the machine what the horse and the dog are to man. He will continue to exist, nay even to improve, and will be probably better off in his state of domestication under the beneficient rule of the machines than he is in his present wild state...

Day by day, however, the machines are gaining ground upon us; day by day we are becoming more subservient to them; more men are daily bound down as slaves to tend them, more men are daily devoting the energies of their whole lives to the development of mechanical life. The upshot is simply a question of time, but that the time will come when the machines hold the real supremacy over the world and its inhabitants is what no person of a truly philosophic mind can for a moment question. Our opinion is that war to the death should be instantly proclaimed against them. Every machine of every sort should be destroyed by the well-wisher of his species. Let there be no exceptions made, no quarter shown; let us at once go back to the primeval condition of the race. If it be urged that this is impossible under the present condition of human affairs, this at once proves that the mischief is already done, that our servitude has commenced in good earnest, that we have raised a race of beings whom it is beyond our power to destroy, and that we are not only enslaved but are absolutely acquiescent in our bondage.

Expand on the thoughts here by looking at Butler's *Erewhon*, which also urges the destruction of the machines. Then update this to today's world. How much of Butler's prophecy has come true? Is the only solution to destroy all the "machines," or is he just a crazy old coot? Think about this carefully in light of this as a course in ethics. This expands on some of the ideas you have already written on, but it is not a simple paper.

21. **Kant and freedom:** Building upon the discussion of Kant, and perhaps a look into the *Critique of Practical Reason*, write as clear an exposition as you can of Kant's defense of freedom of the will. This is a difficult philosophical problem, and you should just see what light you can throw on it from Kant's perspective. The question to try to answer with respect to Kant's position is how he reconciles a nonphysical causality (an act of a free will) having an effect in the physical realm; see if you can shed any illumination on that along the way. This is clearly a more purely philosophical topic, and perhaps harder than many of the others, but you may want to tackle it. It is clear that freedom is fundamental for [computer, or any] ethics.

22. **Computers and power:** Look at Chapter 5 (First Edition) or Chapter 8 (Second Edition) of Deborah Johnson's book, *Computer Ethics*, and Herbert Simon's article, "The Consequences of Computers for Centralization and Decentralization" in *The Computer Age: A Twenty-Year View*, and write a

thoughtful paper on the impact of computerization on the location and intensity of political power.

23. **"Would you sell a computer to Hitler?"** Begin with Laurie Nadel's article and expand it into a full-fledged computer ethics paper. (Louise Nadel, "Would You Sell a Computer to Hitler?", *Computer Decisions* 28 (February 1977), 22–27)

24. **Notes from the underground:** Read Dostoevsky's *Notes from the Underground,* and then explain the concerns of its main character with technology, his flirtation with and rejection of utilitarianism, and his affirmation of his own free will. Does this work as a "proof" of free will? Try to update the character to see how he would react to today's computerized world.

25. **"Can a made-up mind be moral?"** This is the title of a chapter in Pamela McCorduck's book, *Machines Who Think,* and it clearly raises a serious question that relates to computer ethics. Begin with McCorduck's chapter, and look also at appropriate sections in Joseph Weizenbaum's book, *Computer Power and Human Reason,* and write a carefully thought-out paper on McCorduck's question, examining both sides.

ACM CODE OF ETHICS AND PROFESSIONAL CONDUCT

On October 16, 1992, the Executive Council of the Association for Computing Machinery voted to adopt a revised Code of Ethics. The following imperatives and explanatory guidelines were proposed to supplement the Code as contained in the new ACM Bylaw 17.

Commitment to ethical professional conduct is expected of every voting, associate, and student member of ACM. This Code, consisting of 24 imperatives formulated as statements of personal responsibility, identifies the elements of such a commitment.

It contains many, but not all, issues professionals are likely to face. Section I outlines fundamental ethical considerations, while Section 2 addresses additional, more specific considerations of professional conduct. Statements in Section 3 pertain more specifically to individuals who have a leadership role, whether in the workplace or in a volunteer capacity, for example with organizations such as ACM. Principles involving compliance with this Code are given in Section 4.

The Code is supplemented by a set of Guidelines, which provide explanation to assist members in dealing with the various issues contained in the Code. It is expected that the Guidelines will be changed more frequently than the Code.

The Code and its supplemented Guidelines are intended to serve as a basis for ethical decision making in the conduct of professional work. Secondarily, they may serve as a basis for judging the merit of a formal complaint pertaining to violation of professional ethical standards.

It should be noted that although computing is not mentioned in the moral imperatives section, the Code is concerned with how these fundamental imperatives apply to one's conduct as a computing professional. These imperatives are expressed in a general form to emphasize that ethical principles which apply to computer ethics are derived from more general ethical principles.

It is understood that some words and phrases in a code of ethics are subject to varying interpretations, and that any ethical principle may conflict with other ethical principles in specific situations. Questions related to ethical conflicts can best be answered by thoughtful consideration of fundamental principles, rather than reliance on detailed regulations.

1. General Moral Imperatives.

As an ACM member 1 will . . .

1.1 Contribute to society and human well-being

This principle concerning the quality of life of all people affirms an obligation to protect fundamental human rights and to respect the diversity of all cultures. An essential aim of computing professionals is to minimize negative consequences of computing systems, including threats to health and safety. When designing or implementing systems, computing professionals must attempt to ensure that the products of their efforts will be used in socially responsible ways, will meet social needs, and will avoid harmful effects to health and welfare.

In addition to a safe social environment, human well-being includes a safe natural environment. Therefore, computing professionals who design and develop systems must be alert to, and make others aware of, any potential damage to the local or global environment.

1.2 Avoid harm to others

"Harm" means injury or negative consequences, such as undesirable loss of information, loss of property, property damage, or unwanted environmental impacts. This principle prohibits use of computing technology in ways that result in harm to any of the following: users, the general public, employees, employers. Harmful actions include intentional destruction or modification of files and programs leading to serious loss of resources or unnecessary expenditure of human resources such as the time and effort required to purge systems of computer viruses.

Well-intended actions, including those that accomplish assigned duties, may lead to harm unexpectedly. In such an event the responsible person or persons are obligated to undo or mitigate the negative consequences as much as possible. One way to avoid unintentional harm is to carefully consider potential impacts on all those affected by decisions made during design and implementation.

To minimize the possibility of indirectly harming others, computing professionals must minimize malfunctions by following generally accepted standards for system design and testing. Furthermore, it is often necessary to assess the social consequences of systems to project the likelihood of any serious harm to others. If system features are misrepresented to users, coworkers, or supervisors, the individual computing professional is responsible for any resulting injury.

In the work environment the computing professional has the additional obligation to report any signs of system dangers that might result in serious personal or social damage. If one's superiors do not act to curtail or mitigate such dangers, it may be necessary to "blow the whistle" to help correct the problem or reduce the risk. However, capricious or misguided reporting of violations can, itself, be harmful. Before reporting violations, all relevant aspects of the incident must be thoroughly assessed. In particular, the assessment of risk and responsibility must be credible. It is suggested that advice be sought from other computing professionals. (See principle 2.5 regarding thorough evaluations.)

1.3 Be honest and trustworthy

Honesty is an essential component of trust. Without trust an organization cannot function effectively. The honest computing professional will not make deliberately false or deceptive claims about a system or system design, but will instead provide full disclosure of all pertinent system limitations and problems.

A computer professional has a duty to be honest about his or her own qualifications, and about any circumstances that might lead to conflicts of interest.

Membership in volunteer organizations such as ACM may at times place individuals in situations where their statements or actions could be interpreted as carrying the "weight" of a larger group of professionals. An ACM member will exercise care to not misrepresent ACM or positions and policies of ACM or any ACM units.

1.4 Be fair and take action not to discriminate

The values of equality, tolerance, respect for others, and the principles of equal justice govern this imperative. Discrimination on the basis of race, sex, religion, age, disability, national origin, or other such factors is an explicit violation of ACM policy and will not be tolerated.

Inequities between different groups of people may result from the use or misuse of information and technology. In a fair society, all individuals would have equal opportunity to participate in, or benefit from, the use of computer resources regardless of race, sex, religion, age, disability, national origin or other such similar factors. However, these ideals do not justify unauthorized use of computer resources nor do they provide an adequate basis for violation of any other ethical imperatives of this code.

1.5 Honor property rights including copyrights and patents

Violation of copyrights, patents, trade secrets and the terms of license agreements is prohibited by law in most circumstances. Even when software is not so protected, such violations are contrary to professional behavior. Copies of software should be made only with proper authorization. Unauthorized duplication of materials must not be condoned.

1.6 Give proper credit for intellectual property

Computing professionals are obligated to protect the integrity of intellectual property. Specifically, one must not take credit for other's ideas or work, even in cases where the work has not been explicitly protected, for example by copyright or patent.

1.7 Respect the privacy of others

Computing and communication technology enables the collection and exchange of personal information on a scale unprecedented in the history of civilization. Thus there is increased potential for violating the privacy of individuals and groups. It is the responsibility of professionals to maintain the privacy and integrity of data describing individuals. This includes taking precautions to ensure the accuracy of data, as well as protecting it from unauthorized access or accidental disclosure to inappropriate individuals. Furthermore, procedures must be established to allow individuals to review their records and correct inaccuracies.

This imperative implies that only the necessary amount of personal information be collected in a system, that retention and disposal periods for that information be clearly defined and enforced, and that personal information gathered for a specific purpose not be used for other purposes without consent of the individual(s). These principles apply to electronic communications, including electronic mail, and prohibit procedures that capture or monitor electronic user data, including messages, without the permission of users or *bona fide* authorization related to system operation and maintenance. User data observed during the normal duties of system operation and maintenance must be treated with strictest confidentiality, except in cases where it is evidence for the violation of law, organizational regulations, or this Code. In these cases, the nature or contents of that information must be disclosed only to proper authorities.

1.8 Honor confidentiality

The principle of honesty extends to issues of confidentiality of information whenever one has made an explicit promise to honor confidentiality or, implicitly, when private information not directly related to the performance of one's duties becomes available. The ethical concern is to respect all obligations of confidentiality to employers, clients, and users unless discharged from such obligations by requirements of the law or other principles of this Code.

2. More Specific Professional Responsibilities.

As an ACM computing professional I will...

2.1 Strive to achieve the highest quality, effectiveness and dignity in both the process and products of professional work

Excellence is perhaps the most important obligation of a professional. The computing professional must strive to achieve quality and to be cognizant of the serious negative consequences that may result from poor quality in a system.

2.2 Acquire and maintain professional competence

Excellence depends on individuals who take responsibility for acquiring and maintaining professional competence. A professional must participate in setting standards for appropriate levels of competence, and strive to achieve those standards. Upgrading technical knowledge and competence can be achieved in several ways: doing independent study; attending seminars, conferences, or courses; and being involved in professional organizations.

2.3 Know and respect existing laws pertaining to professional work

ACM members must obey existing local, state, province, national, and international laws unless there is a compelling ethical basis not to do so. Policies and procedures of the organizations in which one participates must also be obeyed. But compliance must be balanced with the recognition that sometimes existing laws and rules may be immoral or inappropriate and, therefore, must be challenged.

Violation of a law or regulation may be ethical when that law or rule has inadequate moral basis or when it conflicts with another law judged to be more important. If one decides to violate a law or rule because it is viewed as unethical, or for any other reason, one must fully accept responsibility for one's actions and for the consequences.

2.4 Accept and provide appropriate professional review

Quality professional work, especially in the computing profession, depends on professional reviewing and critiquing. Whenever appropriate, individual members should seek and utilize peer review as well as provide critical review of the work of others.

2.5 Give comprehensive and thorough evaluations of computer systems and their impacts, including analysis of possible risks

Computer professionals must strive to be perceptive, thorough, and objective when evaluating, recommending, and presenting system descriptions and alternatives. Computer professionals are in a position of special trust, and therefore have a special responsibility to provide objective, credible evaluations to employers, clients, users, and the public. When providing evaluations the professional must also identify any relevant conflicts of interest, as stated in imperative 1.3.

As noted in the discussion of principle 1.2 on avoiding harm, any signs of danger from systems must be reported to those who have opportunity and/or responsibility to resolve them. See the guidelines for imperative 1.2 for more details concerning harm, including the reporting of professional violations.

2.6 Honor contracts, agreements, and assigned responsibilities

Honoring one's commitments is a matter of integrity and honesty. For the computer professional this includes ensuring that system elements perform as intended. Also, when one contracts for work with another party, one has an obligation to keep that party properly informed about progress toward completing that work.

A computing professional has a responsibility to request a change in any assignment that he or she feels cannot be completed as defined. Only after serious consideration and with full disclosure of risks and concerns to the employer or client, should one accept the assignment. The major underlying principle here is the obligation to accept personal accountability for professional work. On some occasions other ethical principles may take greater priority.

A judgment that a specific assignment should not be performed may not be accepted. Having clearly identified one's concerns and reasons for that judgment, but failing to procure a change in that assignment, one may yet be obligated, by contract or by law, to proceed as directed. The computing professional's ethical judgment should be the final guide in deciding whether or not to proceed. Regardless of the decision, one must accept the responsibility for the consequences. However, performing assignments "against one's own judgment" does not relieve the professional of responsibility for any negative consequences.

2.7 Improve public understanding of computing and its consequences

Computing professionals have a responsibility to share technical knowledge with the public by encouraging understanding of computing, including the impacts of computer systems and their limitations. This imperative implies an obligation to counter any false views related to computing.

2.8 Access computing and communication resources only when authorized to do so

Theft or destruction of tangible and electronic property is prohibited by imperative 1.2—"Avoid harm to others." Trespassing and unauthorized use of a computer or communication system is addressed by this imperative. Trespassing includes accessing communication networks and computer systems, or accounts and/or files associated with those systems, without explicit authorization to do so. Individuals and organizations have the right to restrict access to their systems so long as they do not violate the discrimination principle (see 1.4).

No one should enter or use another's computing system, software, or data files without permission. One must always have appropriate approval before using system resources, including .rm57 communication ports, file space, other system peripherals, and computer time.

3. Organizational Leadership Imperatives.

As an ACM member and an organizational leader, I will . . .

3.1 Articulate social responsibilities of members of an organizational unit and encourage full acceptance of those responsibilities

Because organizations of all kinds have impacts on the public, they must accept responsibilities to society. Organizational procedures and attitudes oriented toward quality and the welfare of society will reduce harm to members of the public, thereby serving public interest and fulfilling social responsibility. Therefore, organizational leaders must encourage full participation in meeting social responsibilities as well as quality performance.

3.2 Manage personnel and resources to design and build information systems that enhance the quality of working life

Organizational leaders are responsible for ensuring that computer systems enhance, not degrade, the quality of working life. When implementing a computer system, organizations must consider the personal and professional development, physical safety, and human dignity of all workers. Appropriate human-computer ergonomic standards should be considered in system design and in the workplace.

3.3 Acknowledge and support proper and authorized uses of an organization's computing and communications resources

Because computer systems can become tools to harm as well as to benefit an organization, the leadership has the responsibility to clearly define appropriate and inappropriate uses of organizational computing resources. While the number and scope of such rules should be minimal, they should be fully enforced when established.

3.4 Ensure that users and those who will be affected by a system have their needs clearly articulated during the assessment and design of requirements. Later the system must be validated to meet requirements

Current system users, potential users and other persons whose lives may be affected by a system must have their needs assessed and incorporated in the statement of requirements. System validation should ensure compliance with those requirements.

3.5 Articulate and support policies that protect the dignity of users and others affected by a computing system

Designing or implementing systems that deliberately or inadvertently demean individuals or groups is ethically unacceptable. Computer professionals who are in decision-making positions should verify that systems are designed and implemented to protect personal privacy and enhance personal dignity.

3.6 Create opportunities for members of the organization to learn the principles and limitations of computer systems

This complements the imperative on public understanding (2.7). Educational opportunities are essential to facilitate optimal participation of all organizational members. Opportunities must be available to all members to help them improve their knowledge and skills in computing, including courses that familiarize them with the consequences and limitations of particular types of systems. In particular, professionals must be made aware of the dangers of building systems around oversimplified models, the improbability of anticipating and designing for every possible operating condition, and other issues related to the complexity of this profession.

4. Compliance with the Code.

As an ACM member I will . . .

4.1 Uphold and promote the principles of this Code

The future of the computing profession depends on both technical and ethical excellence. Not only is it important for ACM computing professionals to adhere to the principles expressed in this Code, each member should encourage and support adherence by other members.

4.2 Treat violations of this code as inconsistent with membership in the ACM

Adherence of professionals to a code of ethics is largely a voluntary matter. However, if a member does not follow this code by engaging in gross misconduct, membership in ACM may be terminated.

This code and the supplemental Guidelines were developed by the Task Force for the Revision of the ACM Code of Ethics and Professional Conduct: Ronald E. Anderson, chair, Gerald Engel, Donald Gotterbarn, Grace C. Herlein, Alex

Hoffman, Bruce Jawer, Deborah G. Johnson, Doris K. Lidtke, Joyce Currie Little, Dianne Martin, Donn B. Parker, Judith A. Perrolle, and Richard S. Rosenberg. The Task Force was organized by ACM/SIGCAS and funding was provided by the ACM SIG Discretionary Fund.

Source: Communications of the ACM 32, 2 (February 1993), 100–105. It can also be accessed online at: **www.acm.org**

Appendix C

IEEE CODE OF ETHICS

We, the members of the IEEE, in recognition of the importance of our technologies in affecting the quality of life throughout the world, and in accepting a personal obligation to our profession, its members and the communities we serve, do hereby commit ourselves to the highest ethical and professional conduct and agree:

1. to accept responsibility in making engineering decisions consistent with the safety, health and welfare of the public, and to disclose promptly factors that might endanger the public or the environment;
2. to avoid real or perceived conflicts of interest whenever possible, and to disclose them to affected parties when they do exist;
3. to be honest and realistic in stating claims or estimates based on available data;
4. to reject bribery in all its forms;
5. to improve the understanding of technology, its appropriate application, and potential consequences;
6. to maintain and improve our technical competence and to undertake technological tasks for others only if qualified by training or experience, or after full disclosure of pertinent limitations;
7. to seek, accept, and offer honest criticism of technical work, to acknowledge and correct errors, and to credit properly the contributions of others;

8. to treat fairly all persons regardless of such factors as race, religion, gender, disability, age, or national origin;
9. to avoid injuring others, their property, reputation, or employment by false or malicious action;
10. to assist colleagues and co-workers in their professional development and to support them in following this code of ethics.

Note: This Code was adopted in August 1990. It can also be accessed at:

www.ieee.org

Bibliography

Adam, Alison. *Artificial Knowing: Gender and the Thinking Machine.* London: Routledge, 1998.

Albus, James S. *Brains, Behavior, and Robotics.* Peterborough, NH: Byte Books, 1981.

Albus, James S. "The Robot Revolution: An Interview with James Albus." *Communications of the ACM* (March 1983), 179–80.

Arbib, Michael A. "Man-Machine Symbiosis and the Evolution of Human Freedom." *American Scholar* 43 (1973), 38–54.

Arendt, Hannah. *The Origins of Totalitarianism.* New York: Harcourt Brace Jovanovich, 1973.

Aristotle. *Nicomachean Ethics, Eudemian Ethics.*

Baer, Robert M. *The Digital Villain.* Reading, MA: Addison-Wesley, 1972.

Baird, Robert M., Reagan Ramsower, and Stuart E. Rosenbaum, eds. *Cyberethics: Social and Moral Issues in the Computer Age.* Amherst, NY: Prometheus Books, 2000.

Baumrin, Bernard H., and Benjamin Freedman, eds. *Moral Responsibility and the Professions.* New York: Haven, 1983.

Bayles, Michael D. *Professional Ethics.* Belmont, CA: Wadsworth, 1981.

Bellin, David, and Gary Chapman, eds. *Computers in Battle—Will They Work?* Boston, MA: Harcourt Brace Jovanovich, 1989.

Benedikt, Michael, ed. *Cyberspace: First Steps.* Cambridge, MA: MIT Press, 1991.

Beniger, James R. *The Control Revolution.* Cambridge, MA: Harvard University Press, 1986.

Bergin, Thomas J. "Teaching Ethics, Teaching Ethically," *Computers & Society* 21, nos. 2, 3, 4 (October 1991), 33–39.

Bequai, August. *Computer Crime*. Lexington, MA: D.C. Heath, 1978.

Berners-Lee, Tim (with Mark Fischetti). *Weaving the Web: The Original Design and Ultimate Destiny of the World Wide Web by Its Inventor*. San Francisco: Harper SF, 1999.

Bliss, Edwin C., and Isamu S. Aoki. *Are Your Employees Stealing You Blind?* Amsterdam, Netherlands: Pfeiffer & Co., 1993.

Bloombecker, Jay, ed. *Computer Crime, Computer Security, Computer Ethics*. National Center for Computer Crime, 1986.

BloomBecker, J. J. Buck. "Computer Ethics: An Antidote to Despair," in *Computers & Society* 16, 4 (October 1986), 3–11.

Boden, Margaret A., ed. *The Philosophy of Artificial Life*. New York: Oxford University Press, 1996.

Boettinger, Henry M. "Humanist Values: What Place in the Computer Age?" *Financial Executive* (March 1970), 44–46.

Bolter, J. David. *Turing's Man: Western Culture in the Computer Age*. Chapel Hill, NC: University of North Carolina Press, 1984.

Bowyer, Kevin W., ed. *Ethics and Computing: Living Responsibly in a Computerized World*, 2nd ed. New York: IEEE Press, 2001.

Boyle, James. *Shamans, Software, and Spleens: Law and the Construction of the Information Society*. Cambridge, MA: Harvard University Press, 1996.

Brand, Stewart. *The Clock of the Long Now: Time and Responsibility/The Ideas Behind the World's Slowest Computer*. New York: Basic Books, 1999.

Brod, Craig. *Technostress: The Human Cost of the Computer Revolution*. Reading, MA: Addison-Wesley, 1984.

Brown, Geoffrey. *The Information Game: Ethical Issues in a Microchip World*. Atlantic Highlands, NJ: Humanities Press, 1990.

Brown, Geoffrey. "Is There an Ethics of Computing?" *Journal of Applied Philosophy* 8, 1 (1991), 19–26.

Bunnell, David. *Making the CISCO Connection: The Story Behind the Real Internet Power*. New York: Wiley, 2000.

Burnham, David. *The Rise of the Computer State*. New York: Vintage, 1984.

Butchvarov, Panayot. *Skepticism in Ethics*. Bloomington, IN: University of Indiana Press, 1989.

Bynum, Terrell Ward, ed. *Computers and Ethics*. October 1985 Issue of *Metaphilosophy*. Oxford, England: Blackwell, 1985.

Byte Magazine.

Center for Philosophy and Public Policy. "Privacy in the Computer Age." QQ-Report, vol. 4. University of Maryland.

Clark, Jim (with Owen Edwards). *Netscape Time: The Making of the Billion-Dollar Start-up that Took on Microsoft.* New York: St. Martin's, 1999.

Communications of the ACM.

Computer Crime and Computer Security: Hearing Before the Subcommittee on Crime, U.S. House of Representatives, May 23, 1985. Washington, DC: Government Printing Office, 1986.

Computers and Society.

Computerworld.

Cusumano, Michael A., and David B. Yoffie. *Computing on Internet Time.* New York: Free Press, 1998.

Dalai Lama. *Ethics for the New Millennium.* New York: Riverbank Books, 1999.

DeCew, Judith Wagner. *In Pursuit of Privacy.* Ithaca, NY: Cornell University Press, 1997.

DeLanda, Manuel. *War in the Age of Intelligent Machines.* New York: Zone Books, 1991.

Dennett, Daniel C. *Brainstorms: Philosophical Essays on Mind and Psychology.* Montgomery, VT: Bradford Books, 1978.

Dennett, Daniel C. *Consciousness Explained.* Boston, MA: Little, Brown, 1991.

Dennett, Daniel C. *The Intentional Stance.* Cambridge, MA: MIT Press/Bradford, 1987.

Dertouzos, Michael L., and Joel Moses, eds. *The Computer Age: A Twenty-Year View.* Cambridge, MA: MIT Press, 1980.

Deweese, J. Taylor. "Giving the Computer a Conscience." *Harper's Magazine* (November 1973), 14–17.

Diffie, Whitfield, and Susan Landau. *Privacy on the Line: The Politics of Wiretapping and Encryption.* Cambridge, MA: MIT Press, 1998.

Dretske, Fred I. *Knowledge and the Flow of Information.* Cambridge, MA: MIT Press, 1982.

Dreyfus, Hubert L. *What Computers Can't Do.* New York: Harper & Row, 1979.

Dreyfus, Hubert L. *What Computers Still Can't Do.* Cambridge, MA: MIT Press, 1993.

Dreyfus, Hubert L., and Stuart E. Dreyfus. *Mind Over Machine: Human Intuition and Expertise in the Era of the Computer.* New York: Free Press, 1986.

Dunlop, Charles, and Rob Kling, eds. *Computerization and Controversy: Value Conflicts and Social Choices.* Boston, MA: Academic Press, 1991.

Ermann, M. David, Claudio Gutierrez, and Mary B. Williams, eds. *Computers, Ethics, and Society.* New York: Oxford University Press, 1990.

Feigenbaum, Edward A., and Julian Feldman, eds. *Computers and Thought.* New York: McGraw-Hill, 1963. A classic.

Ford, Daniel. *The Button: The Pentagon's Strategic Command and Control System.* New York: Simon & Schuster, 1985.

Forester, Tom, and Perry Morrison. *Computer Ethics: Cautionary Tales and Ethical Dilemmas in Computing,* 2nd ed. Cambridge, MA: MIT Press, 1990.

Fox, Richard M., and Joseph P. DeMarco. *Moral Reasoning: A Philosophic Approach to Applied Ethics.* New York: Holt, 1990.

Friedman, Batya, and Terry Winograd, eds. *Computing and Social Responsibility: A Collection of Course Syllabi.* Palo Alto, CA: Computer Professionals for Social Responsibility, 1990.

Friedman, Benjamin. "A Meta-Ethics for Professional Morality." *Ethics* 89 (1978), 1–19.

Garfinkel, Simson. *Database Nation: The Death of Privacy in the 21st Century.* Sebastopol, CA: O'Reilly, 2000.

Gerschenfeld, Neil. *When Things Start to Think.* New York: Holt, 1999.

Gibson, William. *Neuromancer.* New York: Ace Books, 1984.

Godwin, Mike. *CyberRights: Defending Free Speech in the Digital Age.* New York: Random House/Times Books, 1998.

Goldkind, Stuart. "Machines and Mistakes." *Ratio* 24 (1982), 173–84.

Goldman, Alan. *The Moral Foundations of Professional Ethics.* Totowa, NJ: Rowman and Littlefield, 1980.

Goldstein, Robert C., and Richard L. Nolan. "Personal Privacy Versus the Corporate Computer." *Harvard Business Review* 53 (March–April 1975), 62–70.

Gordon, Gil E., and Marcia M. Kelly. *Telecommuting: How to Make It Work for You and Your Company.* Englewood Cliffs, NJ: Prentice-Hall, 1986.

Gould, Carol C., ed. *The Information Web: Ethical and Social Implications of Computer Networking.* Boulder, CO: Westview Press, 1988.

Hafner, Katie, and Matthew Lyon. *Where Wizards Stay Up Late: The Origins of the Internet.* New York: Simon & Schuster, 1996.

Haraway, Donna. "A Manifesto for Cyborgs: Science, Technology, and Socialist Feminism in the 1980s." *Socialist Review* 15 (1985), 65–107.

Hester, D. Micah, and Paul J. Ford, eds. *Computers and Ethics in the Cyber-age.* Upper Saddle River, NJ: Prentice-Hall, 2001.

Hoffman, W. Michael, and Jennifer Mills Moore, eds. *Ethics and the Management of Computer Technology: Proceedings of the Fourth National Conference on Business Ethics.* Cambridge, MA: Oelgeschlager, Gunn, & Hain Publishers, 1982.

Hollander, Patricia A. *Computers in Education: Legal Liabilities and Ethical Issues Concerning their Use and Misuse.* Asheville, N.C.: College Administration Publications, Inc., 1986.

Hussain, Donna S., and Khateeb M. Hussain. *The Computer Challenge: Technology, Applications, and Social Implications.* Santa Rosa, CA: Burgess Communications, 1986.

James, William. *Pragmatism.* 1907.

Johnson, Deborah G. *Computer Ethics.* 3rd ed. Englewood Cliffs, NJ: Prentice-Hall, 2001.

Johnson, Deborah G., and Helen Nissenbaum, eds. *Computers, Ethics, and Social Values.* Englewood Cliffs, NJ: Prentice-Hall, 1995.

Johnson, Deborah G., and John W. Snapper, eds. *Ethical Issues in the Use of Computers.* Belmont, CA: Wadsworth, 1985.

Johnson, Douglas W. *Computer Ethics: A Guide for the New Age.* Elgin, IL: Brethren Press, 1984.

Kahin, Brian, and Charles Nesson, eds. *Borders in Cyberspace: Information Policy and the Global Information Infrastructure.* Cambridge, MA: MIT Press, 1997.

Kant, Immanuel. *Foundations of the Metaphysics of Morals.*

Keplinger, Michael S. "Computer Software—Its Nature and Protection." *Emory Law Journal* 30 (Spring 1981), 483–512.

Kidder, Tracy. *The Soul of a New Machine.* Boston, MA: Little, Brown, 1981.

Kizza, Joseph M. *Ethics in the Computer Age: ACM Conference Proceedings (November 11–13, 1994).* New York: ACM, 1994.

Kleiner, Art. "The Ambivalent Miseries of Personal Computing." *Whole Earth Review* (January 1985), 6–10.

Koepsell, David R. *The Ontology of Cyberspace: Philosophy, Law, and the Future of Intellectual Property.* Chicago, IL: Open Court, 2000.

Kurzweil, Ray. *The Age of Spiritual Machines: When Computers Exceed Human Intelligence.* New York: Viking, 1999.

Langford, Duncan, ed. *Internet Ethics.* New York: St. Martin's Press, 2000.

Larson, Erik. *The Naked Consumer: How Our Private Lives Become Public Commodities.* New York: Holt, 1992.

Laudon, Kenneth C. *Dossier Society: Value Choices in the Design of National Information Systems*. New York: Columbia University Press, 1986.

Lawyers on Line: Ethical Perspectives in the Use of Tele-computer Communication. American Bar Association, 1986.

Lessig, Larry. *Code and Other Laws of Cyberspace*. New York: Basic Books, 1999.

Lessig, Lawrence. *The Future of Ideas: The Fate of the Commons in a Connected World*. New York: Random House, 2001.

Mander, Jerry. *In the Absence of the Sacred: The Failure of Technology and the Survival of the Indian Nation*. San Francisco, CA: Sierra Club Books, 1991.

Maner, Walter. "Unique Ethical Problems in Information Technology." *Science and Engineering Ethics* 2, 2 (1996), 137–54.

Mathews, Walter, ed. *Monster or Messiah: The Computer's Impact on Society*. Jackson, MS: University of Mississippi Press, 1980.

McCorduck, Pamela. *Machines Who Think*. San Francisco, CA: W. H. Freeman, 1979.

McCracken, Daniel D. et al. "A Problem-List of Issues Concerning Computers and Public Policy: A Report of the ACM Committee on Computers and Public Policy." *Communications of the ACM* 17 (September 1974), 495–503.

Mill, John Stuart. *Utilitarianism*.

Mitcham, Carl. *Thinking Through Technology: The Path Between Engineering and Philosophy*. Chicago, IL: University of Chicago Press, 1994.

Moor, James H. "Are There Decisions Computers Should Never Make?" *Nature and System* 1 (1979), 217–29.

Moore, G.E. *Principia Ethica*.

Moravec, Hans. *Mind Children*. Cambridge, MA: Harvard University Press, 1988.

Mowshowitz, Abbe. *Conquest of Will: Information Processing in Human Affairs*. Reading, MA: Addison-Wesley, 1976.

Nadel, Laurie, and Hesh Wiener. "Would You Sell a Computer to Hitler?" *Computer Decisions* 28 (February 1977), 22–27.

National Conference on Business Ethics Staff. *Ethics and the Management of Computer Technology*. Cambridge, MA: Oelgeschlager, Gunn, & Hain, 1982.

Negroponte, Nicholas. *Being Digital*. New York: Knopf, 1995.

Nurminen, Markku. *People or Computers: Three Ways of Looking at Information Systems*. Krieger, 1988.

Nycum, Susan. "Legal Protection for Computer Programs." *Computer/Law Journal*, Vol. 1 (1978), 1–88.

Orwant, Carol J. "Computer Ethics—Part of Computer Science?", in *Computers & Society*, 21, nos. 2, 3, and 4 (October 1991), 40–45.

Orwell, George. *1984*.

Pagels, Heinz. *The Dreams of Reason*. New York: Simon & Schuster, 1988.

Parker, Donn B. *Crime by Computer*. New York: Scribner, 1976.

Parker, Donn B. *Ethical Conflicts in Computer Science and Technology*. AFIPS Press, 1981.

Parker, Donn B. *Fighting Computer Crime*. New York: Scribner, 1983.

Parkhill, D. F., and P. H. Emslow, Jr., eds. *So This Is Nineteen Eighty-Four: Some Personal Views by Governors of the International Council for Computer Communication*. New York: Elsevier, 1984.

Parnas, David L. "SDI: A Violation of Professional Responsibility." *Abacus* 4, 2 (1987), 46–52.

Pecorino, Philip A., and Walter Maner. "The Philosopher As Teacher: A Proposal for a Course on Computer Ethics." *Metaphilosophy* 16, 4 (October 1985), 327–35. In Bynum, 1985.

Perrolle, Judith A. *Computers and Social Change: Information, Property, and Power*. Belmont, CA: Wadsworth, 1987.

Peterson, I. *Fatal Defect: Why Computers Fail*. New York: Random House, 1995.

Pool, Ithiel de Sola. *Technologies of Freedom: On Free Speech in an Electronic Age*. Cambridge, MA: Belknap Press of Harvard University Press, 1983.

Power, Richard. *Tangled Web: Tales of Digital Crime in the Shadows of Cyberspace*. Indianapolis, IN: Que/Macmillan, 2000.

Rifkin, Jeremy. *The End of Work: The Decline of the Global Labor Force and the Dawn of the Post-Market Era*. New York: G. P. Putnam's Sons, 1996.

Robinett, Jane, and Ramon Barquin, eds. *Computers and Ethics: A Sourcebook for Discussions*. Brooklyn, NY: Polytechnic Press, 1989.

Rochlin, Gene I. *Trapped in the Net: The Unanticipated Consequences of Computerization*. Princeton, NJ: Princeton University Press, 1997.

Rosen, Jeffrey. *The Unwanted Gaze: The Destruction of Privacy in America*. New York: Random House, 2000.

Roszak, Theodore. *The Cult of Information: The Folklore of Computers and the True Art of Thinking*. New York: Pantheon Books, 1986.

Rothfeder, Jeffrey. *Privacy for Sale*. New York: Simon & Schuster, 1992.

Ruse, Michael, ed. *Philosophy of Biology*. New York: Macmillan, 1989.

Savage, John E., Susan Magidson, and Alex M. Stein. *The Mystical Machine: Issues and Ideas in Computing*. Reading, MA: Addison-Wesley, 1986.

Schwartau, Winn. *Information Warfare: Chaos on the Electronic Superhighway*. New York: Thunder's Mouth Press, 1994.

Simon, Herbert A. "The Consequences of Computers for Centralization and Decentralization." In Michael L. Dertouzos and Joel Moses, eds., *The Computer Age: A Twenty-Year View.* Cambridge, MA: MIT Press, 1979, pp. 212–28.

Simons, Geoff. *Eco-Computer: The Impact of Global Intelligence.* New York: Wiley, 1987.

Simons, G.L. *Privacy in a Computer Age.* Manchester, England: National Computing Centre, 1982.

Smith, Brian Cantwell. *Limits of Correctness in Computers.* (Presented at a Symposium on Unintentional Nuclear War at the Fifth Congress of the International Physicians for the Prevention of Nuclear War, Budapest, Hungary, June 28–July 1, 1985.) Stanford, CA: Center for the Study of Language and Information, 1985. Reprinted in Dunlop and Kling, pp. 632–46.

Spector, Robert. *Amazon.com: Get Big Fast.* New York: HarperCollins, 2000.

Spinello, Richard A. *Cyberethics: Morality and Law in Cyberspace.* Sudbury, MA: Jones and Bartlett, 2000.

Spinello, Richard A. *Ethical Aspects of Information Technology.* Englewood Cliffs, NJ: Prentice-Hall, 1995.

Spinello, Richard A., and Herman T. Tavani, eds. *Readings in Cyberethics.* Sudbury, MA: Jones and Bartlett, 2001.

SRI International Staff. *Ethical Conflicts in Information and Computer Science, Technology, and Business.* Wellesley, MA: QED Information Sciences, 1990.

Steinke, Gerhard, and Gilbert Hamann. "Ethics and Computers: Can Universities Set the Standards?" In *Advances in Computing and Information—ICCI '90.* New York: Springer-Verlag, 1990.

Stoll, Cliff. *The Cuckoo's Egg.* New York: Bantam, 1990.

Stoll, Clifford. *Silicon Snake Oil: Second Thoughts on the Information Highway.* New York: Doubleday, 1995.

Talingdan, Arsenio B. "Implications of Computer Use in Politics." *Technology and Society* 2 (September 1980), 8–11.

Turing, Alan. "Can A Machine Think?" *Mind* 59, No. 236 (October 1950), 433–60. Also found in James R. Newman, ed., *The World of Mathematics,* vol. 4 (New York: Simon & Schuster, 1956), pp. 2099–123; Feigenbaum and Feldman (1963), pp. 11–35; Alan Ross Anderson, ed., *Minds and Machines* (Englewood Cliffs, NJ: Prentice-Hall, 1964), pp. 4–30; Douglas R. Hofstadter and Daniel C. Dennett, eds., *The Mind's I* (New York: Basic Books, 1981), pp. 53–67.

Turkle, Sherry. *Life on the Screen: Identity in the Age of the Internet*. New York: Simon & Schuster, 1995.

U.S. Department of Health, Education, and Welfare. *Records, Computers, and the Rights of Citizens: Report of the Secretary's Advisory Committee on Automated Personal Data*. DHEW Publication No. (OS) 73-97, 1973.

Van Tassel, Dennie L., and Cynthia L. Van Tassel. *The Compleat Computer*. 2nd ed. Chicago, IL: SRA, 1983.

Vincent, Phillip Fitch, and Thomas Milton Kemnitz. *Computer Ethics: A Philosophical Problem Book*. New York: Trillium Press, 1983.

Vonnegut, Kurt. *Player Piano*. New York: Laurel/Dell/Bantam, [1952] 1980.

Waldrop, M. Mitchell. *Man-Made Minds: The Promise of Artificial Intelligence*. New York: Walker, 1987.

Wallace, Jonathan, and Mark Mangan. *Sex, Laws, and Cyberspace*. New York: Holt, 1997.

Weckert, John. *Computer and Information Ethics*. Westport, CT: Greenwood Press, 1997.

Weil, Vivian, and John Snapper, eds. *Owning Scientific and Technical Information: Value and Ethical Issues*. New Brunswick, NJ: Rutgers University Press, 1989.

Weizenbaum, Joseph. *Computer Power and Human Reason: From Judgment to Calculation*. New York: W. H. Freeman, 1976.

Wertheim, Margaret. *The Pearly Gates of Cyberspace*. New York: Norton, 1999.

Wessel, Milton R. *Freedom's Edge: The Computer Threat to Society*. Reading, MA: Addison-Wesley, 1974.

Whiteside, Thomas. "Dead Souls in the Computer-I & II." *New Yorker*, August 22, 1977 and August 29, 1977.

Wiener, Norbert. *Cybernetics: Or Control and Communication in the Animal and the Machine*. Cambridge, MA: MIT Press, 1961 [1948].

Wiener, Norbert. *God and Golem, Inc*. Cambridge, MA: MIT Press, 1964.

Wiener, Norbert. *The Human Use of Human Beings*. Boston, MA: Houghton Mifflin, 1950.

Index